# INDUSTRIAL BIOTECHNOLOGY

*Current Progress and Novel Technologies*

# INDUSTRIAL BIOTECHNOLOGY

*Current Progress and Novel Technologies*

**Prakash Kumar Sarangi, PhD**
**Akhilesh Kumar Singh, PhD**
**Rajesh Kumar Srivastava, PhD**
**Brijesh Pandey, PhD**
*Editors*

AAP | APPLE ACADEMIC PRESS

First edition published 2027

**Apple Academic Press Inc.**
1265 Goldenrod Circle, NE,
Palm Bay, FL 32905 USA

760 Laurentian Drive, Unit 19,
Burlington, ON L7N 0A4, Canada

**CRC Press**
2385 NW Executive Center Drive,
Suite 320, Boca Raton FL 33431

4 Park Square, Milton Park,
Abingdon, Oxon, OX14 4RN, UK



**Library and Archives Canada Cataloguing in Publication**

CIP data on file with Canada Library and Archives

**Library of Congress Cataloging-in-Publication Data**

CIP data on file with US Library of Congress

ISBN: 978-1-77964-222-6 (hbk)
ISBN: 978-1-77964-223-3 (ebk)

DOI: 10.1201/9781779642233

# About the Editors

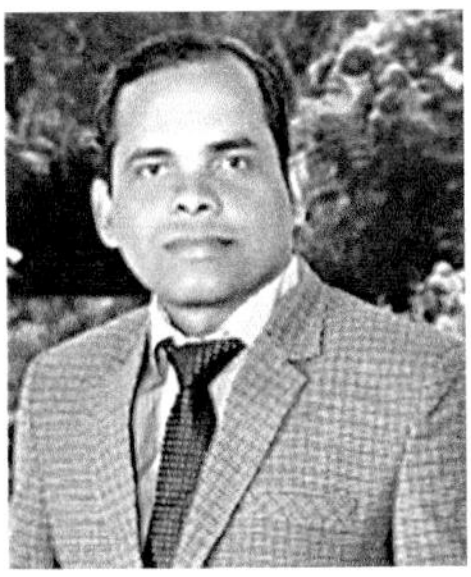

**Prakash Kumar Sarangi, PhD**
*Scientist (Microbiology), Central Agricultural University, Imphal, Manipur, India*

Prakash Kumar Sarangi, PhD, is a Scientist with specialization in Microbiology at the Central Agricultural University in Imphal, India. Dr. Sarangi's research is focused on bioprocess engineering, biochemicals, biomaterials, and sustainable development. His expertise is in bioconversion of biomass into biofuels, biochemicals, and nutraceuticals, as well as environmental waste remediation. He has taken leading roles as the principal investigator in different R&D projects on biomass conversion and microbial biodegradation into value-added products. He has more than 15 years of teaching and research experience in biochemical engineering, microbial biotechnology, downstream processing, food microbiology, and molecular biology. He is serving as an editorial board member for many international journals, including *PLOS One, 3 Biotech,* and *Biofuels, Bioproducts and Biorefining*. He is also serving as guest editor of the journals *Biomass Conversion and Biorefinery, Chemical Engineering and Technology,* and *Biofuels, Bioproducts and Biorefining*. He has published more than 130 research articles in peer-reviewed journals and authored more than 75 book chapters. He has presented at many national and international conferences. He is associated with many scientific societies as a fellow member (Society for Applied Biotechnology) and life member (Biotech Research Society of India, Society for Biotechnologists of India, Association of Microbiologists of India, Indian Science Congress Association, Forum of Scientists, Engineers and Technologists, and International Association of Academicians and Researchers). He has published many books on the field of biomass conversion and value addition. Dr. Sarangi has a PhD degree in Microbial Biotechnology from the Ravenshaw University, India, and MTech degree from the Department of Agriculture and Food Engineering, Indian Institute of Technology Kharagpur, India.

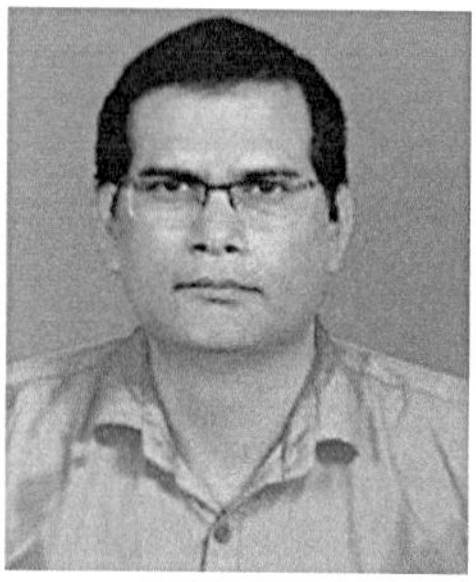

**Akhilesh Kumar Singh, PhD**
*Assistant Professor, Department of Biotechnology, Mahatma Gandhi Central University (MGCU), Motihari, Bihar, India*

Akhilesh Kumar Singh, PhD, is currently an Assistant Professor in the Department of Biotechnology, Mahatma Gandhi Central University (MGCU), Motihari, Bihar, India. Before joining MGCU, Dr. Singh worked as a faculty at the Amity Institute of Biotechnology, Amity University Uttar Pradesh, Lucknow Campus, Lucknow, India (September 2008 to October 2019). He has over 16 years of experience in teaching and multidisciplinary research, focusing on microbial physiology, industrial biotechnology, and nanobiotechnology. His research focuses on the production of polyhydroxyalkanoate bioplastics, metallic nanobiotechnology, and nitric oxide signaling. Dr. Singh holds a PhD in agricultural and food engineering and an MTech in agricultural biotechnology from the prestigious Indian Institute of Technology (IIT), Kharagpur, India, with a master's degree in biotechnology from another prestigious institute, i.e., IIT, Roorkee, India. He has qualified Graduate Aptitude Test in Engineering (GATE) in Life Science conducted by IIT Kanpur on behalf of the Ministry of Human Resource Development (MHRD), Government of India. He was awarded the prestigious Council of Scientific and Industrial Research (CSIR)-University Grants Commission (UGC) Junior Research Fellowship (CSIR-UGC JRF) by the Council of Scientific and Industrial Research, India. In addition, Dr. Singh has also qualified the Indian Council of Agriculture Research (ICAR)-National Eligibility Test (NET), i.e., ICAR-NET in Agricultural Biotechnology, conducted by ICAR, India. He has been credited with four patents, 35 research papers, 35 review articles in high-repute international journals, and 60 chapters in reputed books. He has also edited the book titled *Nanobiotechnology: Mitigation of Abiotic Stress in Plants*, published by Springer. Dr. Singh has been on the editorial board as well as the panels of reviewers of several reputed journals of Elsevier, Springer Nature, John Wiley & Sons, and so on. Dr. Singh has also supervised several PhD, MTech, MSc, and BTech students.

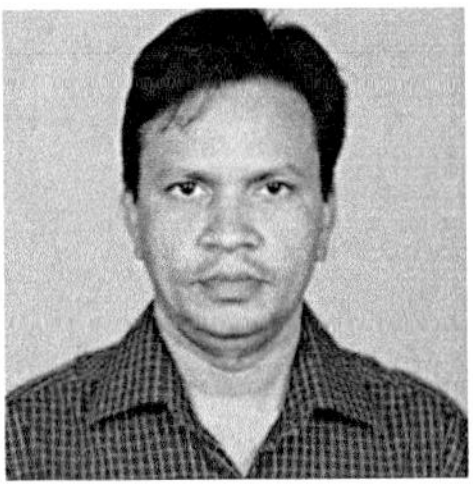

**Rajesh Kumar Srivastava, PhD**
*Senior Assistant Professor,*
*Department of Biotechnology, School of Core Engineering, GITAM (Deemed to be University), Visakhapatnam, Andhra Pradesh, India*

Rajesh Kumar Srivastava, PhD, is a Senior Assistant Professor in the Department of Biotechnology, School of Core Engineering, GITAM (Deemed to be University), Visakhapatnam, Andhra Pradesh, India. He focuses his research on applied microbiology, industrial biotechnology, and fermentative production synthesis. He has published 48 papers in international and national journals, 13 book chapters in international books, and five book chapters in national books, with several papers and book chapters currently in progress. He has also published two national-level books. He is a reviewer for the *Journal of Applied Microbiology, Archives of Microbiology*, *PLOS One*, and *Biomass Conversion and Biorefinery*. He received his PhD degree in fermentation technology from IIT Bombay, Mumbai, in 2009. Before this degree, he completed his MSc in Microbiology and MTech in Biochemical Engineering (from IIT BHU, Varanasi, UP). After earning his PhD degree, he had a postdoctoral fellowship from the University of Amsterdam, Netherlands.

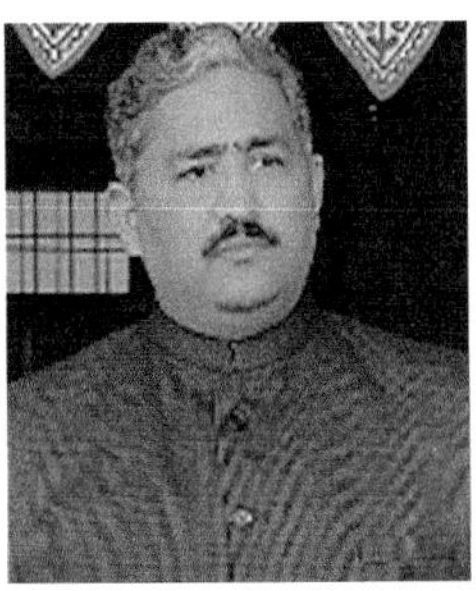

**Brijesh Pandey, PhD**
*Professor, Department of Biotech, School of Life Sciences, Mahatma Gandhi Central University, Motihari, Bihar, India*

Brijesh Pandey, PhD, specializes in secondary metabolism and genetic engineering for regulatory manipulation of secondary metabolic pathways. He is a Professor in the Department of Biotechnology, School of Life Sciences at Mahatma Gandhi Central University, Motihari, Bihar, India. His research focuses on metabolic regulation and assessment of the therapeutic and industrial importance of secondary metabolites. He has more than three dozen international publications to his credit. He is a life member of the Indian

Science Congress and the Association, Society of Biological Chemists (I) and a founding member of the Florafauna Science Foundation, aimed at enabling entrepreneurial villages. He has more than 15 years of teaching and research experience at the university level. He received his PhD degree in Biochemistry from the University of Lucknow in India.

# Contents

# Contributors

**Nitin Bhardwaj**
Department of Zoology and Environmental Sciences, Gurukula Kangri (Deemed to be University), Haridwar, Uttarakhand, India

**Harish Chandra**
Department of Botany and Microbiology, Gurukula Kangri (Deemed to be University), Haridwar, Uttarakhand, India

**Ravi Deshwal**
Institute of Bioscience and Technology, Sri Ramswaroop Memorial University, Lucknow, Uttar Pradesh, India

**Kartikey Kumar Gupta**
Department of Botany and Microbiology, Gurukula Kangri (Deemed to be University), Haridwar, Uttarakhand, India

**Rahul Gupta**
Amity Institute of Biotechnology, Amity University Uttar Pradesh, Lucknow Campus, Lucknow, India

**Swinder Jeet Singh Kalra**
Department of Chemistry, DAV College, Kanpur, Uttar Pradesh, India

**Arjun Singh Kohli**
Amity Institute of Biotechnology, Amity University Uttar Pradesh, Lucknow Campus, Lucknow, Uttar Pradesh, India

**Abhishek Kumar**
Parul Institute of Management and Research, Parul University, Vadodara, Gujarat, India

**Pradeep Kumar**
Department of NMR and MRI Facility, All India Institute of Medical Sciences, New Delhi, Delhi, India

**Virendra Kumar**
Department of NMR and MRI Facility, All India Institute of Medical Sciences, New Delhi, Delhi, India

**Babli Kumari**
Department of Biotechnology, School of Life Sciences, Mahatma Gandhi Central University, Motihari, Bihar, India

**Priti Pal**
Amity Institute of Biotechnology, Amity University Uttar Pradesh, Lucknow Campus, Lucknow, India

**Brijesh Pandey**
Department of Biotechnology, School of Life Sciences, Mahatma Gandhi Central University, Motihari, Bihar, India

**Paras Porwal**
Amity Institute of Biotechnology, Amity University Uttar Pradesh, Lucknow Campus, Lucknow, Uttar Pradesh, India

**Anand Prakash**
Department of Biotechnology, School of Life Sciences, Mahatma Gandhi Central University, Motihari, Bihar, India

**Om Prakash**
Department of Biotechnology, School of Life Sciences, Mahatma Gandhi Central University, Motihari, Bihar, India

**Saurabh Singh Rathore**
Department of Biotechnology, School of Life Sciences, Mahatma Gandhi Central University, Motihari, Bihar, India

**Kalpana Sagar**
Department of Botany and Microbiology, Gurukula Kangri (Deemed to be University), Haridwar, Uttarakhand, India

**Somali Sanyal**
Amity Institute of Biotechnology, Amity University Uttar Pradesh, Lucknow Campus, Lucknow, Uttar Pradesh, India

**Prakash Kumar Sarangi**
College of Agriculture, Central Agricultural University, Imphal, Manipur, India

**Laxuman Sharma**
Department of Horticulture, Sikkim University, Gangtok, Sikkim, India

**Akhilesh Kumar Singh**
Department of Biotechnology, School of Life Sciences, Mahatma Gandhi Central University, Motihari, Bihar, India

**Alok Kumar Singh**
ICAR–National Bureau of Agriculturally Important Microorganisms (NBAIM), Mau, Uttar Pradesh, India; Amity Institute of Biotechnology, Amity University Uttar Pradesh, Lucknow Campus, Lucknow, Uttar Pradesh, India

**Rishi Kumar Singh**
School of Biosciences, IMS Institute, University Courses Campus, Ghaziabad, Uttar Pradesh, India

**Sujeet Pratap Singh**
Amity Institute of Biotechnology, Amity University Uttar Pradesh, Lucknow Campus, Lucknow, Uttar Pradesh, India

**Sashi Sonkar**
Department of Botany, Bankim Sardar College, Tangrakhali, West Bengal, India

**Alok Kumar Srivastava**
ICAR–National Bureau of Agriculturally Important Microorganisms (NBAIM), Mau, Uttar Pradesh, India

**Rajesh Kumar Srivastava**
Senior Assistant Professor, Department of Biotechnology, School of Core Engineering, GITAM (Deemed to be University), Visakhapatnam, Andhra Pradesh, India

**Vikram Srivastava**
Department of Biomedical Sciences, College of Veterinary Medicine, Iowa State University, Ames, Iowa, USA

**Mala Trivedi**
Amity Institute of Biotechnology, Amity University Uttar Pradesh, Lucknow Campus, Lucknow, Uttar Pradesh, India

**Archana Yadav**
Department of Microbiology, Institute of Biosciences and Biotechnology, C.S.J.M. University, Kanpur, Uttar Pradesh, India

# Abbreviations

| | |
|---|---|
| AA | arachidonic acid |
| ABE | acetone-butanol-ethanol |
| AD | Alzheimer's disease |
| ADHD | attention deficit hyperactivity disorder |
| AI | artificial intelligence |
| BC | bacterial cellulose |
| BD | bulk density |
| BMP-2 | bone morphogenetic protein-2 |
| BNC | bacterial nanocellulose |
| BOD | biological oxygen demand |
| BSA | bovine serum albumin |
| CBB | Calvin-Benson-Bassham |
| CCCP | carbonyl cyanide m-chlorophenylhydrazone |
| CLEA | cross-linked enzyme aggregate |
| CMC | carboxymethylcellulose |
| CNS | central nervous system |
| COD | chemical oxygen demand |
| CPS | capsular polysaccharides |
| CRL | *Candida rugosa* lipase |
| CSID | congenital sucrase-isomaltose deficiency |
| CVD | cardiovascular dysfunction |
| DAC | dialdehyde cellulose |
| DGLA | dihomo-γ-linolenic acid |
| DHA | docosahexaenoic acid |
| DMSO | dimethyl sulfoxide |
| DNA | divergence from nucleic acids |
| ECM | extracellular matrix |
| ED | Entner-Doudoroff |
| EFA | essential fatty acid |
| EMA | European Medicines Agency |
| EPA | eicosapentaenoic acid |
| EPS | exo-polysaccharides |
| ER | endoplasmic reticulum |
| FAEE | fatty acid ethyl ester |
| FAME | fatty acid methyl ester |
| FBP | fungal biomass protein |

| | |
|---|---|
| FDA | Food and Drug Administration |
| FFA | free fatty acid |
| FMT | fluorescence molecular tomography |
| GC-MS | gas chromatography-mass spectrometry |
| GDH | glucose dehydrogenase |
| GH | growth hormone |
| GM | genetically modified |
| GMP | good manufacturing practices |
| GO | graphene oxide |
| GRAS | generally recognized as safe |
| HA | hyaluronic acid |
| HMF | hydroxymethylfurfural |
| HOFA | hyper-oxygenated fatty acids |
| HTS | high-throughput screening |
| IBC | initial biomass concentration |
| IL | ionic liquid |
| LIMS | laboratory information management systems |
| MBC | metabolically engineered bacterial cellulose |
| MFC | microbial fuel cells |
| MMT | million metric tons |
| MRI | magnetic resonance imaging |
| MS | mass spectrometry |
| MSC | mesenchymal stem cell |
| MW-CNT | multi-walled carbon nanotube |
| NAG | N-acetylglucosamine |
| NAM | N-acetylmuramic acid |
| NDP-sugars | nucleoside diphosphate sugars |
| NMR | nuclear magnetic resonance |
| NO | nitric oxide |
| NSAID | non-steroidal anti-inflammatory medication |
| OD | optical density |
| OGP | osteogenic growth peptide |
| PBR | photobioreactor |
| PDMS | poly-di-methyl-siloxane |
| PEM | proton exchange membrane |
| PET | positron emission tomography |
| PGA | phosphoglycerate |
| PGDB | pathway/genome database |
| PGP | plant growth promoting |
| PGPM | plant growth-promoting microorganism |
| PGPR | plant growth promoting rhizobacteria |
| PHA | polyhydroxyalkanoates |

| | |
|---|---|
| PKS | polyketide synthase |
| PM | particulate matter |
| PTM | posttranslational modification |
| PUFA | polyunsaturated fatty acids |
| QCM | quartz crystal microbalance |
| QMS | quality management system |
| ROS | reactive oxygen species |
| RSM | response surface methodology |
| SA | succinic acid |
| SANS | small-angle neutron scattering |
| SCO | single-celled microorganism |
| SERS | surface-enhanced raman scattering |
| SmF | submerged fermentation |
| SMRT | single-molecule real-time |
| SOD | superoxide dismutase |
| SPI | soy protein isolate |
| SSF | solid-state fermentation |
| SUB | single-use bioreactor |
| TA | teichoic acids |
| TC | transmembrane cellulose |
| TNF | tumor necrosis factor |
| UDP-Glc | uridine diphosphate glucose |
| ULSD | low-sulfur diesel fuel |
| VFA | volatile fatty acid |
| VS | volatile solid |
| ZN | zein protein nanoparticle |

# Preface

The prime focus of this book is on industrial biotechnological processes for the production of value-added industrial compounds in the food, fuel, and other related sectors. Various fermentation processes and systems are key highlights of this book. Bioconversion technologies to recover energy and fuel from plant-based non-edible biomass and other organic wastes are also discussed. This book serves as a platform to showcase breakthrough research in understanding the roles of biotechnological tools and mechanisms in biorefinery applications, available fermentation technologies, and advanced engineering for large-scale biomass processing. The book is dedicated to advancing new developments and approaches in bioreactor design and characterization. The chapters in this book make a widespread impact on current microbial research and development. It provides information on recent advances in the fields of biotechnology, catalysis, bioprocess engineering, and downstream processing for the environmentally friendly production of valuable biochemicals. This book also serves as an instructive introduction for research in microbiology and the efficient utilization of microbial community interventions. It can offer ideas for research and graduate-level work, as well as serve as a reference for scientists, engineers, and scholars already active in the field and related areas.

The editors are grateful to all the authors for contributing their valuable chapters to this book. The editors are also grateful to Ashish Kumar and Sandra Jones Sickels of Apple Academic Press, Inc. for their kind support and coordination throughout the entire project.

—***Editors***

## CHAPTER 1

# Bioprocess Engineering for Enzyme Production: Experience from Microbes

PRITI PAL,[1] AKHILESH KUMAR SINGH,[2,*] SAURABH SINGH RATHORE,[2] BRIJESH PANDEY,[2] ANAND PRAKASH,[2] SUJEET PRATAP SINGH,[1] PRAKASH KUMAR SARANGI,[3,*] and RAHUL GUPTA[1]

[1]*Amity Institute of Biotechnology, Amity University Uttar Pradesh, Lucknow Campus, Lucknow, India*

[2]*Department of Biotechnology, School of Life Sciences, Mahatma Gandhi Central University, Motihari, Bihar, India*

[3]*College of Agriculture, Central Agricultural University, Imphal, Manipur, India*

*Corresponding author

### ABSTRACT

Microorganisms are rich metabolic systems capable of synthesizing a wide array of industrially important enzymes. These microbial enzymes function as highly efficient biocatalysts, offering benefits such as reduced processing time, high catalytic efficiency, operational stability, cost-effectiveness, and environmentally friendly performance compared to plant- or animal-derived enzymes. By optimizing fermentation parameters, microbes can be tailored to produce enzymes with desirable functional characteristics, while the use of low-cost agricultural residues as substrates further enhances process economics. Microbial enzymes are extensively employed in industrial and medical sectors due to their non-toxic nature, ease of handling, and adaptability to diverse conditions. They play a crucial role in degrading hazardous compounds

Industrial Biotechnology: Current Progress and Novel Technologies.
Prakash Kumar Sarangi, Akhilesh Kumar Singh, Rajesh Kumar Srivastava, and Brijesh Pandey (Eds.)


DOI: 10.1201/9781779642233-1

present in industrial and household wastes, including phenolics, nitriles, and amines. Large-scale enzyme production depends on controlled microbial growth through advanced fermentation technologies. Modern molecular tools, such as recombinant DNA technology, enable the overproduction of enzymes with improved substrate specificity, thermal stability, and activity. Additionally, strategies like genetic fusion and post-translational modifications support the development of hybrid enzymes with enhanced performance. This chapter discusses microbial sources, strain improvement techniques, fermentation processes, and downstream methods that improve enzyme yield, purity, and recovery. It also highlights emerging technologies for optimizing industrial-scale microbial enzyme production.

## 1.1 INTRODUCTION

More than 60% of all biomass on Earth is made up of microbes. It is considered to be greater than that fixed by green plants, the quantity of carbon fixed by microbial activities (Singh et al., 2016). Enzymes, also known as biocatalysts, are biological molecules that aid in the process and particularity of numerous chemical reactions and physiological processes (Anbu et al., 2017). Every bacterium generates enzymes that conduct numerous metabolic processes such as hydrolysis, oxidation, and reduction. Microorganisms are the major source of enzymes because of their wide accessibility, fast growth rate, capacity to culture large quantities of enzymes in a short period, and enhancing bacterial cell viability through genetic engineering to increase the desired properties yield of targeted enzyme synthesis (Anbu et al., 2013). Yeasts and molds account for more than half of all industrial enzymes. Similarly, industrial enzymes are mostly produced by bacteria, which make up 30% of them. Mammals make up 8% of them, and plants make up roughly 4%. Microbial enzymes are expected to be more stable and active than enzymes originating from plants and mammals, providing greater performance across a variety of physiological and chemical circumstances (Raveendran et al., 2018). It also has diverse biodiversity that may be studied to find novel enzymes utilizing cutting-edge methods such as metagenomics and genome mining. Almost 90% of commercial enzymes are designed (Adrio et al., 2014). Furthermore, effective downstream processing and immobilization procedures have greatly improved the enzymes' stability, purity, and reusability.

Natural biocatalysts can be found all around and in great abundance in nature. The screening and identification of hundreds of enzymes from various bacteria have been substantially improved by conventional methods combining conventional microbiological procedures with whole-genome sequencing and proteomics.

Microbial enzymes are being employed in the manufacture of over 500 commercial goods across a wide variety of biotechnological applications (Imchen et al., 2017). The majority of hydrolytic enzymes (about 65%) are used in a variety of industrial applications, including agrochemical intermediates, textiles, laundry detergents, starch, pulp, and paper, leather, and personal care products. Approximately 25% of microbial enzymes are utilized in food processing, with the remaining 10% provided as animal feed additives (Koutsandreas et al., 2019). Hydrolases are frequently used in the biodegradation of natural polymers such as starch, cellulose, proteins, and other substances due to their flexibility (Jemli et al., 2016). Protease is the most prevalent hydrolytic enzyme when it comes to using in physiology and biotechnology, making up about 57% of the market for industrial enzymes (Koutsandreas et al., 2019). Lipase, xylanase, amylase, ligninase, isomerase, pullulanase, cellulose, laccase, and catalase are a few of the additional enzymes (May, 2019). More than 75% of all enzymes produced on a big scale are hydrolases. In the global enzyme sector, companies including Novozymes, Dupont, DSM, and Roche are leaders (Liu and Kokare, 2016). The market for industrial enzymes is expected to grow steadily and reach $7.0 billion by 2023 (Wellesly, 2018).

## 1.2 MICROORGANISMS: SOURCES OF ENZYMES

Commercial enzymes have been identified from bacteria ranging from *Actinoplanes* to *Zymomonas*, as well as spinach and snake venom. A major aspect of a bio-based economy is the widespread use of microorganisms like bacteria, yeast, fungi, molds, and their enzymes as biological catalysts. The marketing of enzymes as a potential substitute for chemical catalysts highlights their increased catalytic power, effective stereo-selectivity, and specificity (Zhang et al., 2016). Several enzymes are very important because they are widely used in biochemical analysis and clinical diagnostics. Microbial sources of enzymes are preferred over non-microbial sources for a variety of industrial applications because their production costs are lower, raw materials are readily available and of constant composition, as needed, and due to rapid microbial growth and a well-defined cellular metabolism. Microbial enzyme production is in high demand due to its superior activities and remarkable performance in several industrial sectors (Srinivasan et al., 2019). Enzymes are also produced by bacteria from the genera, *Pseudomonas, Streptomyces, Acinetobacter, Staphylococcus, Fusarium, Penicillium, Mucor*, and *Trichoderma*. Microorganisms such as bacteria, fungi, and yeasts have mostly been used to produce enzymes tailored to specific industrial purposes. The two microorganisms that Novozymes most frequently utilized for the production of enzymes are the bacterium *Bacillus subtilis* and the fungus *Aspergillus oryzae*, a multinational biotechnology business. Industrially relevant proteases, for example, have been bio-synthesized mostly by bacteria such as *Bacillus, Clostridium,* and *Pseudomonas*. Amylases are another key family of industrially essential enzymes generated mostly by *Bacillus* sp. Cellulases of commercial importance have been isolated from *Aspergillus, Basidiomycetes, Polyporus, Pleurotus*, and *Trichoderma* species (Rathi and Kumar, 2021). Keratinases have been generated mostly by Actinomycetes and a few fungal strains. Many *Aspergillus* sp., *Candida* sp., *Penicillium* sp., *Rhizopus,* and *Mucor* fungus and yeast strains generate industrially useful lipases. Xylanases, which have important uses in the paper and pulp industries, are generated by fungal species from the genera *Aspergillus, Penicillium,* and *Trichoderma* and have been shown to have high catalytic efficiency and stability across a wide temperature range (Sarmah et al., 2018). Furthermore, with the constant advancements in recombinant DNA technology and protein engineering, manipulating enzymatic activities inside a microorganism to fulfill rising industrial needs has become simple and approachable. Enzymes derived from microbial sources may be significantly modified to meet the needs of complicated industrial applications through gene modification.

## 1.3 BIOPROSPECTING: IDENTIFICATION OF INDUSTRIAL ENZYME-PRODUCING MICROBES

Nature is a wide and plentiful source of natural biocatalysts. Hundreds of enzymes from various bacteria have been discovered and screened using standard approaches that combine conventional microbiological procedures with whole-genome sequencing and proteomics. These strains are accessible in a variety of international culture collections (ATCC, NCTC, NCIMB, NCYC, CCM, JCM, and so on). Programs like the Earth Microbiome Project (Gilbert et al., 2014), the Fungal genome project (Grigoriev et al., 2014), the Microbial genome sequencing project (Fraser et al., 2000), the Human microbiome project (Koppel and Balskus, 2016), and the Plant genome project are seeking to gather data on huge metagenomes with the emergence of next-generation sequencing. The coordinated approach that combines metagenomics with 'Omics' information (Miyauchi et al., 2016), and structural and biochemical data has opened up the potential of exploring newer and more diverse microorganism genomes and discovering new enzymes with improved characteristics. Using a metagenomic approach, several hydrolytic enzymes from uncultured microorganisms and extremophiles have been discovered (Berini et al., 2017). Glycan microarrays were used to identify Carbohydrate-Active enZymes (CAZymes) from marine metagenomic data (Salmeán et al., 2018). From the Carbohydrate-Active enZymes (CAZy) database, fungal esterases were identified through genome mining (Dilokpimol et al., 2018). Additionally, the Medema group is developing and using computational techniques to identify secondary metabolite gene clusters and biosynthetic pathways in plants and microorganisms (Medema, 2018).

Numerous databases contain regulated data on genomes, operons, gene regulatory networks, omics data, metabolic pathways, differential expression, protein properties, and structural information. Websites like www.biocyc.org, a collection of Pathway/Genome Databases (PGDBs) with analytical tools, are a few instances of these databases (Karp et al., 2019). The webpage http://mbgd.genome.ad.jp/ is a database for microbial genomes used in comparative genomic studies (Uchiyama et al., 2019). Carbohydrate-active enzyme's genetic, structural, and biochemical data are available at www.cazy.org (Henrissat, 2013). The webpage www.ebi.ac.uk/merops/ uses graded, structure-based cataloging of peptidases (Rawlings et al., 2018). The webpage www.genome.jp/kegg/annotation/enzyme KEGG's database of enzymes can be utilized as the primary identifier when reconstructing metabolic pathways from entire genomes (Kanehisa, 2017). The webpage www.led.biocatnet.de is a lipase and esterase engineering database (Bauer et al., 2020). These databases assist researchers in their studies, comparisons, analyses, and formulation of experimental designs.

## 1.4 STRAIN IMPROVEMENT OF MICROBIAL ENZYME

Strain improvement using enzyme technology is the most crucial stage of bioprocess exploitation. It is a rapidly developing engineering that is used to produce customized enzymes that aid in large-scale, financially sustainable, and industrial enzyme production. Generally speaking, natural enzymes are unable to tolerate the harsh industrial conditions that obstruct efficient bioprocessing. To improve the efficiency and sustainability of natural enzymes, strategies like directed evolution, rational or semi-rational design, and metabolic engineering have been employed (Chowdhury et al., 2020). The improvement of enzyme features, including kinetic efficiency, thermostability, higher tolerance to pH and organic solvents, elimination of allosteric regulation, increased enzyme-substrate specificity, the enzyme's broad substrate range, and enhanced stereoselectivity of the product, has been greatly aided by protein structure data in combination with computational methods and bioengineering. Many recent publications have considered genetic engineering approaches for increasing hydrolytic enzyme properties (Manisha and Yadav, 2017). Recombinant DNA technology (Gao et al., 2019), recombination protoplast fusion (Li et al., 2018), and mutations-site-directed mutagenesis (Xu et al., 2018) are a few approaches related to the strain enhancement process. The effectiveness of these procedures is boosted by raising the dose of gene concentration, which increases the product activity, which contains one or more genes, such as enzymes. Recent developments in computational biology and rDNA technology have made it possible to customize *de novo* enzymes (Vaissier and Head-Gordon, 2019), the construction of multifunctional chimeric enzymes (Gilmore et al., 2020), the use of synthetic amino acids, and the development of enzymes with desired characteristics (Narancic et al., 2019). Metabolic engineering is another significant advancement in strain improvement (Chae et al., 2017). Access to omics data has made it possible to repurpose metabolic pathways, regulate gene expression, edit multiple genes, and design novel synthetic routes for the mass production of durable biomolecules. These advancements have been made possible by *in silico* tools and cutting-edge tailoring techniques like the CRISPR-Cas system (Donohoue et al., 2018).

## 1.5 OPTIMIZATION OF PROCESS VARIABLES FOR MAXIMAL PRODUCTION OF MICROBIAL ENZYMES

Incubation duration, beginning pH, concentration, inoculum, agitation/shaking, temperature, carbon supply, metal ions, and nitrogen source are all important elements in the manufacture of enzymes by microorganisms (Table 1.1). The adjustment of these process parameters is important in increasing commercial enzyme production. To manufacture enzymes in sufficient quantities, optimization of a media component, culture factors, and fermentation state is required. The process variables are typically optimized one at a time while maintaining all other variables constant, and the ideal condition or factor is employed in subsequent tests sequentially. Optimizing a variety of physicochemical properties, nutritional traits, and fermentation factors has the advantage of assisting in the creation of a fermentation process that is affordable (Niyonzima and More, 2013). Statistical approaches for optimizing process parameters are also utilized to enhance the output of enzymes in less time. The Plackett-Burman and Box-Behnken designs were used to improve nutritional factors (such as C, N, and P sources) and Physico-chemical variables (such as inoculum age, incubation period, and temperature), and *Mucor circinelloides* F6–3–12 was found to produce more tanas (El-Refai et al., 2017). Using response surface methodology (RSM), *Staphylococcus arlettae* JPBW-1 produced an acceptable quantity of lipase (Chauhan et al., 2013). To maximize amylase production in *Bacillus subtilis* DM-03 and *Bacillus licheniformis* AS08E, Roy and Mukherjee (2013) use statistical techniques. A 2-level factorial Plackett-Burman concept was used, accompanied by a central composite design to improve the culture conditions for *Trichoderma estonicum*'s protease production (Saravanakumar and Kathiresan, 2012).

### 1.5.1 *IMPACT OF TIME ON MICROBIAL ENZYME PRODUCTION*

The time spent incubating is crucial to the production of enzymes by bacteria and fungus. For bacterial species, the ideal period for commercial enzyme synthesis ranged from 24 to 48 hours (Hussain et al., 2017). The expense of the fermentation process is decreased by the shorter incubation period suggested for the majority of enzyme synthesis. Additionally, incubation durations of 60–96 hours for the production of the

**TABLE 1.1** Process Variables that are Ideal for the Microbial Synthesis of Enzymes

| Type of Microbe | Enzyme Produced | pH | Temperature (°C) | Agitation (rpm) | Inoculum Size (%) | Incubation Period | Carbon Source | Preferred Nitrogen Source | References |
|---|---|---|---|---|---|---|---|---|---|
| Acinetobacter calcoaceticus 1-7 | Lipase | 9 | 37 | 180 | 0.6 | 48 h | Starch, olive oil | Corn flour, bean flour | Wang et al. (2012) |
| *Bacillus halodurans* | CGTase | 10.5 | 37 | Not specified | Not specified | 48 h | Soluble starch | Yeast extract and peptone | More et al. (2012) |
| *Bacillus* cereus GA6 | Amylase | 10 | 20 | 120 | 1 | 96 h | Glycerol | Ammonium acetate | Roohi et al. (2013) |
| *Bacillus flexus* XJU-1 | Lipase | 11 | 37 | 100 | 2 | 36 h | Cotton seed oil | Yeast extract | Niyonzima and More (2013) |
| *Bacillus subtilis* | Pectinase | 8.5 | 37 | Not specified | Not specified | 24 h | Glucose | Yeast extract | Mathur et al. (2014) |
| *Sphingobacterium* sp. SaH-05 | Xylanase | 8 | 37 | 150 | Not specified | 24 h | Wheat bran | Ammonium sulfate | Ghasemi et al. (2014) |
| *Bacillus* cereus | Pullulanase | 6 | 50 | 200 | Not specified | 48 h | Soluble pullulan | Tryptone | Waleed et al. (2015) |
| *Aspergillus* sp. GM4 | Tannase | 4 | 30 | ns | Not specified | 4 days | Jamun leaves /tannate | Potassium nitrate | Souza et al. (2015) |
| *Bacillus lehensis* MLB2 | Phytase | 5.5 | 30 | 100 | 2 | 24 h | Rice bran | Potassium nitrate | More et al. (2015) |
| *Bacillus* cereus FT9 | L-glutaminase | 7 | 37 | 150 | Not specified | 24 h | Malt extract | Peptone | Sinha et al. (2016) |
| *Penicillium* sp. | Cellulase | 5 | 30 | ns | Not specified | 7 days | lactose | Yeast extract | Prasanna et al. (2016) |
| *Fusarium* sp. XPF-5 | Xylanase | 8 | 47 | 160 | Not specified | 4 days | Xylan | NS | Sharma et al. (2016) |

**TABLE 1.1** *(Continued)*

| Type of Microbe | Enzyme Produced | pH | Temperature (°C) | Agitation (rpm) | Inoculum Size (%) | Incubation Period | Carbon Source | Preferred Nitrogen Source | References |
|---|---|---|---|---|---|---|---|---|---|
| *Bacillus flexus* MSBC2 | CGTase | 10 | 37 | ns | Not specified | 120 h | Corn starch | Peptone with yeast extract | Shwetha et al. (2017) |
| *Bacillus megaterium* BMS4 | Cellulase | 7 | 37 | 120 | Not specified | 24 h | Sucrose | LB medium BHM medium | Hussain et al. (2017) |
| *Mucor circinelloides* F6-3-12 | Tannase | 5.5 | 30 | 200 | 2 | 7 days | Green tea leaves powder | Sodium nitrate | El-Refai et al. (2017) |
| *Bacillus cereus* LC13 | L-Glutamines | 7 | 37 | 100 | Not specified | 24 h | Maltose | L-glutamine | Lincoln et al. (2018) |
| *Aspergillus awamori* | Cellulase | 6 | 25 | Not specified | Not specified | 7 days | Carboxymethylcellulose (CMC) | Peptone | Pachauri et al. (2018) |

bacterial enzyme's keratinase, protease, pullulan's, amylase, and lipase have been observed (Roy and Mukherjee, 2013). *Bacillus flexus* MSBC 2 produced cyclodextrin glycosyltransferase (or CGTase) after 120 and 168 hours of incubation, respectively (Shwetha et al., 2017). As a result, the time duration for enzyme production by bacteria differs from species to species. This might be attributed to genetic differences. The fungal enzymes are released at their peak on the fourth or fifth day (Table 1.1) (Niyonzima and More, 2013). There have been reports of fermentation times of 2 and 3 days, respectively, for the production of invertases from *Saccharomyces cerevisiae* and L-asparaginase from *Trichoderma viride* Pers: SF Grey. In contrast, the production of tanas by *Mucor coccinellids* isolate F6-3-12 (El-Refai et al., 2017), pectinases by *Aspergillus niger*, cellulases by *Penicillium* sp. and *Aspergillus awamori*, laccases by *Scytalidium lignicola*, and tanas by *Mucor circinelloides* isolate required a longer incubation time (Sidhu et al., 2017). Similar to this, Usha et al. (2014) discovered that *Stereum ostrea* could manufacture laccase in sufficient quantities for 12 days. In general, bacteria produce more enzymes as the incubation time increases. However, beyond the optimal incubation period, there is a decrease in commercial enzyme production. This reduction in enzyme synthesis was linked to decreased food availability and toxic metabolite release or breakdown of an industrial enzyme by protease (Anandan et al., 2007). The reduction in industrial lipase was attributed to the buildup of fatty acids and glycerol as a result of lipolysis. The decline in amylase output for most commercial enzymes, such as amylases, was caused by enzyme denaturation caused by the interaction of the enzyme generated with the medium components (Niyonzima and More, 2015). Variations in growth and metabolic activity can be linked to changes in enzyme synthesis by bacteria and fungi (Niyonzima and More, 2015).

### 1.5.2 INFLUENCE OF PH ON PRODUCTION OF MICROBIAL ENZYMES

The synthesis of microbial enzymes is significantly influenced by the initial pH of the culture and fermentation media. It might affect how nutrients are delivered or how different nutrient components are transported across bacterial or fungal membranes, which promotes microbial growth and, as a result, the production of enzymes (Niyonzima and More, 2015). The most common beginning pH range seen for bacterial enzymes is 6 to 10 (Hussain et al., 2017). *Chryseobacterium* sp. produced amylase at a low pH of 5.0 (Hasan et al., 2017). Moreover, *Bacillus lehensis* MLB2 produces phytase (More et al., 2015). *Bacillus halodurans* produced industrial CGTase at a higher pH of 10.5 (More et al., 2012). The variation in genomes might also explain why bacteria that produce enzymes have varied beginning pH needs. The optimal pH reported for the formation of fungal enzymes spans from acidic to basic, namely pH 5 to 9 (Prasanna et al., 2016). *Aspergillus terreus* gr. was employed by Niyonzima and More (2013) to produce an alkaline protease active at pH 10.0. The best starting pH for *Aspergillus* species in the production of tanas, phytase, and pectinases was also demonstrated to be between 4 and 4.5 (Sandhya et al., 2015). The specificity of the bacterial or fungal strains may be responsible for the variation in commercial enzyme output at different starting pH requirements. Any deviation from the ideal initial pH led to a reduction in enzyme secretion. This has to do with how the bacterial or fungal barrier, which restricts the release of enzymes, interferes with transport activities.

### 1.5.3 EFFECT OF TEMPERATURE ON MICROBIAL ENZYME PRODUCTION

Microorganisms produce enzymes in response to environmental factors, one of which is temperature. It could affect the development of bacteria and fungus and, as with initial pH, the resulting generation of bacterial or fungal enzymes. The optimal temperature for bacterial enzyme production is between 30 and 50°C. In most situations, 37°C was shown to be the best production temperature (Table 1.1) (Wang et al., 2012). *Bacillus* species produced industrial amylase and lipase at low optimal temperatures of 20 and 28°C, respectively (Roohi et al., 2013). The optimal temperature for fungal species ranges from 25 to 47°C (Niyonzima and More, 2013). However, 60°C was shown to be the optimal fermentation temperature for *Penicillium nigricans* α-amylase synthesis (Uday et al., 2103). Due to the thermostability of enzymes or denaturing of the structure of the enzyme at the active site, the yield of industrial enzyme synthesis is poor at higher incubation temperatures.

### 1.5.4 IMPACT OF INOCULUM SIZE ON MICROBIAL ENZYME PRODUCTION

Inoculum concentration is one of the most crucial culture parameters for microbial development and, subsequently, for the manufacture of commercial enzymes. It was shown that different inoculum concentrations between 0.6 and 4% were ideal for encouraging microorganisms to produce bacterial enzymes (Table 1.1) (More et al., 2015). However, Chauhan et al. (2013) found that *Staphylococcus arlettae* JPBW-1 produces detergent lipase at a larger inoculum size of 10%. To maximize the production of enzymes by various fungi, different inoculum quantities were found. For the production of tannase by *Mucor circinelloides isolate* F6-3-12 and protease by *Aspergillus terreus* gr, a 2% inoculum level was ideal (Niyonzima and More, 2013). For *Scopulariopsis* sp. protease secretion, a 3% inoculum size was ideal. At a 9% inoculum level, Lincoln and More (2018) identified industrial invertase from *Aspergillus sojae* JU12. Therefore, the type of microorganism, inoculum load, and size and type of the bacterial or fungal organism may all have an impact on the influence of inoculum on enzyme production. In general, an increase in inoculum concentration was linked to an increase in enzyme synthesis by microorganisms until the ideal inoculum size was reached because of rapid substrate breakdown (Niyonzima and More, 2013). Indeed, at lower inoculum levels, enzyme production by microorganisms is typically high; yet, once the inoculum size has been reached, a low industrial enzyme yield is observed. Similar to this, Hasan et al. (2017) found that at greater inoculum levels, output was poor because the bacteria were not receiving enough total dissolved oxygen and nutrients.

### 1.5.5 EFFECT OF CARBON SOURCE ON MICROBIAL ENZYME PRODUCTION

The primary energy source for bacterial and fungal growth, and consequently for the production of enzymes, comes from carbon sources. For the manufacture of bacterial enzymes, carbon sources such as starch, glucose, soluble pullulan, malt extract, maltose, pullulan, sucrose, and carboxymethylcellulose are employed (Hasan et al., 2017). Soybean oil, olive oil, and cotton seed oil served as carbon sources. In some cases, a variety of carbon sources, such as corn flour and bean flour, glucose and skim milk, and glucose and sesame oil, are used to produce bacterial enzymes. The production of industrial fungal enzymes uses a variety of carbon sources, including starch, glucose, maltose, sucrose, lactose, carboxymethylcellulose, pectin, and tannate (Roy and Mukherjee, 2013). Many inexpensive materials, including wheat bran, Jamun leaves, green tea leaves, and orange peel soaked with molasses, were used as carbon sources for the manufacture of industrial enzymes by a fungus (Chauhan et al., 2013). Microorganisms with low carbon source concentrations are commonly used to manufacture industrial enzymes. This reduces the overall cost of production. In some cases, carbon source repression is accomplished when a sizable amount of the carbon source is consumed. Due to restrictions on oxygen transport, enzyme production declines when a substantial amount of carbon source is consumed; this leads to poor bacterial or fungal growth.

### *1.5.6 EFFECT OF NITROGEN SOURCES ON MICROBIAL ENZYME PRODUCTION*

As a secondary energy source for microbial growth and, subsequently, for the manufacture of enzymes, nitrogen sources were utilized. They aid in the synthesis of amino acids, peptides, proteins (including enzymes used in industry), nucleotides, and nucleic acids in the majority of bacteria (Chauhan et al., 2013). To create bacterial enzymes, tryptone, peptone, yeast extract, and beef extract are used (Table 1.1). Optimal commercial enzyme synthesis is sometimes found when nitrogen sources, such as peptone and yeast extract, are combined (Narancic et al., 2019). Additionally, bacteria employ inexpensive organic nitrogen sources like maize flour, bean flour, and soybean meal to produce enzymes. The production of fungal enzymes uses organic nitrogen sources, similar to those used by bacteria, such as peptone, tryptone, urea, yeast extract, beef extract, and L-asparagine. In general, enzyme production is at its highest when organic nitrogen sources are present in the production medium. A variety of minerals, vitamins, amino acids, peptides, and growth factors may be present in enzyme-producing microorganisms, which may account for their preference for organic nitrogen sources (Table 1.1) (Niyonzima and More, 2013). To create commercial keratinase, *Bacillus megaterium* employed feather meal as a source of carbon and nitrogen. After a certain point, nitrogen metabolite suppression is observed. Nitrogen inputs boost enzyme production. Complex organic nitrogen sources, which are often rich in short peptides and amino acids (such as glycine and valine), may block enzymes when utilized in significant quantities. As a result, a greater nitrogen supply concentration inhibits enzyme production by bacteria or fungi. Although it is uncommon to find inorganic nitrogen sources to encourage enzyme synthesis, they have been demonstrated to do so under certain conditions. For instance, significant enzyme production was observed when bacteria exploited the output of ammonium acetate, potassium nitrate, and ammonium sulfate. Similar to this, fungi produced enzymes using inorganic nitrogen sources such as ammonium nitrate, potassium nitrate, sodium nitrate, and sodium nitrite.

### *1.5.7 EFFECT OF AGITATION ON THE ENZYMES PRODUCTION*

Microorganisms that produce enzymes are often cultivated in shaking conditions. Shaking at 100 to 200 rev/min is commonly used in the synthesis of bacterial enzymes (Table 1.1). For example, 100 rpm was optimal for *Bacillus* species producing enzymes, whereas 200 rpm was also optimal for other bacterial species. Similarly, fungi were agitated in the 120 to 200 rev/min range while producing enzymes. For example, 120 rpm, 150 rpm, 160 rpm, 180 rpm, and 200 rpm were discovered to be appropriate shaking conditions for fungal species. The moderate agitation of the culture flasks provides for excellent nutrient availability to the microorganisms as well as optimum aeration, encouraging the generation of significant numbers of enzymes.

## 1.6 APPROACHES FOR INDUSTRIAL PRODUCTION OF MICROBIAL ENZYME

After strain selection, improvement, and medium optimization, fermentation technology is the crucial element in enzyme synthesis. By reducing complicated substrates to simple molecules, microorganisms can evolve and metabolize them, creating a range of enzymes and byproducts in the process. For the large-scale production of the bioactive compounds, submerged fermentation (SMF) and solid-state fermentation (SSF) procedures are used (Figure 1.1).

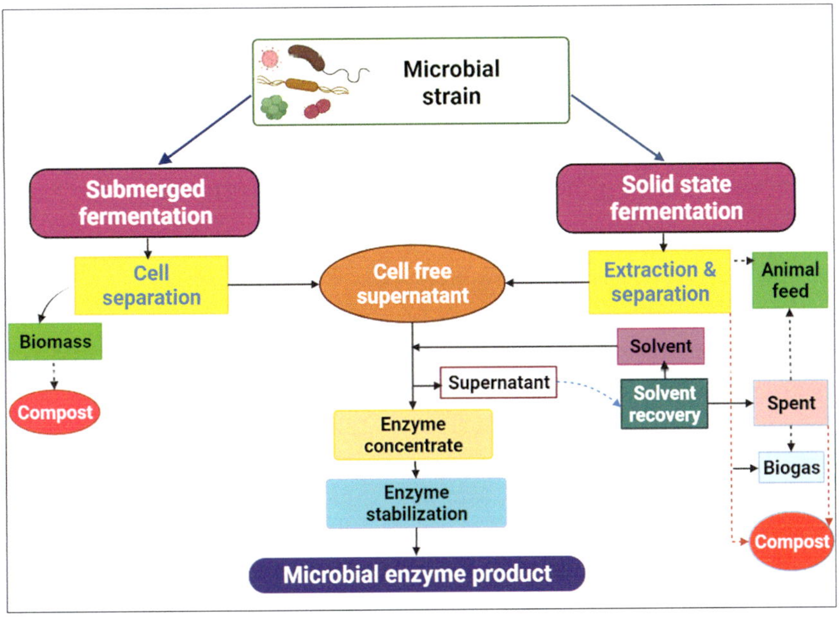


**FIGURE 1.1** An overview on the production process of microbial enzymes.

### 1.6.1 *SUBMERGED FERMENTATION*

The technique with the highest adoption rate, known as SMF, involves the controlled growth of microbes in liquid substrates like broth, a nutritive medium with high oxygen availability and ideal pH, temperature, and carbon dioxide levels. An aerobic submerged culture in a stirred-tank reactor is a typical commercial technology for enzyme production using microorganisms that produce an extracellular enzyme (Singh et al., 2016). Large-scale SMF fermenters with volumes ranging from thousands to hundreds of thousands of liters have no issues with mass transfer or heat removal. Microorganisms continue to be in contact with the liquid medium in the SMF. The SMF requires an oxygen supply, which is provided by a sparger. In these fermenters, stirrers and impellers are critical for blending gas, biomass, and suspended particles (Sivamani and Baskar, 2018). The microorganisms in the SMF can be grown in four different methods. There are four types of culture: batch culture, fed-batch culture, perfusion batch culture, and continuous culture. Microorganisms are injected into a predetermined volume of media in batch culture. In the case of fed-batch culture, the concentrated nutrient components are gradually delivered to the batch culture. In the perfusion batch culture, the culture is added, and an equivalent amount of used cell-free media is withdrawn. Fresh medium is added to the batch system at the exponential stage of microbial development, and then the medium containing the product is removed. A nearly balanced development with little change in nutrients, metabolites, cell counts, or biomass is the consequence of continuous culture.

### 1.6.2 SOLID STATE FERMENTATION

SSF uses solid substrates with low or no moisture content, such as agro-industrial waste. SSF has recently become the favored fermentation method due to its ease of use, low cost, and environmentally friendly nature. The benefits of SSF include increased enzyme synthesis, the utilization of nutrient-rich agro-waste as complete media, reduced catabolic suppression in the presence of surplus substrate, decreased effluent waste and foam production, and quick and straightforward end-product purification (Thomas et al., 2013b). The key factors that affect microbial enzyme production in an SSF system are as follows: pre-treatment of the substrate, particle size (interparticle spacing and surface area), water content and water activity, relative humidity, type and size of the inoculum, temperature control of fermenting matter/removal of metabolic heat, culture duration, homogeneity in the SSF system's environment, and the gaseous atmosphere, that is, oxygen consumption rate and carbon dioxide concentration. SSF bioreactors' design and operation have changed significantly over the past 10 years to address problems with things like oxygen circulation, heat dissipation, moisture management, agitation aeration, scale-up, and so on (Singhania et al., 2015). As a result of its resemblance to their natural environment, SSF was first designed as a fermentation medium for fungus. However, recent studies have revealed that other microorganisms, including yeast and bacteria, may also thrive on SSF, making it a preferable choice for biomolecule synthesis. Several compounds, including industrially significant enzymes like proteases, cellulases, ligninases, xylanases, pectinases, amylases, and glucoamylases, are being synthesized using its potential; Additionally, efforts are being made to investigate

SSF processes for the production of antibiotics, organic acids, phenolic compounds, biofuels, phytases, inulinases, tannases, phenolic acid esterases, microbial rennet, aryl-alcohol oxidases, oligosaccharide oxidases, tannin acyl hydrolase, and a-L-arabinofuranosidase (Lizardi et al., 2017). The great achievement of SSF in enzyme synthesis has demonstrated its applicability in the enzyme market. In recent years, Novozymes (Otto et al., 2005), Biocon Ltd., and Japan Enzymes have all branched out into SSF-based specialty enzyme manufacturing. PlaFractor, a new SSF bioreactor, was created by Biocon thanks to early R&D investments. Similar to this, He and Chen (2013) used an enhanced SSF fermenter that was built for industrial scale to produce 2.5 times more hydrolytic enzymes at the pilot scale (800 liters). With so many advantages associated with SSF, research on bioreactor design is quickly advancing and revolutionizing the technology for improved, flexible, and substantial bioprocessing.

## 1.7 DOWNSTREAM PROCESSING AND PRODUCTION

### *1.7.1 PURIFICATION*

Purity is a significant factor in enzyme activity, stability, applicability, and commercial value. The isolation and purification procedure uses procedures such as flocculation, filtering, precipitation, and chromatography (Mukherjee, 2019). Industries are always looking for methods to minimize the number of purification processes, which have a direct impact on both manufacturing and product cost. Among these is the secretion of extracellular biomolecules. As a result, a lot of research is devoted to finding new microbes that secrete extracellular enzymes, as well as enzyme engineering techniques like adding a secretory tag to the target protein, altering the entire secretory machinery, or fine-tuning secretory system regulation networks for improved extracellular secretion (Burdette et al., 2018).

### *1.7.2 ENZYME IMMOBILIZATION*

The production process is inhibited because free enzymes are usually denatured after prolonged contact with extreme conditions. To address these issues, enzyme immobilization was developed, which not only allows for the reuse of enzymes but also boosts their activity and stability

(Bernal et al., 2018). Additionally, the purifying procedure is made simpler by mounting the catalyst on a sturdy base, enabling successful manufacture. The typical techniques for immobilizing enzymes on biocompatible, thermostable, and nontoxic carrier materials are adsorption, trapping, and encapsulation, as well as covalent binding/cross-linking (Figure 1.2), with natural biopolymers (Bilal et al., 2019) and nanomaterials rapidly gaining popularity (Bhavaniramya et al., 2019). Before choosing the biomaterial, a thorough examination of the carrier material must be carried out because not all carrier materials are compatible with every enzyme and have a significant impact on enzyme properties. Immobilized hydrolytic enzymes are widely used in the food, pharmaceutical, and biofuel industries (Verma et al., 2016).

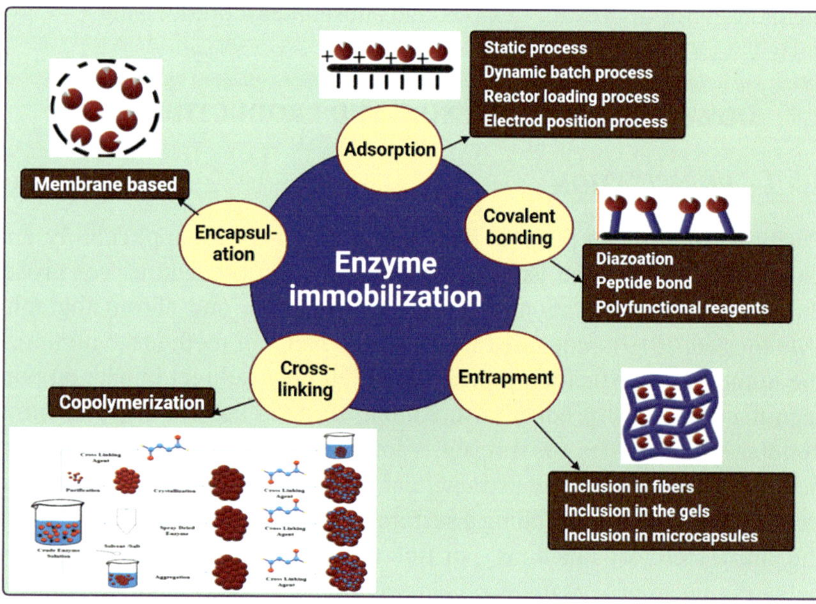


**FIGURE 1.2** Various approaches of enzyme immobilization.

### 1.7.3 WHOLE-CELL BIOCATALYSIS

The next major development that is gaining traction is whole-cell biocatalysis. Enzymes perform best in physiologically ideal conditions that are provided by intact cells. Additionally, they make it unnecessary to add cofactors to the process and allow for the complete omission of steps like cell lysis and purification, which reduces the cost of production (de Carvalho, 2017). The co-expression of numerous enzymes in a single cell has been made possible via metabolic engineering, turning it into an independent, fully functional factory that can successfully perform biotransformation (Aalbers and Fraaije, 2019). Furthermore, a stable, reusable catalyst with a long shelf life may be created by immobilizing whole cells on biopolymers or catalytic biofilms that have been successfully used to produce biofuels, food additives, and other things (Polakovic et al., 2017). It is an appealing technology with the ability to push the manufacturing process well beyond industry norms. Cell surface display technology is a superior alternative to whole-cell biocatalysis. To achieve high productivity through concerted catalysis, one or many proteins are tethered to the cell's surface. The attached enzymes are stabilized by the cell membrane and may be easily produced by simply cultivating the cells (Han et al., 2018). Biofuel generation is one application that benefits from this technique. In a single fermenter, yeast with cell surface expression of lignocellulose-degrading enzymes can directly produce a large number of biofuels (Sakuragi et al., 2011). Similar research found multienzyme cascades to be involved in the augmented synthesis of endoglucanase and β-glucosidase tethered to glycosylphosphatidylinositol anchor proteins (Inokuma et al., 2016). Guirimand et al. (2016) demonstrated direct xylitol synthesis by expressing four distinct enzymes on the yeast surface: xylose reductase, β-glucosidase, xylosidase, and xylanase. These studies demonstrate the technology's promise and ease of use.

### 1.7.4 HYDROLYTIC ENZYMES

A family of approximately 200 enzymes, known as hydrolases (EC3), catalyzes the dissociation of large molecules into smaller parts when they are in the presence of water. It is necessary to hydrolyze complex substrates in bioprocessing and the production of several products with value additions. These enzymes play a crucial role in the production of biofuel, animal feed, paper and pulp, textiles, coffee, and juice extraction, all of which require lignocellulosic biomass as a raw material. There are about 20 hydrolytic enzymes produced on a truly industrial basis. These enzymes are mostly derived from native or engineered fungi and bacteria. A recent analysis highlighted the technical improvement in the enzyme industry by citing many patented and commercially available enzymes strengthened through engineering and immobilization (Prasad and Roy, 2018). A comprehensive approach that considers all aspects of upstream and downstream production is beneficial for the development of the entire bioprocess for industrial-scale hydrolytic enzyme production. Pilot-scale (300–800) trials, conducted after strain development and medium optimization, help us comprehend the scale-up constraints. The large-scale synthesis of these enzymes is driven by the combination of the necessary conditions, once they have been determined, and technological proficiency. The entire description of the process development, operating procedures, engineering and design of bioreactors, economics, and regulatory difficulties in industrial-scale fermentation is provided in a recent book chapter (Meyer et al., 2016). Investing in R&D and fine-tuning enzyme process technologies will result in a significant rise in both the number and supply of industrial enzymes.

## 1.8 APPLICATIONS OF MICROBIAL ENZYMES IN INDUSTRIAL PROCESSES

The speed and specificity of different biotechnological reactions and metabolic activities are significantly increased by microbial enzymes. This covers all processes, including digestion and DNA synthesis (Chapman et al., 2018). Some of the commercially exploited microbial enzymes include proteases, cellulases, xylanases, amylases, and lipases. The great majority of commercial enzymes are hydrolytic (used for the disintegration of natural compounds). Proteases account for roughly 60% of the global enzyme market. This section covered a range of enzyme applications in different industrial processes, from detergents to pharmaceuticals (Table 1.2).

### *1.8.1 ANIMAL FEED INDUSTRY*

Microbial enzymes have long been used in animal nutrition. Feed enzymes generally boost feed utilization efficiency and nutrient digestibility. Carbohydrase's, for example, improve carbohydrate digestibility, increasing the efficiency of animal feeds. The amount of non-protein nitrogen additions

**TABLE 1.2** Various Applications of Industrially Produced Microbial Enzymes

| Sl. No. | Types of Microbes | Types of Enzymes | Fermentation Method | Industrial Applications | Industry |
|---|---|---|---|---|---|
| 1. | *Penicillium* sp. | Penicillin oxidase | SmF | Antibiotic synthesis | Pharmaceuticals |
| 2. | *Bacillus* sp. | Amylase | SSF and SmF | Increase the bread shelf life | Baking industry |
| 3. | *Bacillus* sp. | Amylase | SmF | Starch hydrolysis | Beverages industry |
| 4. | *Bacillus* sp. | Xylanase | SSF and SmF | Augmentation of pulp | Paper and Pulp industry |
| 5. | *Bacillus subtilis* | Laccase | SmF | Fabric dyeing | Textile industry |
| 6. | *Bacillus subtilis, Trametes versicolor* | laccase | SmF | Hair dye | Cosmetics |
| 7. | *Bacillus* sp. | Alpha-amylase | SmF | Digestive disorders | Pharmaceuticals |
| 8. | *Bacillus* sp. | Amlyase | SmF | Cleanliness of paper | Paper and Pulp industry |
| 9. | *Aspergillus niger* | Phytase | SSF | Hydrolyze phytic acid to release phosphorous | Animal feed |
| 10. | *Aspergillus niger, A. oryzae* | limoninase | SSF and SmF | Debittering | Beverages industry |
| 11. | *Aspergillus* sp. | Acid proteinase | SmF | Milk coagulation | Dairy industry |
| 12. | *Aspergillus* sp., *Bacillus subtilis* | Amylase | SSF and SmF | Fiber splitting | Leather industry |
| 13. | *Aspergillus* sp. | Catalase | SSF | Bleach termination | Textile industry |
| 14. | *Aspergillus* sp., *Bacillus subtilis* | Amylase | SSF and SmF | Carbohydrate stain removal | Detergent |
| 15. | *Aspergillus niger* | Amyloglucosidase | SSF | Starch hydrolysis for bioremediation | Waste management |
| 16. | *Aspergillus* sp., *Bacillus* sp. | Xylanase | SSF and SmF | Enhanced digestibility of starch | Animal feed |
| 17. | *Clostridium* sp. | Cellulase | SSF and SmF | Stability and texture | Beverages industry |
| 18. | *Streptococci* sp. | Streptokinase | SmF | Anticoagulants | Pharmaceuticals |
| 19. | *Pseudomonas* sp. | Peroxidase | SSF | Formation of cross-links | Polymer industry |
| 20. | *Pseudomonas* sp., *Rhodococcus* sp. | Oxygenase | SSF and SmF | Degradation of halogenated contaminants | Waste management |
| 21. | *Aspergillus niger, A. flflavus, Bacillus subtilis* | Protease | SSF and SmF | Removal of dead skin | Cosmetics |

**TABLE 1.2** *(Continued)*

| Sl. No. | Types of Microbes | Types of Enzymes | Fermentation Method | Industrial Applications | Industry |
|---|---|---|---|---|---|
| 22. | *Aspergillus oryzae, A. Flavus* | Lipase | SSF | Fat stain elimination | Detergent |
| 23. | *Candida* sp. | Lipase | SSF | Degreasing to remove fats | Leather industry |
| 24. | *Streptoverticillium* sp. | Transglutaminase | SmF | Enhance flour quality | Baking industry |
| 25. | *Aspergillus niger* | $\beta$-glucanase | SSF and SmF | Digestive aid | Animal feed |
| 26. | *Streptoverticillium* sp. | Transglutaminase | SmF | Protein polymerization | Dairy industry |
| 27. | *Clostridium perfringens* | Collagenase | SSF and SmF | Skin ulcers | Pharmaceuticals |
| 28. | *Candida* sp. | Lipase | SSF | Polyester preparation | Polymer industry |
| 29. | *Candida Antarctica* | Lipase | SSF | Pitch control | Paper and Pulp industry |
| 30. | *Fusarium solani f. pisi* | Cutinase | SSF and SmF | Degradation of plastics, Polycaprolactone | Waste management |
| 32. | *Acinetobacter* | Galactosidase | – | Antitumor activity | Pharmaceuticals |
| 33. | *Lactobacillus* sp. | Lactase | SmF | Sweetness to milk | Dairy industry |
| 34. | *Bacillus* sp., *Aspergillus* sp. | Proteases | SSF and SmF | Softness, supple, pliable | Leather industry |
| 35. | *Fusarium solani f. pisi* | Cutinase | SSF and SmF | Triglyceride removal | Detergent |
| 36. | *Pseudomonas* sp. | Cutinase | SSF and SmF | Cotton scouring | Textile industry |
| 37. | *Candida lipolytica* | Lipase | SSF | Dough stability | Baking industry |
| 38. | *Trichoderma reesei* | Tyrosinase | SmF | Polymerization of lignin and chitosan | Polymer industry |
| 39. | *B. licheniformis, Aspergillus sp* | Amylase | SSF and SmF | Bioremediation of vegetable wastes | Waste management |

SmF, Submerged fermentation; SSF, Solid state fermentation.

in animal diets is reduced by the use of feed proteases (Morin et al., 2019). Around 85–90% of the natural plant phosphorus in cereal-based feed for monogastric animals is bound in phytic acid. Current commercially available feed enzymes include phytases, proteases, subtilisin, α-galactosidase, xylanase, glucanase, α-amylase, and polygalacturonase. The swine and poultry industries are the main users of these feed enzymes (Bajaj and Mahajan, 2019).

### 1.8.2 FOOD PROCESSING INDUSTRY

Food bio-molecule enzymes are a useful tool for optimizing food quality and production, as well as other food attributes like flavor, texture, digestibility, fragrance, functionality, and nutritional value (Tavano et al., 2018). Some of the most popular food enzymes used in food processing are cellulase, protease, lipase, amylase, and pectinase. These food enzymes are largely employed in the starch processing, baking, wine and beer making, juice production, dairy (cheese manufacture), and baking sectors. There are now roughly nine recombinant microorganisms that are deemed Generally Recognized as Safe (GRAS), according to FDA standards. Microbial lipases are important for retailing vegetable oils because they are regiospecific and fatty acid specific. Lipases were previously used in bio-lipolysis to refine rice flavor, modify soybean milk, improve aroma, and stimulate apple wine fermentation (Baudrexl et al., 2019). Brewing enzymes aid in the control of the overall process, resulting in higher quality beer and other beverages. The beverage industry uses the most microbial enzymes, followed by the dairy industry. The most crucial enzymes utilized in the brewing sector are proteases, pentosanes, α-amylases, and β-guanase's (Jia et al., 2017). The main purposes of dairy enzymes are to extend the shelf life and improve the quality of dairy products. Cheese, yogurt, and other dairy products are frequently made using chymosin, lipases, and lysozymes. Milk products' allergenicity is reduced by proteases (Struch et al., 2016). Other enzymes, such as proteases, decrease bread's gluten strength, mix time, dough consistency, and protein concentration (Ge et al., 2020). Enzymes can increase the effectiveness of processes like peeling, extraction, maceration, juicing, and clarifying in juice manufacturing in addition to improving sensory qualities. Pectinases enhance total juice output while amylases are employed to hydrolyze starch into glucose and clarify murky juice (such as that produced while making apple juice).

### 1.8.3 POLYMER AND TEXTILE INDUSTRY

Environmentally sustainable and secure alternatives to chemical and physical polymer modification are enzymatic polymer modification and enzymatic monomer synthesis/polymerization. The apex of biopolymers with industrial applications is the development of polylactide (PLA) from lactic acid fermentation and the production of genetically designed eco-friendly polyester. Numerous biomedical sectors, including orthopedic devices, tissue engineering, drug delivery, vaccine adjuvants, and therapeutic methods, use biopolymers in a variety of ways. For instance, clinically utilized surgical sutures and implants are made of degradable polymers. The main enzymes employed in polymer manufacturing include transglutaminase, laccase, peroxidase, and lipase. Lipase is a naturally occurring renewable biocatalyst. Developed polyesters based on lipases are frequently regarded as highly valuable products for biomedical and pharmaceutical applications (Nisha, 2016). Without the usage of $H_2O_2$, laccases are flexible organic synthesis biocatalysts that are utilized to create polymers in the air. Acrylamide is radically polymerized by laccases both with and without a mediator. The textile industry is one of the most significant polluters of the environment (Chiliveri et al., 2016). Hydrolase and oxidoreductase are the two types of enzymes that are most frequently used in the textile industry. Enzymes called hydrolases are employed in the removal of starch size, cotton softening, enhancement of color and surface vividness, wrinkle resistance, and treatment of wool in addition to biopolishing and bioscouring of fabric.

### 1.8.4 PAPER AND PULP INDUSTRY

In the paper and pulp sectors, the use of different enzymes has rapidly increased. Enzymes are used to enhance waste treatment, bleaching, and de-inking. Enzymes can also speed up operations while using less energy and hazardous chemicals (Mitrofanova et al., 2017). The wood pulp that has been pretreated with laccase benefits from cleaner, milder delignification, and whitening processes. Pulp grafting and deinking are two other possible applications for bacterial and fungal laccases. In the pulp and paper business, lipases are used to de-ink pulping procedures and enhance pitch control.

### *1.8.5 DETERGENT INDUSTRY*

One of the greatest industrial uses of enzymes is in the detergent sector. Enzymes in laundry detergents aid to improve fabric whiteness and color, softening cotton, and increasing stain removal efficiency. The chosen enzymes should be stable at low temperatures, have high catalytic activity, and have an alkaline pH (Mohandas et al., 2018). Hydrolases make up the majority of the enzymes used in laundry detergents. Examples of such enzymes include the cold-active serine protease (CP70) from *Flavobacterium balustinum* and the cold-active alkaline protease from *Stenotrophomonas maltophilia*. The stability and compatibility of proteases with washing detergents (Pivnenko et al., 2015). Enzymes are used in detergent manufacturing because they contain fewer bleaching agents and phosphates than traditional surfactants, which benefit the environment and the general population. Amylases are utilized in dishwashing to remove insoluble starch residues, while cutinize is mainly found in laundry detergents and lipase helps to remove lipid stains from fabric surfaces.

### *1.8.6 PHARMACEUTICAL INDUSTRY AND MEDICINE*

Enzymes are utilized as therapeutic medications to treat digestive problems and enzymatic deficiencies. In clinical diagnostic processes like ELISA and diabetes testing kits, enzymes are crucial. Microbes are significant biocatalysts with numerous uses in the pharmaceutical and biotechnology sectors (Anbu et al., 2017). Microbial lipases are an effective biocatalyst for the production of bioactive compounds and are beneficial in the manufacture of chiral synthons. Examples of these include alumina in kidney dialysis patients, acne, malaria, prion disorders, diabetes, obesity, ulcers, and even prion diseases (Singh and Singh, 2016). *Streptomyces* is the most common gram-negative soil bacteria. *Castanospermine,* a potent anti-AIDS medication, is regioselectivity modified using lipases. To diagnose serious medical disorders, the amount of lipase in blood serum can be utilized as a diagnostic tool (Hasin et al., 2017). Enzymes are used to treat burns, thrombosis, and cardiovascular diseases. Cholesterol oxidase has the potential to be used in cholesterol testing and control. Putrescine oxidase aids in the identification of biogenic amines such as food spoilage (Bush et al., 2020). The enzyme tyrosinase (EC 1.14.18.1) is necessary for the production of L-dihydroxyphenyl alanine (l-DOPA), which is a precursor to dopamine. Parkinson's disease and myocardial neurogenic damage can both be effectively treated with dopamine. A storehouse of substances with biological activity is a sponge. Marine cyanobacteria help to produce a variety of chemical compounds and drugs with antiviral, antibacterial, and anticancer properties. The utilization of microbial enzymes in medicines and human medicine still requires novel strategies.

### 1.8.7 BIOFUEL INDUSTRY

The carbon-rich biodegradable material known as lignocellulosic biomass is created by plants. Additionally, it can be discovered in wastewater treatment facilities, municipal and industrial trash, and forest residues. As an environmentally friendly feedstock for the biofuel industry, biomass has received a lot of attention (Lancaster et al., 2018). Biomass can be transformed into feedstock chemicals using cellulolytic enzymes produced by various cellulolytic and xylanolytic bacteria, fungi, and microorganisms. Bacterial species that can effectively hydrolyze the components of plant cell walls can be found in the soil, the sea, and the intestines of herbivorous animals (Qu et al., 2020). For a variety of industrial biofuel applications, custom cellulases and xylanases can be created by engineering microbial enzymes. An essential step in the effective hydrolysis of polysaccharides is the pretreatment of lignin. In order to detoxify lignocellulosic hydrolysates, a new laccase isolated from the white rot fungus (*Ganoderma lucidum*) was utilized (Rao et al., 2017). Hemicellulose hydrolysis necessitates the involvement of several functional enzymes, as well as complementary activities at various levels. During the hydrolysis of cellulose, the cooperative action of endoglucanases and cellobiohydrolases is essential. Several hydrolytic enzymes, including endoxylanases, beta-xylosidases, and arabinofuranosidases, must work together to hydrolyze xylan. The creation of more effective competitive enzyme cocktails is one of the emerging strategies for isolating these multi-functional enzymes to boost saccharification efficiency in biomass conversion.

## 1.9 CONCLUSION AND FUTURE PROSPECTS

The possibilities of industrial usage of microbial enzymes have greatly increased in the 21st century and continue to develop because enzymes provide enormous potential for many industries to meet the needs of a continually expanding population while coping with resource exhaustion. The current chapter provides an overview of microbial enzyme production and optimization of nutritional and physical factors. Because microbial enzymes are in constant demand, the current information can assist other researchers in cost effectively optimizing microbial enzyme production. Enzymes have been shown to offer enormous promise in a range of industrial fields, including medicine, food, feed, beverages, detergents, leather processing, and paper and pulp. Alternatively, these biomolecules might be employed continually to fulfill the ever-increasing need for food supply. Microbial enzymes offer tremendous promise in waste management and, as a result, in the creation of a green environment. Enzymes are effectively utilized in many industries to produce outputs of greater quality at a faster rate of reaction, with less pollution, and at a lower cost. Despite advancements in technology, we are just now starting to grasp the potential of enzymes. We have released enormous power thanks to our expertise in rDNA technology, computational biology, biostatistics, biopolymer sciences, and other areas. Today, we can separate novel strains from inhospitable microorganisms, create enzymes with specific properties that are made to order, reroute metabolic pathways in microbes, increase enzyme output by changing conditions, and enhance enzyme stability and reusability by immobilization and whole-cell use. However, there is still more to be developed in terms of bioprocess design. Biocatalysis will undergo a revolution because of ongoing research into new enzymes, the creation of novel upstream and downstream processing mechanisms, and a multidisciplinary approach.

## KEYWORDS

- **bioprocess engineering**
- **enzyme production**
- **fermentation**
- **microbial enzymes**
- **recombinant technology**
- **strain improvement**

## REFERENCES

Aalbers, F. S., & Fraaije, M. W. (2019). Enzyme fusions in biocatalysis: coupling reactions by pairing enzymes. *Chembiochem: European Journal of Chemical Biology, 20*, 20–28.

Adrio, J. L., & Demain, A. L. (2014). Microbial enzymes: tools for biotechnological processes. *Biomolecules, 4*, 117–139.

Anandan, D., Marmer, W. N., & Dudley, R. L. (2007). Isolation, characterization, and optimization of culture parameters for production of an alkaline protease isolated from *Aspergillus tamarii*. *Journal of Industrial Microbiology and Biotechnology, 34*(5), 339–347.

Anbu, P., Gopinath, S. C. B., Chaulagain, B. P., & Lakshmipriya, T. (2013). Microbial enzymes and their applications in industries and medicine. *BioMed Research International*, 204014. https://doi.org/10.1155/2017/2195808 (accessed on 5th November 2025).

Anbu, P., Gopinath, S. C. B., Chaulagain, B. P., & Lakshmipriya, T. (2017). Microbial enzymes and their applications in industries and medicine. *BioMed Research International*, *2016*, 1–3. https://doi.org/10.1155/2017/2195808 (accessed on 5th November 2025).

Bajaj, P., & Mahajan, R. (2019). Cellulase and xylanase synergism in industrial biotechnology. *Applied Microbiology and Biotechnology, 103*, 8711–8724. https://doi.org/10.1007/s00253-019-10146-0 (accessed on 5th November 2025).

Baudrexl, M., Schwarz, W. H., Zverlov, V. V., & Liebl, W. (2019). Biochemical characterization of four rhomboideus from thermophilic bacteria of the genera *Thermotoga, Caldicellulosiruptor,* and *Thermoclostridium*. *Scientific Reports, 9*, Article No. 15924. https://doi.org/10.1038/s41598-019-52251-0 (accessed on 5th November 2025).

Bauer, T. L., Buchholz, P. C. F., & Pleiss, J. (2020). The modular structure of α/β-hydrolases. *FEBS Journal, 287*, 1035–1053.

Berini, F., Casciello, C., Marcone, G. L., & Marinelli, F. (2017). Metagenomics: novel enzymes from non-culturable microbes. *FEMS Microbiology Letters, 364*(21).

Bernal, C., Rodríguez, K., & Martínez, R. (2018). Integrating enzyme immobilization and protein engineering: an alternative path for the development of novel and improved industrial biocatalysts. *Biotechnology Advances, 36*, 1470–1480.

Bhavaniramya, S., Vanajothi, R., Vishnupriya, S., Premkumar, K., AlAboody, M. S., Vijayakumar, R., & Baskaran, D. (2019). Enzyme immobilization on nanomaterials for biosensors and biocatalyst in food and biomedical industry. *Current Pharmaceutical Design, 25*, 2661–2676.

Bilal, M., & Iqbal, H. M. N. (2019). Naturally-derived biopolymers: potential platforms for enzyme immobilization. *International Journal of Biological Macromolecules, 130*, 462–482.

Burdette, L. A., Leach, S. A., Wong, H. T., & Tullman-Ercek, D. (2018). Developing gram-negative bacteria for the secretion of heterologous proteins. *Microbial Cell Factories, 17*, 196.

Bush, C. L., Blumberg, J. B., El-Sohemy, A., Minich, D. M., Ordovás, J. M., Reed, D. G., & Behm, V. A. Y. (2020). Toward the definition of personalized nutrition: a proposal. *Journal of the American College of Nutrition, 39*, 5–15. https://doi.org/10.1080/07315724.2019.1685332 (accessed on 5th November 2025).

Carvalho de, C. C. C. R. (2017). Whole-cell biocatalysts: essential workers from nature to the industry. *Microbial Biotechnology, 10*, 250–263.

Chae, T. U., Choi, S. Y., Kim, J. W., Ko, Y. S., & Lee, S. Y. (2017). Recent advances in systems metabolic engineering tools and strategies. *Current Opinion in Biotechnology, 47*, 67–82.

Chapman, J., Ismail, A. E., & Dinu, C. Z. (2018). Industrial applications of enzymes: recent advances, techniques, and outlooks. *Catalysts, 8*, 238.

Chauhan, M., Chauhan, R. S., & Garlapati, V. K. (2013). Evaluation of a new lipase from *Staphylococcus* sp. for detergent additive capability. *BioMed Research International*, 374967.

Chiliveri, S. R., Koti, S., & Linga, V. R. (2016). Retting and degumming of natural fibers by pectinolytic enzymes produced from *Bacillus tequilensis* SV11-UV37 using solid state fermentation. *SpringerPlus, 5*(1). https://doi.org/10.1186/s40064-016-2173-x (accessed on 5th November 2025).

Chowdhury, R., & Maranas, C. D. (2020). From directed evolution to computational enzyme engineering—a review. *AIChE Journal, 66*, e16847.

Dilokpimol, A., Mäkelä, M. R., Cerullo, G., Zhou, M., Varriale, S., Gidijala, L., Brás, J. L. A., Jütten, P., Piechot, A., Verhaert, R., et al. (2018). Fungal glucuronoxylan esterases: genome mining-based enzyme discovery and biochemical characterization. *New Biotechnology, 40*, 282–287.

Donohoue, P. D., Barrangou, R., & May, A. P. (2018). Advances in industrial biotechnology using CRISPR-Cas systems. *Trends in Biotechnology, 36*, 134–146.

El-Refai, H. A., Abdel-Naby, M. A., & Mostafa, H. (2017). Statistical optimization for Tanase production by *Mucor circinelloides* isolate F6-3-12 under submerged and solid-state fermentation. *Current Trends of Biotechnology and Pharmacy, 11*, 167–180.

Fraser, C. M., Eisen, J. A., & Salzberg, S. L. (2014). Microbial genome sequencing. *Nature, 406*, 799–803.

Gao, S., Lu, Y., Li, Y., Huang, R., & Zheng, G. (2019). Enhancement in the catalytic activity of *Sulfolobus solfataricus* P2 (+)-γ-lactamase by semi-rational design with the aid of a newly established high-throughput screening method. *Applied Microbiology and Biotechnology, 103*, 251–263.

Ge, J., Jiang, X., Liu, W., et al. (2020). Characterization, stability improvement, and bread baking applications of a novel cold-adapted glucose oxidase from *Cladosporium neopsychrotolerans* SL16. *Food Chemistry, 310*, Article ID: 125970. https://doi.org/10.1016/j.foodchem.2019.125970 (accessed on 5th November 2025).

Ghasemi, Y., Sadeghi, H., Gholami, A., Mohkam, M., & Kargar, M. (2014). Isolation and identification of highly xylanase producing bacterium *Sphingobacterium* sp. SaH-05 from soil. *International Journal of Scientific and Engineering Research, 5*, 205–209.

Gilbert, J. A., Jansson, J. K., & Knight, R. (2014). The Earth microbiome project: successes and aspirations. *BMC Biology, 12*, 69.

Gilmore, S. P., Lillington, S. P., Haitjema, C. H., de Groot, R., & O'Malley, M. A. (2020). Designing chimeric enzymes inspired by fungal celluloses. *Synthetic and Systems Biotechnology, 5*, 23–32.

Grigoriev, I. V., Nikitin, R., Haridas, S., Kuo, A., Ohm, R., Otillar, R., Riley, R., Salamov, A., Zhao, X., Korzeniewski, F., et al. (2014). MycoCosm portal: gearing up for 1000 fungal genomes. *Nucleic Acids Research, 42*, D699–D704.

Guirimand, G., Sasaki, K., Inokuma, K., Bamba, T., Hasunuma, T., & Kondo, A. (2016). Cell surface engineering of *Saccharomyces cerevisiae* combined with membrane separation technology for xylitol production from rice straw hydrolysate. *Applied Microbiology and Biotechnology, 100*, 3477–3487.

Han, L., Zhao, Y., Cui, S., & Liang, B. (2018). Redesigning of microbial cell surface and its application to whole-cell biocatalysis and biosensors. *Applied Biochemistry and Biotechnology, 185*, 396–418.

Hasan, M. M., WalMarzan, L., Hosna, A., AlHakim, & Azad, A. K. (2017). Optimization of some fermentation conditions for the production of extracellular amylases by using *Chryseobacterium* and *Bacillus* isolates from organic kitchen wastes. *Journal of Genetic Engineering and Biotechnology, 15*, 59–68.

Hasin, Y., Seldin, M., & Lusis, A. (2017). Multi-omics approaches to disease. *Genome Biology, 18*, 1–15. https://doi.org/10.1186/s13059-017-1215-1 (accessed on 5th November 2025).

He, Q., & Chen, H. (2013). Pilot-scale gas double-dynamic solid-state fermentation for the production of industrial enzymes. *Food and Bioprocess Technology, 6*, 2916–2924.

Henrissat, B. (2013). The carbohydrate-active enzymes database (CAZy). *Nucleic Acids Research, 42*, 490–495. https://doi.org/10.1093/nar/gkt1178 (accessed on 5th November 2025).

Hussain, A. A., Abdel-Salam, M. S., & Abo-Ghalia, H. H. (2017). Optimization and molecular identification of novel cellulose degrading bacteria isolated from Egyptian environment. *Journal of Genetic Engineering and Biotechnology, 15*, 77–85.

Imchen, M., Kumavath, R., Barh, D., Avezedo, V., Ghosh, P., Viana, M., & Wattam, A. R. (2017). Searching for signatures across microbial communities: metagenomic analysis of soil samples from mangrove and other ecosystems. *Scientific Reports, 7*(1), 1–13.

Inokuma, K., Bamba, T., Ishii, J., Ito, Y., Hasunuma, T., & Kondo, A. (2016). Enhanced cell-surface display and secretory production of cellulolytic enzymes with *Saccharomyces cerevisiae* Sed1 signal peptide. *Biotechnology and Bioengineering, 113*, 2358–2366.

Jemli, S., Ayadi-Zouari, D., Ben H., & Bejar, S. (2016). Biocatalysts: application and engineering for industrial purposes. *Critical Reviews in Biotechnology, 36*, 246–258. https://doi.org/10.3109/07388551.2014.950550 (accessed on 5th November 2025).

Jia, X., Lin, X., Tian, Y., Chen, J., & You, M. (2017). High production, purification, biochemical characterization and gene analysis of a novel catalase from the thermophilic bacterium *Ureibacillus thermosphaericus* FZSF03. *International Journal of Biological Macromolecules, 103*, 89–98. https://doi.org/10.1016/j.ijbiomac.2017.05.034 (accessed on 5th November 2025).

Kanehisa, M. (2017). Enzyme annotation and metabolic reconstruction using KEGG. *Methods in Molecular Biology, 1611*, 135–145.

Karp, P. D., Ivanova, N., Krummenacker, M., Kyrpides, N., Latendresse, M., Midford, P., Ong, W. K., Paley, S., & Seshadri, R. (2019). A comparison of microbial genome web portals. *Frontiers in Microbiology, 10*, 208.

Koppel, N., & Balskus, E. P. (2016). Exploring and understanding the biochemical diversity of the human microbiota. *Cell Chemical Biology, 23*, 18–30.

Koutsandreas, T., Ladoukakis, E., Pilalis, E., Zarafeta, D., Kolisis, F. N., Skretas, G., & Chatziioannou, A. A. (2019). An automated metagenomic analysis pipeline for novel enzyme discovery exploiting next generation sequencing data. *Frontiers in Genetics, 10*, 1–15. https://doi.org/10.3389/fgene.2019.00469 (accessed on 5th November 2025).

Lancaster, L., Abdallah, W., Banta, S., & Wheeldon, I. (2018). Engineering enzyme microenvironments for enhanced biocatalysis. *Chemical Society Reviews, 47*, 5177–5186. https://doi.org/10.1039/c8cs00085a (accessed on 5th November 2025).

Li, G., Chen, Y., Fang, X., Su, F., Xu, L., & Yan, Y. (2018). Identification of a hotspot to enhance *Candida rugosa* lipase thermostability by rational design methods. *RSC Advances, 8*, 1948–1957.

Lincoln, L., & More, S. S. (2018). Purification and biochemical characterization of β-d-fructofuranosidase from *Bacillus subtilis* LYN12. *Journal of Food Biochemistry, 42*(18), e12592.

Liu, X., & Kokare, C. (2016). Chapter 11: Microbial enzymes of use in industry. In *Industrial Biotechnology: Microbial Enzymes* (pp. 267–298).

Lizardi-Jiménez, M. A., & Hernández-Martínez, R. (2017). Solid state fermentation (SSF): diversity of applications to valorize waste and biomass. *3 Biotech, 7*, 44.

Manisha, & Yadav, S. K. (2017). Technological advances and applications of hydrolytic enzymes for valorization of lignocellulosic biomass. *Bioresource Technology, 245*, 1727–1739.

Mathur, A., Kushwaha, A., Singh, A. K., & Katiyar, A. (2014). Isolation, purification and characterization of alkaline pectinase from *Bacillus subtilis* isolated from soil. *Journal of Pharmaceutical Sciences, 5*, 1–6.

May, O. (2019). Industrial enzyme applications–overview and historic perspective. In *Industrial Enzyme Applications* (pp. 1–24). John Wiley & Sons, Ltd.

Medema, M. H. (2018). Computational genomics of specialized metabolism: from natural product discovery to microbiome ecology. *mSystems, 3*. https://doi.org/10.1128/msystems.00182-17 (accessed on 5th November 2025).

Meyer, H. P., Minas, W., & Schmidhalter, D. (2016). Industrial-scale fermentation. In *Industrial Biotechnology* (pp. 1–53). Edited by Wittmann, C., & Liao, J. C. Wiley Online Library.

Mitrofanova, O., Mardanova, A., Evtugyn, V., Bogomolnaya, L., & Sharipova, M. (2017). Effects of *Bacillus* serine proteases on the bacterial biofilms. *BioMed Research International, 2017*(6), 1–10. https://doi.org/10.1155/2017/8525912 (accessed on 5th November 2025).

Miyauchi, S., Navarro, D., Grigoriev, I. V., Lipzen, A., Riley, R., Chevret, D., Grisel, S., Berrin, J. G., Henrissat, B., & Rosso, M. N. (2016). Visual comparative omics of fungi for plant biomass deconstruction. *Frontiers in Microbiology, 7*, 1335.

Mohandas, A., Raveendran, S., Parameswaran, B., Abraham, A., Athira, R. S. R., Mathew, A. K., & Pandey, A. (2018). Production of pectinase from *Bacillus sonorensis* MPTD1. *Food Technology and Biotechnology, 56*(1), 110–116. https://doi.org/10.17113/ftb.56.01.18.5477 (accessed on 5th November 2025).

More, S. S., Niraja, R., Evelyn, C., Byadgi, A. M., Shwetha, V., & Mangaraj, S. D. (2012). Isolation, purification and biochemical characterization of CGTase from *Bacillus halodurans*. *Croatian Journal of Food Technology, Biotechnology and Nutrition, 7*, 26–33.

More, S. S., Shrinivas, S., Agarwal, A., Chikkanna, A., Janardhan, B., & Niyonzima, F. N. (2015). Purification and characterization of phytase from *Bacillus lehensis* MLB2. *Biological, 70*, 294–304.

Morin-Crini, N., Lichtfouse, E., Torri, G., & Crini, G. (2019). Applications of chitosan in food, pharmaceuticals, medicine, cosmetics, agriculture, textiles, pulp and paper, biotechnology, and environmental chemistry. *Environmental Chemistry Letters, 17*, 1667–1692. https://doi.org/10.1007/s10311-019-00904-x (accessed on 5th November 2025).

Mukherjee, S. (2019). Chapter 2–Isolation and purification of industrial enzymes: Advances in enzyme technology. In *Advances in Enzyme Technology* (pp. 41–70). Edited by Singh, R. S., Singhania, R. R., Pandey, A., & Larroche, C. Elsevier.

Narancic, T., Almahboub, S. A., & O'Connor, K. E. (2019). Unnatural amino acids: production and biotechnological potential. *World Journal of Microbiology and Biotechnology, 35*, 67.

Nisha, M. K. (2016). Process optimization for bio scouring of cotton fabrics with pectinase obtained from *Paecilomyces variotii*. *International Journal of Current Microbiology and Applied Sciences, 5*(6), 292–299. https://doi.org/10.20546/ijcmas.2016.506.033 (accessed on 5th November 2025).

Niyonzima, F. N., & More, S. S. (2013). Optimization of fermentation culture conditions for alkaline protease production by *Scopulariopsis* sp. *Applied Biological Research, 15*, 66–69.

Niyonzima, F. N., & More, S. S. (2013). Screening and optimization of cultural parameters for an alkaline protease production by *Aspergillus terreus* gr. under submerged fermentation. *International Journal of Pharma and Bio Sciences, 4*, 1016–1028.

Niyonzima, F. N., & More, S. S. (2015). Purification and characterization of detergent compatible alkaline protease from *Aspergillus terreus* gr. *3 Biotech, 5*, 61–70.

Otto, E., & Escovar-Kousen, J. (2005). Ethanol production by simultaneous saccharification and fermentation (SSF). *US Patent App. 10/713,182, Google Patents* US20050026261A1.

Pachauri, P., More, S., Aranganathan, V., & Sullia, S. B. (2018). Kinetic study and characterization of cellulase enzyme from isolated *Aspergillus niger* subsp. *awamori* for cellulosic biofuels. *Journal of Science and Industrial Research, 77*, 55–60.

Pivnenko, K., Eriksson, E., & Astrup, T. F. (2015). Waste paper for recycling: overview and identification of potentially critical substances. *Waste Management, 45*, 134–142. https://doi.org/10.1016/j.wasman.2015.02.028 (accessed on 5th November 2025).

Polakovic, M., Švitel, J., Bučko, M., Filip, J., Nedela, V., Ansorge-Schumacher, M. B., & Gemeiner, P. (2017). Progress in biocatalysis with immobilized viable whole cells: systems development, reaction engineering and applications. *Biotechnology Letters, 39*, 667–683.

Prasad, S., & Roy, I. (2018). Converting enzymes into tools of industrial importance. *Recent Patents on Biotechnology, 12*, 33–56.

Prasanna, H. N., Ramanjaneyulu, G., & Reddy, B. R. (2016). Optimization of cellulase production by *Penicillium* sp. *3 Biotech, 6*, 162–172.

Qu, G., Li, A., Acevedo-Rocha, C. G., Sun, Z., & Reetz, M. T. (2020). The crucial role of methodology development in directed evolution of selective enzymes. *Angewandte Chemie International Edition, 59*, 13204–13231. https://doi.org/10.1002/anie.201901491 (accessed on 5th November 2025).

Rao, T. E., Imchen, M., & Kumavath, R. (2017). Marine enzymes: production and applications for human health. *Advances in Food and Nutrition Research, 80*, 149–163. https://doi.org/10.1016/bs.afnr.2016.11.006 (accessed on 5th November 2025).

Rathi, B. S., Kumar, P. S., & Show, P. L. (2021). A review on effective removal of emerging contaminants from aquatic systems: current trends and scope for further research. *Journal of Hazardous Materials, 409*, 124413. https://doi.org/10.1016/j.jhazmat.2020.124413 (accessed on 5th November 2025).

Raveendran, S., Parameswaran, B., Ummalyma, S. B., Abraham, A., Mathew, A. K., Madhavan, A., Rebello, S., & Pandey, A. (2018). Applications of microbial enzymes in food industry. *Food Technology and Biotechnology, 56*, 16–30. https://doi.org/10.17113/ftb.56.01.18.5491 (accessed on 5th November 2025).

Rawlings, N. D., Barrett, A. J., Thomas, P. D., Huang, X., Bateman, A., & Finn, R. D. (2018). The MEROPS database of proteolytic enzymes, their substrates and inhibitors in 2017 and a comparison with peptidases in the PANTHER database. *Nucleic Acids Research, 46*, D624–D632.

Roohi, R., Kuddus, M., & Saima, S. (2013). Cold-active detergent-stable extracellular α-amylase from *Bacillus cereus* GA6: biochemical characteristics and its perspectives in laundry detergent formulation. *Journal of Biochemical Technology, 4*(4), 636–644.

Roy, J. K., & Mukherjee, A. K. (2013). Applications of a high maltose forming, thermostable α-amylase from an extremely alkalophilic *Bacillus licheniformis* strain AS08E in food and laundry detergent industries. *Biochemical Engineering Journal, 77*, 220–230.

Sakuragi, H., Kuroda, K., & Ueda, M. (2011). Molecular breeding of advanced microorganisms for biofuel production. *Journal of Biomedicine and Biotechnology, 2011*, Article ID: 416931.

Salmeán, A. A., Guillouzo, A., Duffieux, D., Jam, M., Matard-Mann, M., Larocque, R., Pedersen, H. L., Michel, G., Czjzek, M., Willats, W. G. T., et al. (2018). Double blind microarray-based polysaccharide profiling enables parallel identification of uncharacterized polysaccharides and carbohydrate-binding proteins with unknown specificities. *Scientific Reports, 8*(1), 2500.

Sandhya, A., Sridevi, A., & Narasimh, G. (2015). Production and optimization of phytase by *Aspergillus niger*. *Der Pharmacia Lettre, 7*, 148–153.

Saravanakumar, K., & Kathiresan, K. (2012). Statistical optimization of protease production by mangrove-derived *Trichoderma estonicum* and its potential on blood stain removal. *International Journal of Biotechnology and Molecular Biology Research, 3*, 15–21.

Sarmah, N., Revathi, D., Sheelu, G., Yamuna Rani, K., Sridhar, S., Mehtab, V., & Sumana, C. (2018). Recent advances on sources and industrial applications of lipases. *Biotechnology Progress, 34*, 5–28.

Sharma, P., Kaushik, N., Sharma, S., & Kumar, V. (2016). Isolation, screening, characterization and optimization of xylanase production from thermostable alkalophilic *Fusarium* sp. XPF5. *Journal of Biochemical Technology, 7*, 1089–1092.

Shwetha, V., More, S. S., & Uday, M. (2017). Screening, optimization and production of a novel β-cyclodextrinase by *Bacillus flexus* MSBC 2. *Current Trends in Biotechnology and Pharmacy, 11*, 136–143.

Sidhu, A. K., Darade, S. B., Bhavsar, P. P., Vishwas, B., Gaikwad, & Patil, S. N. (2017). Isolation, screening and optimization for laccase production by *Scytalidium lignicola* pesante under submerged fermentation. *International Journal of Current Microbiology and Applied Sciences, 6*, 2477–2491.

Singh, R. S., & Singh, R. P. (2016). Indulines. In *Current Developments in Biotechnology and Bioengineering: Production, Isolation, and Purification of Industrial Products* (pp. 423–446). https://doi.org/10.1016/B978-0-444-63662-1.00018-X (accessed on 5th November 2025).

Singh, R., Kumar, M., Mittal, A., & Mehta, P. K. (2016). Microbial enzymes: industrial progress in 21st century. *3 Biotech, 6*, 174.

Singhania, R. R., Saini, R., Adsul, M., Sain, J. K., Mathur, A., & Tuli, D. (2015). An integrative process for bio-ethanol production employing SSF produced cellulase without extraction. *Biochemical Engineering Journal, 102*, 45–48.

Sinha, S., & Nigam, V. K. (2016). Production and characterization of L-glutaminase by *Bacillus* sp. *International Journal of Pharmaceutical Sciences and Research, 7*, 1620–1626.

Sivamani, S., & Baskar, R. (2018). Process design and optimization of bioethanol production from cassava bagasse using statistical design and genetic algorithm. *Preparative Biochemistry and Biotechnology, 48*, 834–841.

Souza, P. N. C., Maia, N. C., Souza, L. H. G., Resende, M. L. V., & Cardoso, P. G. (2015). Optimization of culture conditions for Tanase production by *Aspergillus* sp. gm4 in solid state fermentation. *Acta Scientiarum, 37*, 23–30.

Srinivasan, S., Sadasivam, S. K., Gunalan, S., Shanmugam, G., & Kothandan, G. (2019). Application of docking and active site analysis for enzyme linked biodegradation of textile dyes. *Environmental Pollution, 248*.

Struch, M., Krahe, N., Linke, D., Mokoonlall, A., & Berger, R. G. (2016). Dose dependent effects of a milk ion tolerant laccase on yogurt gel structure. *LWT–Food Science and Technology, 65*, 1144–1152. https://doi.org/10.1016/j.lwt.2015.10.004 (accessed on 5th November 2025).

Tavano, O. L., Berenguer-Murcia, Á., Secundo, F., & Fernandez-Lafuente, R. (2018). Biotechnological applications of proteases in food technology. *Comprehensive Reviews in Food Science and Food Safety, 17*(2), 412–436. https://doi.org/10.1111/1541-4337.12326 (accessed on 5th November 2025).

Thomas, L., Larroche, C., & Pandey, A. (2013b). Current developments in solid-state fermentation. *Biochemical Engineering Journal, 81*, 146–161.

Uchiyama, I., Mihara, M., Nishide, H., Chiba, H., & Kato, M. (2019). MBGD update 2018: microbial genome database based on hierarchical ortholog relations covering closely related and distantly related comparisons. *Nucleic Acids Research, 47*, D382–D389.

Uday, M. M., Bennur, R. S., Veena, S. M., Niyonzima, F. N., & More, S. S. (2013). Isolation and characterization of β-amylase from *Penicillium nigricans*. *Biotechnology: An Indian Journal, 7*, 85–88.

Usha, K. Y., Praveen, K., & Reddy, B. R. K. Y. (2014). Enhanced production of ligninolytic enzymes by a mushroom *Stereum ostrea*. *Biotechnology Research International, 2014*(2), 815495.

Vaissier Welborn, V., & Head-Gordon, T. (2019). Computational design of synthetic enzymes. *Chemical Reviews, 119*, 6613–6630.

Verma, M. L., Puri, M., & Barrow, C. J. (2016). Recent trends in nanomaterials immobilized enzymes for biofuel production. *Critical Reviews in Biotechnology, 36*, 108–119.

Waleed, M., Faiza, A., & Nizar, I. (2015). Production optimization of pullulan's enzyme produced by *Bacillus cereus* isolated from Syrian sources. *International Food Research Journal, 22*, 1824–1830.

Wang, H., Zhong, S., Ma, H., Zhang, J., & Qi, W. (2012). Screening and characterization of a novel alkaline lipase from *Acinetobacter calcoaceticus* 1–7 isolated from Bohai Bay in China for detergent formulation. *Brazilian Journal of Microbiology, 43*, 148–156.
Wellesly, M. A. (2018). *Global Markets for Enzymes in Industrial Applications*. USA: BCC Publishing.
Xu, L. H., & Du, Y. L. (2018). Rational and semi-rational engineering of cytochrome P450s for biotechnological applications. *Synthetic and Systems Biotechnology, 3*, 283–290.
Zhang, X. F., Yang, G. Y., Zhang, Y., Xie, Y., Withers, S. G., & Feng, Y. (2016). A general and efficient strategy for generating the stable enzymes. *Scientific Reports, 6*, 33797.

## CHAPTER 2

# Engineering Microbial Fuels: Progress and Prospects

PRITI PAL,[1] AKHILESH KUMAR SINGH,[2,*] PRAKASH KUMAR SARANGI,[3] BRIJESH PANDEY,[2] ANAND PRAKASH,[2] SAURABH SINGH RATHORE,[2] PARAS PORWAL,[1] SUJEET PRATAP SINGH,[1] and VIKRAM SRIVASTAVA[4]

[1]*Amity Institute of Biotechnology, Amity University Uttar Pradesh, Lucknow Campus, Lucknow, India*

[2]*Department of Biotechnology, School of Life Sciences, Mahatma Gandhi Central University, Motihari, Bihar, India*

[3]*College of Agriculture, Central Agricultural University, Imphal, Manipur, India*

[4]*Department of Biomedical Sciences, College of Veterinary Medicine, Iowa State University, Ames, Iowa, USA*

*Corresponding author

## ABSTRACT

Microbes are valuable natural resources widely utilized in the production of biofuels such as biogas, bioethanol, biodiesel, and biohydrogen. Efficient microbial systems combined with sustainable raw materials—including crops, biomass residues, and biological wastes—enable biofuel generation through processes like fermentation and anaerobic digestion. Recent advancements have focused on designing improved microbial fuel production systems. Genetically engineered or metabolically modified microorganisms have been developed with enhanced stress tolerance and

Industrial Biotechnology: Current Progress and Novel Technologies.
Prakash Kumar Sarangi, Akhilesh Kumar Singh, Rajesh Kumar Srivastava, and Brijesh Pandey (Eds.)


DOI: 10.1201/9781779642233-2

increased biofuel productivity. Synthetic biology and systems biology approaches further support the creation of microbial cells with tailored genetic modifications, enabling more efficient production of various biofuels using bacteria, yeast, and microalgae. Omics technologies, including genomics, transcriptomics, and metabolomics, play a crucial role in understanding and enhancing microbial lipid synthesis for biodiesel and other fuels. Modern strategies also integrate multiple steps—previously requiring extensive feedstock pretreatment and conversion—into streamlined, single-step microbial processes through metabolic engineering. This chapter provides an overview of microbial-based biofuels, their applications, and recent technological advances. It also discusses current challenges in microbial fuel production and outlines potential solutions for improving efficiency, sustainability, and scalability in future bioenergy systems.

## 2.1 INTRODUCTION

The majority of the biodiversity on Earth is made up of microorganisms, which are also essential to the biosphere process (Das et al., 2020). The economical and environmentally beneficial microbial fuels (biogas, biodiesel, biohydrogen, and so on) are produced from many forms of biomass. Therefore, the best choice to replace the demand for fossil fuels in the near future is biofuels. One potential replacement for conventional fossil fuels is the production of fuels using several kinds of microbes (algae, bacteria, cyanobacteria, fungi, and archaea). Cyanobacteria are one type of microbe that has great promise for making fuel. Additionally, it is possible to manipulate microbes to extract substances with value-added, including lipids (triacylglycerols), carbohydrates, polyunsaturated fatty acids (PUFA), proteins, pigments, antioxidants, different antibacterial chemicals, and so forth. They trade nutrients and metabolites, which boost production and make it easier to commercialize fuel made from microorganisms. Biodiesel, bioelectricity, biohydrogen, and other types of biofuels can all be produced using microbial biomass (Hirokawa et al., 2017). There are many different types of biofuels, but biodiesel is the most popular alternative to petrol-based fuels. Biofuels are categorized into several categories, such as first generation, second generation, third generation, and fourth generation, depending on the sources exploited in their manufacture. Lignocellulosic components of biomass are used to make first- and second-generation biofuels (Dionisi et al., 2014). These biofuels are made from a variety of biomass materials, including plant remains and agricultural waste (Voloshin et al., 2016). The third-generation biofuels are made from biomass from algae or microalgae and are regarded as a good future energy alternative globally. The third-generation biofuel sources serve as the foundation for fourth-generation biofuels (Ananthi et al., 2021). The primary sources of fourth-generation biofuels are genetically modified (GM) microbes (Ananthi et al., 2021). Today, metabolic pathway modification and genetic modification techniques can be used to create an efficient and appropriate microbial system. The improved production of biofuels and benefits to the energy sector is due to the modified genome of the biofuel-producing organism (Liew et al., 2017). Additionally, utilizing metagenomic approaches, relevant microbial communities can be found in environmental sources including soil and water. These biofuels can help lower the number of harmful gases in the atmosphere as well as the health issues that affect living things (Lian et al., 2014). The primary biological fuels used today and having a significant impact on the energy sector are bioethanol and biogas. Future energy resources that could replace fossil fuels include these fuels. Currently, all biogas production depends on naturally occurring methanogen populations, and this situation does not seem to be about to change. Potential fuels made from microalgae, cyanobacteria, and other photosynthetic microorganisms, whether they are produced artificially or naturally, need a lot of work before they can be used on a large scale. The most promising metabolically modified yeasts for the production of bioethanol from starch, pretreated lignocellulose, and other polysaccharides in the near future seem to be those that surface with a variety of hydrolytic enzymes (Singh et al., 2014). Commercialization of the metabolically modified bacterium *Zymomonas mobilis* for the production of bioethanol from pentose sugars has already begun. To manufacture the necessary advanced biofuel, the fuel synthesis pathway must be added to a microbial substrate (Tsegaye et al., 2018b). The choice of microbial substrate is often influenced by a variety of factors, including the carbon source (such as cellulose, lignin, methane, and carbon dioxide), the toxicity of the substrate (or any impurities in it), the toxicity of the fuel itself, and the parameters necessary for converting the substrate into the fuel. Additionally, a variety of methods can be employed to boost the effectiveness of biofuel synthesis, including metabolic engineering to improve substrate consumption, tolerance to inhibitors, and the development of new biosynthetic pathways (Jagadevan et al., 2018). This chapter emphasized microbial fuels, their primary applications, together with the existing potential glitches.

## 2.2 CLASSIFICATION OF BIOFUEL

Biofuels are categorized into two groups: primary and secondary, depending on the technique of development. The primary category of biofuels is derived from natural bioresources such as plants, animal waste, and lignocellulosic materials, whereas secondary biofuel is directly derived from bacteria, microalgae, and fungi (Dutta et al., 2014). There are four generations of secondary biofuel, which are discussed in subsections.

### 2.2.1 FIRST-GENERATION BIOFUELS

A conventional biofuel is another name for first-generation biofuel. The three main categories of first-generation biofuels that are utilized commercially are biodiesel, ethanol, and biogas. These biofuels are crucial to the bioenergy industry, and their production is supported by well-stabilized technology. Transesterification of vegetable oils and fatty acids is the source of the current generation of biofuels. By making a few small adjustments to the diesel engine, biodiesel is utilized as a source of energy. The gaseous fuels biogas and biomethane are essential for the bioenergy industry. Due to the high demand and limited worldwide supply of edible oils and food components, it is extremely difficult to employ them in the manufacturing of biofuels (Atsumi et al., 2008). Some plants have great potential for turning into biofuels. The fact that these crops are grown in barren fields is one of their major features. A widely used oilseed crop called jatropha is grown all over the world to make biodiesel. In comparison to other crops, they may be grown on non-productive land and require fewer supplementary nutrients. Jatropha is thought to be a significant source of biofuels and certain other high-value products (Ko et al., 2020).

### 2.2.2 SECOND-GENERATION BIOFUELS

Biomaterials that are not related to food are used to make second-generation biofuels. These biofuels were made from many types of biomasses, including lignocellulosic biomass, agricultural byproducts, and waste from food crops (Das et al., 2020). Due to the numerous methods utilized to produce these biofuels, they are no longer economically feasible. According to Tahvildari et al. (2015), the cell walls of plants, which can contain up to 75% polysaccharides, make up the majority of their biomass. These polysaccharides have the potential to be used to create biofuels and are excellent sources of valuable sugar. By using cutting-edge techniques and lignocellulosic biomaterials for biofuel production, second-generation biofuel is produced.

### 2.2.3 THIRD-GENERATION BIOFUELS

The biofuels of the third generation, which are produced from planted aquatic feedstock generated from algal biomass, comprise biomethane, biodiesels, bioethanol's, biobutanol, vegetable oil gasoline, jet fuel, and aviation fuels. They provide all living things in many ecosystems with an excellent number of vitamins, proteins, and carbs, as well as 60% of the oxygen they need to survive. Crude oil produced by algae is easily transformed into diesel and gasoline. Microalgae and macroalgae are two subcategories of some algal species. In terms of efficiency, third-generation biofuels have made significant improvements over first- and second-generation biofuels. They use only sustainable energy sources and buy inexpensive materials. These third-generation biofuels are hence economical. Additionally, these energy sources are sustainable and have no negative or adverse consequences on our climate (Qin et al., 2018).

### 2.2.4 FOURTH-GENERATION BIOFUELS

It has two components for the next generation of biofuels and is the most recent biofuel technology. One aspect is based on crops that produce modified biofuels and serve as carbon-capturing devices. The "solar to fuel" theory is the foundation of the second section. The fourth-generation biofuel is favorable since it requires non-arable land and has a high production yield. Electro fuel is one of these biofuels (Hossain et al., 2019). Using $CO_2$ and cyanobacteria, as well as the sun and their existence, the solar to fuel technique works. In this process, flat panels are filled with water, and cyanobacteria are added to them. Similar to solar panels, the panels are oriented toward the sun. The microbes (cyanobacteria) absorb $CO_2$ from the atmosphere while utilizing solar energy from the sun. Compared to third-generation biofuels, this technology is more affordable (Matsakas et al., 2018).

## 2.3 MICROBES AS SUITABLE SOURCES OF BIOFUEL PRODUCTION

Microbes are tiny architects who are essential to recycling and supporting life on Earth. Because they have a high lipid content and a rapid growth rate, microbes are frequently employed for the manufacture of biofuel. Producing biofuels from microorganisms involves the use of cultivation, harvesting, and oil extraction technology (Nikolić et al., 2016). Microbes contribute to reducing global warming because they are highly efficient at photosynthesizing and emit little carbon dioxide into the environment. Microalgae have a rapid pace of growth and can have biomass that contains 60–70% lipids. The amount of lipids varies from species to species and is influenced by several environmental conditions, including temperature, pressure, humidity, and dietary habits. They are able to flourish in unfavorable conditions, which reduces the expense of cultivation. They synthesize, store, and secrete a variety of physiologically active substances, including lipids, amino acids, and carbohydrates (Yao et al., 2014). They could be used to make bioethanol, biodiesel, biomethane, biohydrogen, bioalcohols, and biogas, which are examples of next-generation biofuels (Figure 2.1).

The next-generation biofuels might be accomplished by using bacteria and fungi to convert lignocelluloses into ethanol; as an alternative, microalgae could convert $CO_2$ into biomass; or methane from landfills could be used to produce biofuels. These substrates can be directed to the biosynthetic pathways of various fuel components by adjusting fuel pathways and central metabolism to enhance the production of biofuels (Sahay and Braganza, 2016). Yeast is one type of efficient fermenting microbe that can be utilized to make ethanol from biomass

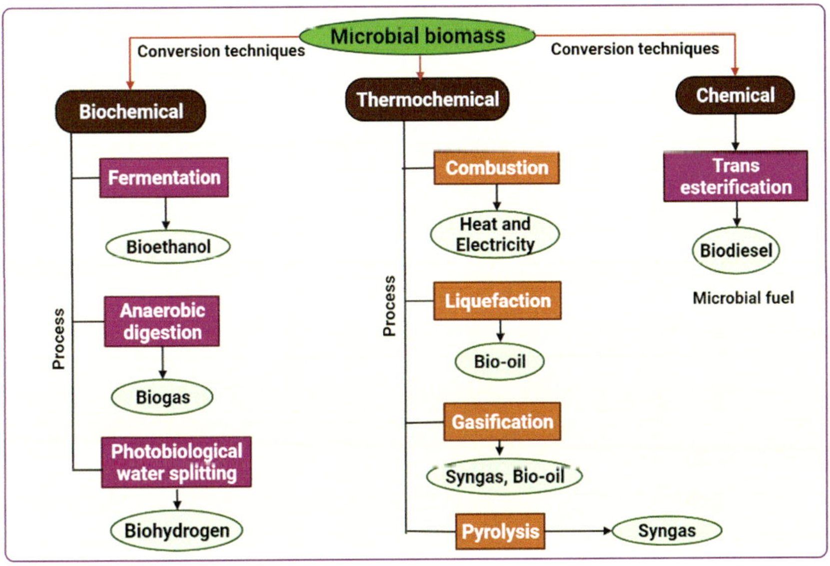


**FIGURE 2.1** Numerous techniques for specifically converting biomass into microbial fuels.

over an extended period of time. The effectiveness of cellulolytic fungal enzymes and biofuel-fermenting strains that can ferment a variety of sugars (6-carbon and 5-carbon) determines how efficiently biofuels may be produced from biomass (Chen et al., 2013). Additionally, bacteria may also release gases as waste products, such as hydrogen, which might be a great alternative to natural gas and be used to make gaseous biofuels. Additionally, several microorganisms can function as fuel cells to generate power; this can be advantageous for the development of batteries. Electrons are created when microorganisms oxidize a variety of substrates. These electrons are then transferred to another electrode to create energy. Biofuels have also been produced using other biological resources such as wheat straw, palm oil, sugarcane crops, and rice straw. Microbes, however, may grow on non-arable and infertile land and have a shorter growth cycle, making them more advantageous (Khalife et al., 2017). Because the size of the production facilities would be cut in half, an increase in the lipid content of microalgal biomass from 20 to 60% would result in a significant decrease in capital expenses associated with cultivation (Agrawal et al., 2017).

## 2.4 APPROACHES FOR MICROBIAL STRAIN IMPROVEMENT

The focus of a recent study has been on the economic advantages of technology as well as the selection and use of effective and affordable techniques (Gaida et al., 2016). Lignocellulosic components from a variety of crops, including maize, are taken into consideration as potential feedstocks for the generation of biofuels. A few difficulties arise, such as choosing the right microbes for the pretreatment process and improving the productivity of biofuel. Because microorganism's express biomass degradation enzymes (extracellularly), they differ in their ability to degrade biomass. For the conversion of biomass, such as the conversion of complicated sugar into simple sugar molecules, perfect creatures have been employed. The effectiveness of microbes at converting biomass is also influenced by many growth variables, including temperature, pH, and nutrient availability. Some inhibitors are created during the process of treating biomass, and these inhibitors have harmful effects that have an impact on the process of converting biomass (Parkash et al., 2016). Therefore, choosing the right microbes is crucial for the generation of biofuel (Liao et al., 2016). In the current study, as a model organism, *E. coli* has been employed to increase the effectiveness of biomass conversion. It has been possible to increase the generation of biofuels by using a variety of metabolic engineering strategies. The change and regulation of metabolic pathways can aid in the process by which microorganisms adapt to physical and biochemical stimuli (Sheng et al., 2017). The majority of enzymes that produce biofuels are not very effective at hydrolyzing waste, which results in reduced biofuel generation. Techniques for protein engineering can be utilized to address these problems. Post-translational modifications in protein molecules are the foundation of protein engineering techniques, and the biofuels industry can utilize these changed proteins (Gaurav et al., 2017).

## 2.5 THE ISOLATION AND CHARACTERIZATION OF MICROORGANISMS USING A METAGENOMIC APPROACH

The identification of novel biofuel enzymes from unculturable microorganisms uses the metagenomic method, which can be culture-dependent or culture-independent. The unique biofuel enzymes are purified from the soil microbial metagenome. It is crucial to choose an adequate environmental location for the gathering of suitable microorganisms that are involved in the biofuel industry when using metagenomics technologies (Gaida et al., 2016). Microorganism isolation and characterization from environmental samples often entails microorganism separation and characterization. In the process of isolating and characterizing microorganisms from various environmental samples, computational biology and molecular biology are heavily involved. The creation of a genomic library of targeted genes responsible for the generation of biofuel enzymes uses genetic engineering techniques. The transformation approach is used to create the targeted gene in the appropriate host (Chen et al., 2017). Additionally, vectors are built for the expression of proteins. As a result, a viable metagenomic library is created for future use. A gene encoding a novel enzyme is extracted from this library (Varman et al., 2013). Novel biofuel enzymes must be isolated and identified using a variety of metagenomic techniques.

### 2.5.1 SAMPLE COLLECTION AND ISOLATION OF GENOMIC DNA

The choice of an appropriate environmental site for the metagenomic sample collection is crucial for the isolation of new enzymes. The initial step in a metagenomic analysis is sample processing, which is also essential. For the production and sequencing of libraries, a significant amount of nucleic acid was acquired together with DNA taken from the ambient sample that represents a cell (Liu et al., 2014).

### 2.5.2 HOST SELECTION AND VECTOR CONSTRUCTION

To host the metagenomic library, an appropriate host bacterium is selected. To maintain a genomic library of metagenomic samples, the necessary DNA fragments are placed into the vector DNA, and the vector is used to transmit the desired DNAs into the host cell (Chen et al., 2015).

### 2.5.3 METAGENOMIC LIBRARY SCREENING

Metagenomics can be developed on sequence and function-driven investigations of the uncultured microbial population. They have been applied to the metagenomic samples to find new biocatalysts. Viruses, fungi, bacteria, and archaea make up microbial communities (Li et al., 2015). For the metagenomic library screening, a variety of screening techniques have been applied, including function-based screening (Hu et al., 2014), sequence-based screening (Yang et al., 2015), and SIGEX screening (Avalos et al., 2013).

### 2.5.4 DNA SEQUENCING FOR METAGENOMIC SAMPLE

Using a variety of sequencing techniques, the region of interest or the subset of the microbial DNAs' genome has been identified. High-throughput sequencing is generally necessary if the gene is fairly large. Illumina HiSeq sequencing will be more effective in this case for sequencing DNA. However, if the needed throughput is smaller and the read length is a key factor, the Illumina MiSeq or perhaps the PacBio may be the best option (Cha et al., 2013). The abundance of DNA serves as the foundation for next-generation sequencing. An extensive investigation of the genes contained in the environmental sample has been conducted using next-generation metagenomic sequencing. Effective library screening is made possible by metagenomic sequencing, which may be feasible for evaluating diverse bacteria and sufficient in various niches. Potential applications for the metagenomic library in the biofuel business include the discovery of novel biocatalysts (Prasad et al., 2020a). The genetic make-up of metagenomic DNAs has been investigated using a variety of sequencing techniques. Oxford Nanopore Technologies created the Oxford Nanopore sequencing technologies (Argyros et al., 2011). Utilizing the low-complexity metagenomic community with MinION sequencing, which may introduce high-quality reads to introduce 99% accurate taxonomic composition, is a developing use in metagenomic taxonomy identification (Vaid et al., 2018). Illumina and Ion Torrent sequencing methods, which generate a lot of short reads (between 150 and 400 bp), are considered second-generation sequencing (Yeong et al., 2018). The first successful second-generation sequencer, or 454 DNA sequences, was created by 454 Life Sciences. A method known as sequencing-by-synthesis results in the production of about one million sequences with reading lengths of 400–500 bp (Oncel and Kose, 2014).

The identification of genomic DNAs also heavily utilizes other crucial sequencing techniques, including single-molecule real-time (SMRT) sequencing, third-generation sequencing, ion torrent, and applied biosystem (Bhandiwad et al., 2014).

## 2.6 METABOLIC ENGINEERING FOR BIOFUEL PRODUCTION

The production of biofuel can be increased by altering native strains' biosynthetic pathways. For instance, *Clostridium thermocellum*'s production of bioethanol was boosted by altering its electron metabolism (Bao et al., 2019). Several metabolically modified microbe strains have been utilized successfully to produce biofuel (Table 2.1). Scientists have successfully produced biofuel and other goods by modifying the genetics and metabolic pathways of microorganisms to increase the production of certain metabolites. Additionally, end products also inhibit pentose-fermenting organisms such as *Pichia stipitis, Candida shehata,* and *Pachysolen tannophilus* (Ko et al., 2020). In contrast to *Saccharomyces cerevisiae*, a well-known indigenous producer of bioethanol, *Zymomonas mobilis* can only efficiently use hexose sugar (glucose), converting it to bioethanol, but not from pentose carbohydrates. Ethanol synthesis requires the bacteria *Bacillus subtilis, Clostridium,* and *E. coli*. By chromosomal insertion of the pyruvate decarboxylase gene from *Z. mobilis* and the alcohol dehydrogenase II gene with the ldh native promoter, *B. subtilis* strain BS35 was created (Park et al., 2020). The *Clostridium acetobutylicum adhE2* gene was fully expressed in *C. cellulovorans*, resulting in significant amounts of n-butanol (1.42 g/L) and ethanol (1.60 g/L) being produced from the crystalline cellulose (Koutra et al., 2018). *Cryptococcus* spp., *Rhodococcus* spp., and *Rhodosporidium* spp., as well as *Candida* spp., *Saccharomyces* spp., and *Kluyveromyces* spp., have all been found to be helpful in the generation of biodiesel, bioalcohol, and biogas, respectively (Silveira et al., 2015). Metabolically modified microbes may produce more products with greater product diversity, yield, concentration, and productivity (Figure 2.2). Furthermore, metabolic engineering may also make it easier to recover a specific biofuel downstream. Furthermore, modifying microbes to utilize inexpensive substrates may lower the cost of fuel generation (Zhang et al., 2021).

**TABLE 2.1** Metabolically modified microorganism strains used to produce biofuel

| Microbes | Microbial Product | Pathway | Substrate | References |
|---|---|---|---|---|
| *E. coli* | 1-butanol, 2-methyl-1-butanol, 3-methyl-1-butanol, 2-phenylethanol | 2-keto acid degradation pathway | Glucose | Atsumi et al. (2008) |
| *Clostridium thermocellum* and *Thermoanaerobacterium saccharolyticum* | Ethanol | Embden-Meyerhof | Cellulose | Argyros et al. (2011) |
| *Synechocystis* sp. | Isobutanol | Ehrlich | Glucose | (Varman et al. 2013) |
| *Caldicellulosiruptor Bescii* | Hydrogen | Glycolytic | Lignocellulose | Cha et al. (2013) |
| *S. cerevisiae* | Isobutanol | Embden-Meyerhof | Synthetic medium | Avalos et al. (2013) |
| *E. coli* | Fatty alcohol | Fatty acyl-ACP reductase-dependent | Synthetic medium | Liu et al. (2014) |
| *Saccharomyces cerevisiae* | 2,3-Butanediol | Butanediol biosynthetic | Glucose, galactose | Lian et al. (2014) |
| *Thermoanaerobacterium saccharolyticum* | n-Butanol | n-butanol | Xylose | Bhandiwad et al. (2014) |
| *Methylobacterium extorqens* | 1-Butanol | Ethyl malonyl-CoA | Ethylamine | Hu and Lidstrom (2014) |
| *Enterobacter cloacae* | 2,3-Butanediol | Pentose phosphate | Lignocellulose | Li et al. (2015) |
| *C. cellulovorans* | Ethanol, n-Butanol | Fatty acyl-ACP reductase-dependent | Cellulose | Yang et al. (2015) |
| *Clostridium Tyrobutyricum* | n-Butanol | Xylose metabolic pathway | Glucose and Xylose | Yu et al. (2015) |
| *C. cellulolyticum* | n-Butanol | CoA-dependent | Cellulose | Gaida et al. (2016) |
| *S. cerevisiae* | n-Butanol | Clostridial acetoacetyl-CoA-derived pathway | Synthetic minimal | Schadeweg and Boles (2016) |
| *Corynebacterium glutamicum* | 3-Hydroxypropic acid | Glycerol | Glucose, xylose | Chen et al. (2017) |
| *Clostridium autoethanogenum* | Ethanol | Ferredoxin oxidoreductase | Synthetic medium | Liew et al. (2017) |
| *S. elongates* | 1,3-Propanediol | Synthetic metabolic pathway | Synthetic medium | Hirokawa et al. (2017) |
| *Klebsiella pneumoniae* | 2-Butanol | Meso-2,3-butanediol synthesis | Glucose | Chen et al. (2017) |
| *S. cerevisiae strain* XUSAE57 | Ethanol | Xylose-isomerase pathway | Xylose and Glucose | Ko et al. (2020) |
| *Clostridium acetobutylicum and Saccharomyces cerevisiae* | n-Butanol | Clostridial acetoacetyl-CoA-derived pathway | Glucose, corn, starch, and corn stover | Das et al. (2020) |

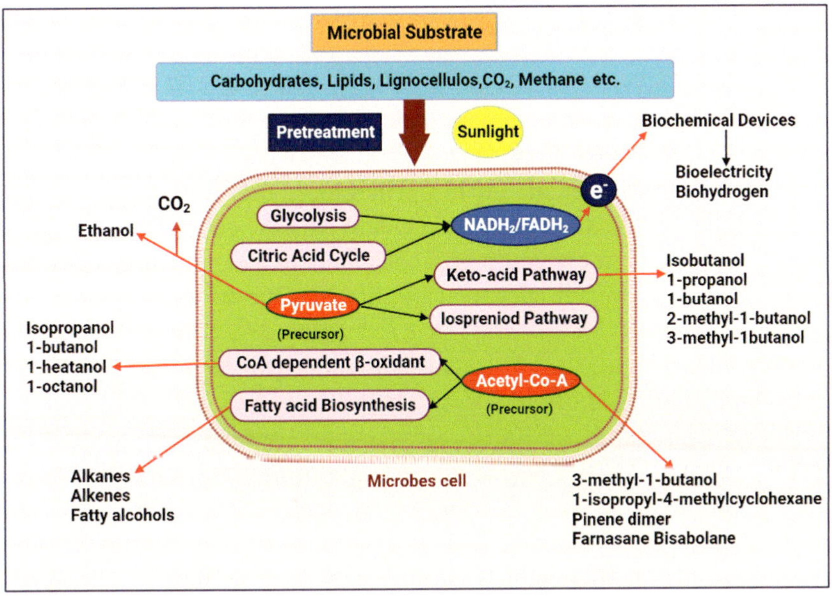


**FIGURE 2.2** A summary of microbial metabolic pathways used in microbial biofuel production.

## 2.7 PRODUCTION OF MICROBIAL FUEL

### *2.7.1 SOLID BIOFUEL*

Solid biofuels can be categorized into several types, which are discussed in subsections.

#### *2.7.1.1 SOLID BIOMASSES*

Solid biomasses, which include agricultural waste, forestry waste, crop waste, and solid waste, are the raw solid biomass feedstocks used in the synthesis of biofuels. Raw, solid biomass feedstocks are another source of biofuel production. Solid biomasses that can be used to make biofuel directly or as a conversion product include oil crops, lignocellulosic biomasses, solid garbage, and so forth.

#### *2.7.1.2 BIOCHAR*

Depending on the type of biomass and manufacturing procedures, biochar, a form of pyrogenic carbonaceous substance created by diverse biomass inside an oxygen-limited atmosphere (Singh et al., 2021), has been widely used as electrode materials, supercapacitors, soil ameliorants, and catalysts (Gaurav et al., 2017). While this is going on, the creation of biochar from biomass is regarded as an alternative technique for $CO_2$ capture and storage and contributes significantly to carbon recycling (Agrawal et al., 2017). Therefore, the production of non-condensable biogas and bio-oils in tandem with the generation of biochar from microbial biomass could also contribute to an appealing and useful sustainability approach (Sekar et al., 2021). Due to its simplicity and speed, pyrolysis is one of the most promising procedures for creating biochar. Vohra et al. (2014) found that *Dunaliella tertiolecta* produced between 22 and 36% of biochar and between 39 and 43% of bio-oil at a pyrolysis temperature of 600°C. Slow and fast pyrolysis have both been improved upon and developed into a range of more efficient processes, taking into account the influences of residence time, temperature, and heating rate (Brachi et al., 2017). Torrefaction is a thermochemical conversion process that happens in an anaerobic environment at temperatures between 100 and 300°C. It creates biochar that is higher in calorific value, more hydrophobic, and contains less ash (Tsegaye et al., 2018b). Hydrocar, also known as charred biomass, is typically created through hydrothermal carbonization (HTC) using a range of wet biomass, such as animal wastes, forest, and agricultural leftovers, algal biomass, and so forth. The manufacturing of activated charcoal, soil amendment, and hydrogen storage all make extensive use of hydrocar (Sekar et al., 2021). Zhang et al. (2021) found that hydrocar made by HTC from *Scenedesmus* sp. at 220°C displayed outstanding physicochemical and fuel attributes. Its high heating value of 26.64 MJ/kg was on par with lignite and other medium-high calorific coals.

### 2.7.2 LIQUID BIOFUELS

Liquid biofuels are more widely used because they are easy to store, have a wide range of combustion, do not explode, have greater energy to mass ratio, are stable for longer storage times, are simple to transport, and are economical. Bioethanol, biomethanol, biopropanols, biodiesels, jet fuel, and so forth, are examples of liquid biofuels. The crucial ones among them are discussed in subsections.

### *2.7.2.1 BIOETHANOL*

Bioethanol is also known as ethanol or ethylic alcohol. It has the same chemical component, $CH_3CH_2OH$, that is present in alcoholic beverages. Sugary or starchy compounds are produced by microbial fermentation of many feedstocks, including sugarcane, corn, cereals, agricultural waste, and forestry waste. The bioethanol's can be utilized directly in engines to replace gasoline. In this case, the results were 0.38–0.46 g ethanol/g glucose, which equates to 76 and 92% of the theoretical convention efficiency. Large amounts of lignocellulosic biomass are present, but they are severely constrained by lignin interferences, decreased sugar yields, and biomass pretreatment (Jang et al., 2018). The microalgal dry biomass's carbohydrate component, primarily glucose, starch, cellulose, and hemicellulose, can be used to ferment into bioethanol. The absence of lignin in the structure of microalgae makes them preferable to other feedstocks like corn, sugarcane, and lignocellulosic biomass, even though the fact that they accumulate very little sugar (Brindhadevi et al., 2021). For produce, the purpose of producing carbohydrates, the microalgae *Isochrysis galbana, Porphyridium cruentum, Spirogyra* sp., *Nannochloropsis oculate,* and *Chlorella* sp. are primarily used (Raut et al., 2016). The most well-known native generator of bioethanol is probably the anaerobic bacterium *Zymomonas mobilis*. Because of their well-understood molecular biology, the bacteria *Escherichia coli* and *Bacillus subtilis* have been utilized the most frequently to create strains that produce ethanol. They can use a variety of substrates and are susceptible to metabolic modification for the sole purpose of producing ethanol. From the beginning, *Saccharomyces cerevisiae, Candida* sp., has been the mainstay of sugar-based bioethanol production. native yeasts that ferment xylose. Native xylose-fermenting yeasts like *Pichia stipites* and *Spathaspora passalidarum* have great promise for genetic and metabolic engineering. Utilizing thermotolerant yeasts has significant advantages when producing bioethanol (Rollin et al., 2015), and metabolic engineering can also improve these yeasts. The thermotolerant yeast *Kluyveromyces marxianus* can thrive at temperatures of almost 50°C and ferments glucose to ethanol. Currently, the main ingredients utilized to produce industrial ethanol are cane molasses or enzymatically hydrolyzed starch (Xue et al., 2017). For large-scale ethanol production, yeasts like *Saccharomyces cerevisiae, Kluyveromyces marxianus,* and so forth, are known as the preferred microorganisms.

### *2.7.2.2 BIOBUTANOL*

Numerous studies have been conducted on the microbial synthesis of primary higher alcohols, including 1-propanol, 1-butanol, and other linear-chain fatty alcohols (Schadeweg et al., 2016). The four-carbon primary alcohol butanol ($C_4H_{10}O$), which has a higher energy density than ethanol and lower vapor pressure, as well as being less corrosive and hygroscopic, is thought to be a better fuel than ethanol (Passos et al., 2015). Therefore, gasoline may be directly replaced by butanol and other higher alcohols. Pure butanol has been used as fuel for unaltered gasoline automobile engines for an extended period of time. The acetone-butanol-ethanol (ABE) fermentation, one of the first significant industrial-scale fermentation processes, is the classic method for producing butanol (Abdelaal et al., 2019). Numerous studies have been conducted on bacteria from the genus *Clostridium* that naturally generate butanol (Yu et al., 2015). The intricate metabolic control system and problems in genetically manipulating *clostridial* strains make metabolic engineering difficult (Dornau et al., 2020). GM *E. coli* strains are also drawing more interest as butanol producers in addition to *clostridial* strains (Gao et al., 2016). *Acidogenesis* and *Solventogenesis* are two separate stages in the *Clostridium* fermentation process that results in butanol synthesis. The amino acid biosynthesis pathway's metabolic intermediates, 2-ketoacids, have also been employed to make higher alcohols by other bacteria, such as *Corynebacterium glutamicum* and *Ralstonia eutropha* (Hwang et al., 2016).

### *2.7.2.3 BIODIESEL*

Fatty acid methyl esters (FAME) used in biodiesels are created by trans esterifying oils with alcohols while using catalysts. Lipids that can be used as a feedstock for the synthesis of biodiesel can be accumulated by microbes (Prasad et al., 2020b). Microalgae cultivation, drying of algal biomass, obtaining oil from algal biomass, and transesterification into FAMEs are the main phases in the synthesis of biodiesel from microalgal biomass (Sengmee et al., 2017). Mechanical extraction, solvent extraction, ultrasonic extraction, supercritical extraction, and enzymatic extraction are a few of the techniques utilized to extract lipids from microalgae. Triglyceride or fatty acid and alcohol reactions take place in the presence of catalysts. Transesterification can be carried out with a variety of alcohols, including methanol, ethanol, propanol, butanol, and amyl alcohols. However, because of their low cost and physical and chemical advantages, methanol and ethanol are more frequently utilized in marketed processes. Transesterification processes are carried out using a variety of homogeneous (acid or base), heterogeneous (metallic nanoparticles), or enzymes (lipase) catalysts (ElFar et al., 2020). The production of biodiesel from oils has been reported using a variety of transesterification techniques (supercritical, BIOX cosolvent), as well as bioreactor designs (microtubular microreactors, membrane microreactors, microchannel reactors, microwave reactors, reactive distillation, and centrifugal contactor) (Venkata et al., 2020). Recent studies on various biochemical paths for lignocellulosic biomass conversion into biofuel. The microalgae *Chlamydomonas reinhardtii* produces 505 mg L1 of biofuel from urban garbage, according to a recent study (Heiman et al., 2016). According to a study, *C. vulgaris* removed a higher content of phosphorus from effluent wastewater treatment facilities under a continuous supply of carbon dioxide (Venkata et al., 2020). A brand-new, highly promising method is being used to produce biodiesel with a high yield by combining nanoparticles with microalgae. Previous research has shown that a little amount of colloidal hydrous iron (III) oxide particles can increase microalgae cell suspension by about 100%. Magnetic particles combined with aluminum sulfate can help separate cells from mixed cultures of the microalgae species *Anabaena* and *Aphanizomenon* (Maurya et al., 2015). While calcium-oxide nanoparticles boosted the biodiesel conversion yield through catalytic transesterification by up to 91%, silver nanoparticles applied to *Chlamydomonas reinhardtii* and *Cyanothece* 51142 microalgae harvesting increased biomass productivity by 30% (Boock et al., 2019). Since it is denser than biodiesel, which is continuously removed to boost biodiesel yield or utilized as feed to make biohydrogen, glycerol is produced as a byproduct (Vaid et al., 2018). The length, branching, and degree of unsaturation of the carbon chain in the created biodiesel all affect its physicochemical qualities (cetane number, oxidation stability, iodine value, cold fellow properties, density, and kinematic viscosity) (Arora et al., 2020). The biomass-derived heterogeneous catalysts for transesterification are economical and environmentally beneficial, yielding 95% biodiesel. Other bacteria can also store high lipid levels, like *Mucor circillenous* and *Mortierella isabellina* (Table 2.2). According to Li et al. (2019), *Chlorella vulgaris* had a high FA content (77.3%), including palmitic acid and linolenic acid, which allowed for further conversion into biodiesel with a yield of 0.76 g/g through transesterification by methanol. Fernandez et al. (2021) used ethanol and lipids extracted from *Spirulina* species and

*Nannochloropsis oculata* via a $CaO/Al_2O_3$ catalytic system to generate a yield of ethyl ester type biodiesel that ranged from 90 to 99%. Fatty acid ethyl esters (FAEEs), which share certain similarities with FAEEs, are another potential sustainable advanced biodiesel in the development of bioenergy (Zhang et al., 2019). The availability of the precursor, lipids, and acetyl-CoA during microbial metabolism typically limits the biosynthesis of FAEEs. According to Giannelli and Torzillo (2012), common microalgae like *Chlorella, Dunaliella, Isochrysis, Nannochloris, Nannochloropsis, Neochloris, Phaeodactylum, Porphyridium,* and *Schizochytrium* have lipid contents that range from 20 to 70% of the dry weight of the cell. These contents can be increased to higher levels by adjusting environmental and other growth factors, optimizing the production process, and genetically. Low-Sulfur Diesel fuel (ULSD) blended with biodiesel has the potential to considerably reduce air pollution and carbon dioxide emissions associated with transportation.

### *2.7.3 GAS BIOFUELS*

Gaseous biofuels are more widely used because they have advantages such as being more reactive, using less oxidant, only a simple reactor, being simple to operate, and producing less waste overall. Biogas, biohydrogens, biosynthesis, and other key gaseous biofuels are some examples (Das et al., 2018).

#### *2.7.3.1 BIOGASES (BIOMETHANE)*

The anaerobic digestion of biological fermentation of organic materials, such as liquid manure and other digestible biomass feedstock, results in the production of biogas, also known as biomethane. Methane (95%) and ethane (5%), which make up natural gases, are known to be present in biogases, which typically contain methane (45–65%) and carbon dioxide (30–40%). In comparison to natural gases, biogas has substantially lower energy due to its high carbon dioxide component (30–40%). In most cases, oxygen is not present when producing biogas. In the absence of oxygen, the organic materials break down and release a variety of biogases. Methane is the primary component of the biogases created when methanogenic bacterial species break down organic material (Vuppaladadiyam et al., 2018). The biogas can be utilized as

**TABLE 2.2** Recent Research on Biomass Biochemical Transformation to Microbial Biofuel

| Biochemical Technologies | Feedstock, Biofuel Produced, Compositions, Yield, and Energy Recovery | Specific Operating Conditions | References |
|---|---|---|---|
| Anaerobic digestion | Sewage sludge, methane recovery 181 mL $CH_4$/g VS | Anaerobic incubation temperature 35°C, pH of 7.0, reaction time 10 h | Passos et al. (2015) |
| | Algal biomass from a mixed culture, methane recovery 146 to 171 mL $CH_4$ per g of chemical oxygen demand (COD) | Temperature for anaerobic digestion of sludge 35°C, $NH_4$ level 250 mg/L, reaction time 14 h | Molinuevo-Salces et al. (2016) |
| | Microalgae and bacterial co-cultured biomass, methane recovery 325 mL $CH_4$ per g of volatile solids | Anaerobic incubation temperature 35°C, pretreatment of biomass by CaO at temperature 72°C, duration of reaction time 24 h | Solé-Bundo et al. (2017) |
| Alcoholic fermentation | Microalgae biomass, ethanol recovery 0.18 kg/kg of biomass | Temperature 37°C, pH 5.5, biomass pretreatment by thermal and enzymatic hydrolysis, hydraulic retention time 2.5 days | Hwang et al. (2016) |
| | Microalgae biomass (*Chlorella*), a mixture of acetone butanol, recovery 0.32 g/ L/h, and 0.35 g/ L/h | Acid hydrolysis with 2% $H_2SO_4$ and detoxification of residue by resin L-493, fermentation by yeast under anaerobic condition | Gao et al. (2016) |
| | Pine needle, ethanol yield (0.148 g/g) | *Schizosaccharomyces pombe* CHFY0201 | Vaid et al. (2018) |
| | Pretreated and saccharified rice straw, maximum ethanol recovery 25.3 g L− 1 | Microwave-assisted alkali pretreatment of rice straw by 2% v/w NaOH, fermentation by *P. stipitis* NCIM 3499, fermentation time 72 h | Prasad et al. (2020a, b) |
| Biological $H_2$-production | Microalgae biomass (*Chlamydomonas reinhardtii* CC124), $H_2$- recovery 0.6 mL/L/h | Sulfur-free medium, nanoparticle 40 mg/ L, anaerobic condition, duration of reaction time 72 h | Giannelli et al. (2012) |
| | Microalgae (*Chlamydomonas* sp.), $H_2$-recovery 1.05 mL/L/h and 1.3 mL/L/h | duration of photo fermentation 120 h, Sulfur-free media, light intensity 50 µE/ m2 /second | Oncel et al. (2014) |
| | Microalgae (*Chlorella* sp.), $H_2$-recovery 11.65 mL/L | Temperature 30°C, pH 6.8, anaerobic condition, light intensity 48 µmol per $m^2$ /second, and duration of photo fermentation 24 h | Sengmee et al. (2017) |
| Transesterification | Recycled waste cooking oil, biodiesel recovery: 98.9% | Temperature 55°C for heating of mixture up to 20 min, MgO + CaO added with methanol and warmed to 75°C, total transesterification reaction time 4–6 h | Tahvildari et al. (2015) |
| | *Jatropha curcas oil,* biodiesel recovery 90% | Temperature 60°C, transesterification reaction time 3 h, and catalyst used in oil with methanol mixture | Zhang et al. (2019) |

fuel for automobiles, in the production of power, and the synthesis of heat. The profile of the microbial community structure employed for pretreatment as well as other growth parameters including nutrient availability, temperature, and pH affects how effectively biogas is produced (Molinuevo-Salces et al., 2016). Some microbial species, including *Clostridium cellulolyticum,* may be used to degrade cellulosic material (Fokum et al., 2016). Methane, hydrogen, and biohythane (a mixture of methane and 5–25 percent hydrogen gas) can all be produced from microalgal biomass with efficiency (Fokum et al., 2019). The capacity of biomethane fermentation employing another microalgal biomass, *N. gaditana* of the same genus, as the substrate by a natural microbial consortium from anaerobic sludge was also investigated by Solé-Bundó et al. (2017). Valdivia et al. (2020) used the TSAF technique to convert the microalgal *Chlorella* sp., yielding 8.29 and 434.38 mL/g VS of biohydrogen and biomethane, respectively. The internal furfural level was greatly reduced following the main dark fermentation to enable the subsequent synthesis of biomethane, and it was discovered that the energy consumption efficiency was significantly increased by 146.78% compared to the solitary fermentation.

#### *2.7.3.2 BIOHYDROGEN*

Due to its high calorific value (122 kJ/g) and ability to produce water molecules as a byproduct of burning, hydrogen is a cleaner and more dependable energy source than non-renewable fossil fuels (Muhammad et al., 2021). The most environmentally friendly and biological solution to the world's energy challenges is the production of biohydrogen from third-generation feedstock (microalgae), which can be further enhanced by utilizing metabolic engineering (Kumar et al., 2016). By using various techniques, such as direct and indirect photolysis of water and dark fermentation, microalgal biomass obtained from wastewater treatment can produce biohydrogen and other volatile fatty acids (VFAs) (Abomohra et al., 2021). The carbon and nitrogen sources and their relative ratios, pH, temperature, light/dark cycles, microalgal strain, culture set-up, and pre-treatment methods used are only a few of the variables that determine the rate at which hydrogen is produced (Singh et al., 2017). Numerous microalgae species, including *Chlorella, Scenedesmus,* and *Saccharina,* are widely utilized to produce biohydrogen (Budzianowsk et al., 2017). *Scenedesmus obliquus,* a microalga, demonstrated a 56.8 mL $H_2$ g1vs yield in urban wastewater (Van et al., 2015). In an urban wastewater setting, blue light stimulates the growth of a lot of algae, while purple light stimulates a lot of biohydrogen generation (Bhattacharjya et al., 2021). The oxygen sensitivity of the enzyme, light, and $CO_2$ fixation efficiency in the commercial setup, however, make the low yield a significant obstacle. A study that addressed the $O_2$-sensitivity problem highlighted the need of adding VFAs to synthetic wastewater in the relation to $O_2$-deprivation. In *C. vulgaris* culture cultivated in PBR, the investigation led to a considerable increase in biohydrogen output (65.4 ± 0.3 mol $H_2$ $L^{-1}$ $mM^{-1}$ acetate) (Bensaid et al., 2015). Recent research centered on using low-cost photoreactors and genetic engineering to increase the process economics (Kaushik et al., 2017). Enzymatic pretreatment of dry biomass resulted in seven times more biohydrogen production (1353.11 ml $H_2$ g-VS1) than corresponding untreated biomass (192.94 ml $H_2$ g-VS1), according to research by Sivagurunathan et al. (2017) on the potential of *Chlorella vulgaris* for the production of biohydrogen. On the other hand, because of the enzymatic activity of chloroplast [Fe]-hydrogenase, certain microalgae species, such as *Chlamydomonas reinhardtii,* can create hydrogen in the presence of light. Caspeta et al. (2017) evaluated the effects of light intensity and chlorophyll content on hydrogen production in *Chlamydomonas reinhardtii* and reported that the optimal combination produced 170 mL $L^{-1}$ of hydrogen at 140 μmol photons $m^{-2}$ $s^{-1}$ and 24 mg $L^{-1}$ chlorophyll in an impeller-mixed reactor. According to Milano et al. (2016), the evaluation of the effects of light intensity and chlorophyll content on hydrogen production in *Chlamydomonas reinhardtii* revealed that the optimal combination produced 170 mL $L^{-1}$ of hydrogen at 140 μmol photons $m^{-2}$ $s^{-1}$ and 24 mg $L^{-1}$ chlorophyll in an impeller-mixed reactor. Depending on the bacterial species involved, dark fermentation processes can be either thermophilic or mesophilic. Hydrogen generation has been examined using both wild-type and metabolically modified bacteria. Mesophilic bacteria including *E. coli, Enterobacter aerogenes,* and *Clostridium butyricum* have gotten a lot of attention (Gronenberg et al., 2013). *E. coli* has been genetically altered to produce hydrogen by secretion. *Thermococcus kodakarensis, Pyrococcus furiosus,* and several members of the genera *Clostridium* and *Thermoanaerobacterium* as well as the families *Thermotoga* and *Caldicellulosiruptor* are among the most prevalent thermophilic hydrogen producers (Prasad et al., 2020a). High hydrogen yields are another characteristic of thermophilic bacteria like *Thermotoga elfii* and *Caldicellulosiruptor saccharolyticus*. Muhammad et al. (2021) used the sterilized microalgal *Chlorella* sp. as substrates and a heat-treated (100°C and 15 min) anaerobic sludge as the microbial producer, ultimately achieving a biohydrogen yield of 8.29 mL/g volatile solid (VS). The heat-pretreated anaerobic sludge was also added by Jothibasu et al. (2021) to the fermentation reactor while utilizing mixed algal biomass, that is, for the synthesis of biohydrogen, *Microcystis wesenbergii*, and *M. aeruginosa* serve as the carbon sources. When a hydrothermal treatment (24.96 mL/g VS) was used for biomass pretreatment instead of a steam-acid pretreatment (18.63 mL/g VS), it was found that the yield of biohydrogen was significantly higher. Additionally, using algal biomass as the substrates, microbial fuel cells (MFC) offer an additional affordable and environmentally friendly approach for producing power and biohydrogen together (Correa et al., 2021).

### 2.7.3.3 BIOSYNGAS

Syngas is created through the gasification of biomass, as opposed to biogases and biohydrogen. Hydrocarbons, $H_2$, CO, $N_2$, and $CO_2$ make up biosyngas. Tar, $H_2S$, $NH_3$, and moisture may be present. Depending on the gasification agents utilized, biomass can be gasified using air, oxygen, steam, or $CO_2$. Air gasification is more widely utilized than any other technology since it is easy and readily available. Biogas can thin syngas since it contains nitrogen. Supercritical water, carbon dioxide, oxygen, or steam can be used to enhance the properties of biosynthetic enzymes in place of air oxygens. Steam is also frequently employed. The effects of $N_2$ can be lessened by oxygen, increasing the volume percentage of various gases. However, it is expensive, and there may be more tar in them (Zhang et al., 2019).

### 2.7.3.4 MICROBIAL FUEL CELL (MFC)

The capacity of MFCs to produce green energy from organic waste has drawn a lot of interest. Microorganisms are used in MFCs to break chemical bonds in organic components to extract energy, which is then converted to electricity (Madvarl et al., 2019). An MFC device is a different type of battery in which a proton exchange membrane (PEM) separates the anode from the cathode in an anaerobic chamber. In the anode chamber, microorganisms that typically consist of bacteria or fungus that create a biofilm oxidize an organic substrate. The produced electrons are transmitted to the cathode through an external connection during the oxidative process (Mercer, 2015). Consequently, the anode is made up of two components. The first is the microbe, which acts as a biocatalyst since it can digest organic substances by producing an enzyme. The second is the electrode that receives the electrons produced when bacteria oxidize organic molecules. After the microorganism's catabolism, the protons and electrons they make are coupled with oxygen at the cathode (aerobic) to create water (Ma et al., 2020). Some microorganisms, including *Geobacter, Shewanella, Pseudomonas, Clostridium, Desulfuromonas*, and so forth, are frequently employed in MFCs for the production of electricity and are capable of oxidizing substrates such as acetate, ethanol, lactate, butyrate, and propionate (Losse et al., 2021). To fully utilize MFCs, more research is required on several topics, including electron transport mechanisms, increasing power outputs, reactor advances, and applications.

## 2.8 MAJOR TECHNOLOGICAL CHALLENGES IN MICROBIAL BIOFUELS PRODUCTION

As mentioned above, there are now several prospects for the development of biofuels. Energy is essential for the global economy and societal progress; therefore, by 2040, this demand will have increased to roughly 37%. Petroleum and other associated industries provide more than 80% of the world's energy consumption (Joshi et al., 2019). To meet the world's energy needs, scientists must now look at more effective, alternative, and sustainable renewable energy sources, such as biofuels, due to the depletion and limitation of the natural resources that make up petroleum fuels (Rodionova et al., 2017).

The use of non-edible feedstock, such as lignocellulosic biomass and other organic waste feedstock, production logistics, energy-efficient pretreatment, enzyme hydrolysis, and fermentation technologies, efficient co-product utilization, the establishment of biofuel standards, distribution logistics, acceptance of its social and economic benefits, and minimization of its environmental impact are the major technological challenges in the production of biofuels. These difficult regions need funding, infrastructure, and knowledge in the sciences and allied specialized sectors. The physical characteristics of the biomass, such as its moisture content, particle size, microstructure, elastic properties, and bulk density (BD), have a significant impact on how well it can be converted into biofuels. Because of this, it requires a significant amount of size reduction to have a high conversion through the biochemical process, and the final volume that can be accepted will depend on how the processing system is used (Li et al., 2019). Additionally, because liquid media heat up quickly, biomass conversion using the thermochemical process is less affected by the biomass particle size. Because of this, the size of the particles is less insensitive. However, the biomass sludge needs to be significantly shrunk before being pumped into a continuous system (Jazrawi et al., 2013). The moisture content is the other physical factor that impacts the conversion of biomass waste into biofuel and is the most troublesome one. It can have a direct or indirect impact on the bio-refining processes and the availability of feedstock. For instance, a few studies suggested that higher moisture content during the biological process pretreatment could reduce thermochemical conversion and bio-oil quality and result in lower combustion thermal efficiency (Bridgwater et al., 2012). Other physical characteristics, including microstructure, elastic properties, and BD, have an impact on the conversion of biomass to biofuels in addition to moisture content and particle size. For instance, Muylaert et al. (2015) revealed that the microstructure and elastic properties of the biomass have a significant impact on the conversion of the biomass into fuels and biochemicals. These characteristics can improve the biomass interparticle interactions and compressibility. Furthermore, they asserted that BD has an impact on the processing and transportation of feedstock supplies. The price of transporting the feedstock supply increases with decreasing BD. The quality and composition of high-value compounds produced during the conversion process are also influenced by the chemical characteristics of the biomass. Ash, lignin, and volatile content are the three main chemical characteristics of biomass that have an impact on its conversion to biofuels (Li et al., 2019). For instance, Hegde et al. (2015) described how an increase in ash content during the biological process pretreatment causes a rise in char yield as well as fouling of the processes that transform biomass into energy, such as combustion, pyrolysis, gasification, and liquefaction. However, by creating air classification and leaching, ash content can be eliminated (Lacey et al., 2015). Volatile organics like acetic acid and volatile organic fractions of furan are among the other chemical characteristics that influence the conversion of biomass into biofuel. Rashid et al. (2019) found in another study that a high volatile organic matter content can affect how thermochemically produced bio-oils behave and how much energy they contain. The conversion of biomass into biofuels is also impacted by lignin content. Nevertheless, depending on the procedure type chosen, it has different effects. Removing lignin and hazardous byproducts of biomass pretreatment, such as acetic acid, clavulanic acid, formic acid, furfural, and 5-hydroxymethylfurfural (HMF), is another significant problem (Sheldon et al., 2018). They hinder the microbe and have a negative effect on fermentation and saccharification (Zhang et al., 2019). Some researchers have used strategies to decrease these inhibitors from pretreated hydrolysates before fermentation to alleviate the issue of inhibitors formed during the manufacturing of biofuel (Sheldon et al., 2018). An effective method to improve biofuels may be to screen for effective microorganisms that can tolerate the impacts of inhibitors. In situ detoxification of hydrolysates that have already undergone treatment, as well as effective enzymatic saccharification and fermentation to produce liquid and gaseous biofuels, are further key applications of genetic engineering tools and techniques. The large-scale expansion of the production of biofuels can be aided by the adaptation of these methods (Martín-Pascual et al., 2020). However, additional study is required to produce unique strains by combining the various genetic engineering techniques and maximizing biofuel output.

## 2.9 CONCLUSIONS AND FUTURE PERSPECTIVES

Biofuel is typically created by fermentation or anaerobic digestion using the microbial system from sustainable raw materials. Utilizing complex organic waste or renewable resources has enabled the creation of bioelectricity with the aid of MFCs. It has been discovered that, using genetic or metabolic pathway engineering techniques, microbial communities can be effectively developed for the production of biofuels. The best design and development of synthetic microbial cells (bacterial or yeast species) using synthetic and systems biology can increase biofuel production. According to reports, biodiesel, bioethanol, biobutanol, biohydrogen, and biogas can be produced by using a variety of sustainable resources, including lignocellulosic materials, microalgae, and various kinds of organic waste that are disposed of in wastewater streams and benefit the environment, farmers, and industries. Microalgae have a promising future as a source for the generation of biofuel on an industrial scale. Additionally, using system biological technologies like fluxomic, metabolomics, transcriptomics, and genomics will make it easier to develop, characterize, and integrate new metabolic pathways for the production of microbial biofuel. It is essential to produce renewable fuels on an industrial scale to reduce our dependence on fossil fuels; the biological sciences' ongoing use and development of systemic and comprehensive tools and procedures can only operate to improve concentrations and the production of vastly different types of biofuels from a variety of feedstocks in the future. The use of "omics" techniques can increase the cost-effective biofuel production efficiency of microbial-based biorefineries while also boosting the national economy. As a result, microorganisms may soon serve as a perfect platform for the manufacturing of a variety of bio-products.

## KEYWORDS

- **anaerobic digestion**
- **biofuels**
- **biohydrogen metabolic pathway**
- **feedstock**
- **genetic modification**
- **metabolic engineering**

## REFERENCES

Abdelaal, A. S., Jawed, K., & Yazdani, S. S. (2019). CRISPR/Cas9-mediated engineering of *Escherichia coli* for n-butanol production from xylose in defined medium. *Journal of Industrial Microbiology and Biotechnology, 46*(7), 965–975.

Abomohra, A. F., Zheng, X., Wang, Q., Huang, J., & Ebaid, R. (2021). Enhancement of biodiesel yield through *in-situ* solve-thermal transesterification of wet microalgae with spent coffee grounds. *Bioresource Technology, 323*, 124640. https://doi.org/10.1016/j.biortech.2020.124640 (accessed on 5th November 2025).

Agrawal, M., Dunn, K. L., & Rao, C. V. (2017). *Zymomonas mobilis* for the conversion of lignocellulosic biomass to fuels and chemicals. In *Engineering of Microorganisms for the Production of Chemicals and Biofuels from Renewable Resources* (pp. 67–92). Springer International Publishing.

Ananthi, V., Raja, R., Carvalho, I. S., Brindhadevi, K., Pugazhendhi, A., & Arun, A. (2021). A realistic scenario on microalgae-based biodiesel production: third generation biofuel. *Fuel, 284*, 118965. https://doi.org/10.1016/j.fuel.2020.118965 (accessed on 5th November 2025).

Argyros, D. A., Tripathi, S. A., Barrett, T. F., Rogers, S. R., Feinberg, L. F., Olson, D. G., Foden, J. M., Miller, B. B., Lynd, L. R., & Hogsett, D. A. (2011). High ethanol titers from cellulose by using metabolically engineered thermophilic, anaerobic microbes. *Applied and Environmental Microbiology, 77*(23), 8288–8294.

Arora, S. T. J. M. N., & Mishra, P. (2020). Microbial cellulolytic enzymes: diversity and biotechnology with reference to lignocellulosic biomass degradation. *Reviews in Environmental Science and Bio/Technology, 19*(3), 1–28.

Atsumi, S., Hanai, T., & Liao, J. C. (2008). Non-fermentative pathways for synthesis of branched-chain higher alcohols as biofuels. *Nature, 451*(7174), 86–89.

Avalos, J. L., Fink, G. R., & Stephanopoulos, G. (2013). Compartmentalization of metabolic pathways in yeast mitochondria improves the production of branched-chain alcohols. *Nature Biotechnology, 31*(4), 335.

Bao, T., Zhao, J., Li, J., Liu, X., & Yang, S. T. (2019). n-Butanol and ethanol production from cellulose by *Clostridium cellulovorans* overexpressing heterologous aldehyde/alcohol dehydrogenases. *Bioresource Technology, 285*, 121316.

Bensaid, S., Ruggeri, B., & Saracco, G. (2015). Development of a photosynthetic microbial electrochemical cell (PMEC) reactor coupled with dark fermentation of organic wastes: medium term perspectives. *Energies, 8*, 399–429.

Bhandiwad, A., Shaw, A. J., Guss, A., Guseva, A., Bahl, H., & Lynd, L. R. (2014). Metabolic engineering of *Thermoanaerobacterium saccharolyticum* for n-butanol production. *Metabolic Engineering, 21*, 17–25.

Bhattacharjya, R., Tiwari, A., Marella, T. K., Bansal, H., & Srivastava, S. (2021). New paradigm in diatom omics and genetic manipulation. *Bioresource Technology, 325*, 124708. https://doi.org/10.1016/j.biortech.2021.124708 (accessed on 5th November 2025).

Boock, J. T., Freedman, A. J., Tompsett, G. A., Muse, S. K., Allen, A. J., Jackson, L. A., Castro-Dominguez, B., Timko, M. T., Prather, K. L., & Thompson, J. R. (2019). Engineered microbial biofuel production and recovery under supercritical carbon dioxide. *Nature Communications, 10*(1), 1–12.

Brachi, P., Miccio, F., Ruoppolo, G., & Miccio, M. (2017). Pressurized steam torrefaction of biomass: focus on solid, liquid, and gas-phase distributions. *Industrial & Engineering Chemistry Research, 56*, 12163–12173.

Bridgwater, A. V. (2012). Review of fast pyrolysis of biomass and product upgrading. *Biomass and Bioenergy, 38*, 68–94.

Brindhadevi, K., Mathimani, T., Rene, E. R., Shanmugam, S., Chi, N. T. L., & Pugazhendhi, A. (2021). Impact of cultivation conditions on the biomass and lipid in microalgae with an emphasis on biodiesel. *Fuel, 284*, 119058. https://doi.org/10.1016/j.fuel.2020.119058 (accessed on 5th November 2025).

Budzianowski, W. M., & Brodacka, M. (2017). Biomethane storage: evaluation of technologies, end uses, business models, and sustainability. *Energy Conversion and Management, 141*, 254–273. http://dx.doi.org/10.1016/j.enconman.2016.08.071 (accessed on 5th November 2025).

Caspeta, L., & Castillo, T. (2017). Systems metabolic engineering of *Saccharomyces cerevisiae* for production of biochemicals from biomass. In *Engineering of Microorganisms for the Production of Chemicals and Biofuels from Renewable Resources* (pp. 31–65). Springer International Publishing.

Cha, M., Chung, D., Elkins, J. G., Guss, A. M., & Westpheling, J. (2013). Metabolic engineering of *Caldicellulosiruptor bescii* yields increased hydrogen production from lignocellulosic biomass. *Biotechnology for Biofuels, 6*(1), 85.

Chen, B., Ling, H., & Chang, M. W. (2013). Transporter engineering for improved tolerance against alkane biofuels in *Saccharomyces cerevisiae*. *Biotechnology for Biofuels, 6*, 21.

Chen, Z., Huang, J., Wu, Y., Wu, W., Zhang, Y., & Liu, D. (2017). Metabolic engineering of *Corynebacterium glutamicum* for the production of 3-hydroxypropionic acid from glucose and xylose. *Metabolic Engineering, 39*, 151–158.

Chen, Z., Wu, Y., Huang, J., & Liu, D. (2015). Metabolic engineering of *Klebsiella pneumoniae* for the de novo production of 2-butanol as a potential biofuel. *Bioresource Technology, 197*, 260–265.

Correa, D. F., Beyer, H. L., Possingham, H. P., Fargione, J. E., Hill, J. D., & Schenk, P. M. (2021). Microalgal biofuel production at national scales: reducing conflicts with agricultural lands and biodiversity within countries. *Energy, 215*, 119033. https://doi.org/10.1016/j.energy.2020.119033 (accessed on 5th November 2025).

Das, M., Patra, P., & Ghosh, A. (2020). Metabolic engineering for enhancing microbial biosynthesis of advanced biofuels. *Renewable and Sustainable Energy Reviews, 119*, 109562.

Das, S., Chatterjee, P., & Ghangrekar, M. M. (2018). Increasing methane content in biogas and simultaneous value-added product recovery using microbial electrosynthesis. *Water Science and Technology, 77*(5–6), 1293–1302.

Dionisi, D., Anderson, J. A., Aulenta, F., McCue, A., & Paton, G. (2014). The potential of microbial processes for lignocellulosic biomass conversion to ethanol: a review. *Journal of Chemical Technology and Biotechnology, 90*, 366–383. https://doi.org/10.1002/jctb.4544 (accessed on 5th November 2025).

Dornau, A., Robson, J. F., Thomas, G. H., & McQueen-Mason, S. J. (2020). Robust microorganisms for biofuel and chemical production from municipal solid waste. *Microbial Cell Factories, 19*(1), 1–18.

Dutta, K., Daverey, A., & Lin, J. G. (2014). Evolution retrospective for alternative fuels: first to fourth generation. *Renewable Energy, 69*, 114–122.

ElFar, O. A., Chang, C. K., Leong, H. Y., Peter, A. P., Chew, K. W., & Show, P. L. (2020). Prospects of Industry 5.0 in algae: customization of production and new advance technology for clean bioenergy generation. *Energy Conversion and Management*, 100048. https://doi.org/10.1016/j.ecmx.2020.100048 (accessed on 5th November 2025).

Fernandez, F. G. A., Reis, A., Wijffels, R. H., Barbosa, M., Verdelho, V., & Llamas, B. (2021). The role of microalgae in the bioeconomy. *New Biotechnology, 61*, 99–107.

Fokum, E., Zabed, H. M., Guo, Q., Yun, J., Yang, M., Pang, H., An, Y., Li, W., & Qi, X. (2019). Metabolic engineering of bacterial strains using CRISPR/Cas9 systems for biosynthesis of value-added products. *Food Bioscience, 28*, 125–132.

Gaida, S. M., Liedtke, A., Jentges, A. H. W., Engels, B., & Jennewein, S. (2016). Metabolic engineering of *Clostridium cellulolyticum* for the production of n-butanol from crystalline cellulose. *Microbial Cell Factories, 15*, Article 6. https://doi.org/10.1186/s12934-015-0406-9 (accessed on 5th November 2025).

Gao, K., Orr, V., & Rehmann, L. (2016). Butanol fermentation from microalgae-derived carbohydrates after ionic liquid extraction. *Bioresource Technology, 206*, 77–85.

Gaurav, N., Sivasankari, S., Kiran, G. S., Ninawe, A., & Selvin, J. (2017). Utilization of bioresources for sustainable biofuels: a review. *Renewable and Sustainable Energy Reviews, 73*, 205–214.

Giannelli, L., & Torzillo, G. (2012). Hydrogen production with the microalga *Chlamydomonas reinhardtii* grown in a compact tubular photobioreactor immersed in a scattering light nanoparticle suspension. *International Journal of Hydrogen Energy, 37*, 16951–16961.

Gronenberg, L. S., Marcheschi, R. J., & Liao, J. C. (2013). Next generation biofuel engineering in prokaryotes. *Current Opinion in Chemical Biology, 17*, 462–471. https://doi.org/10.1016/j.cbpa.2013.03.037 (accessed on 5th November 2025).

Hegde, K., Chandra, N., Sarma, S. J., Brar, S. K., & Veeranki, V. D. (2015). Genetic engineering strategies for enhanced biodiesel production. *Molecular Biotechnology, 57*, 606–624.

Heiman, K. (2016). Novel approaches to microalgal and cyanobacterial cultivation for bioenergy and biofuel production. *Current Opinion in Biotechnology, 38*, 183–189.

Hirokawa, Y., Maki, Y., & Hanai, T. (2017). Improvement of 1,3-propanediol production using an engineered cyanobacterium, *Synechococcus elongatus*, by optimization of the gene expression level of a synthetic metabolic pathway and production conditions. *Metabolic Engineering, 39*, 192–199.

Hossain, N., Mahlia, T. M. I., & Saidur, R. (2019). Latest development in microalgae-biofuel production with nano-additives. *Biotechnology for Biofuels, 12*, 125.

Hu, B., & Lidstrom, M. E. (2014). Metabolic engineering of *Methylobacterium extorquens* AM1 for 1-butanol production. *Biotechnology for Biofuels, 7*(1), 156.

Hwang, J. H., Kabra, A. N., Ji, M. K., Choi, J., El-Dalatony, M. M., & Jeon, B. H. (2016). Enhancement of continuous fermentative bioethanol production using combined treatment of mixed microalgal biomass. *Algal Research, 17*, 14–20.

Jagadevan, S., Banerjee, A., Banerjee, C., Guria, C., Tiwari, R., Baweja, M., et al. (2018). Recent developments in synthetic biology and metabolic engineering in microalgae towards biofuel production. *Biotechnology for Biofuels, 11*, 185. https://doi.org/10.1186/s13068-018-1181-1 (accessed on 5th November 2025).

Jang, M. O., & Choi, G. (2018). Techno-economic analysis of butanol production from lignocellulosic biomass by concentrated acid pretreatment and hydrolysis plus continuous fermentation. *Biochemical Engineering Journal, 134*, 30–43.

Jazrawi, C., Biller, P., Ross, A. B., Montoya, A., Maschmeyer, T., & Haynes, B. S. (2013). Pilot plant testing of continuous hydrothermal liquefaction of microalgae. *Algal Research, 2*, 268–277.

Joshi, S., Hadiya, P., Shah, M., & Sircar, A. (2019). Techno-economical and experimental analysis of biodiesel production from used cooking oil. *Biophysical Economics and Resource Quality, 4*(1), 2.

Jothibasu, K., Dhar, D. W., & Rakesh, S. (2021). Recent developments in microalgal genome editing for enhancing lipid accumulation and biofuel recovery. *Biomass and Bioenergy, 150*, 106093. https://doi.org/10.1016/j.biombioe.2021.106093 (accessed on 5th November 2025).

Kaushik, A., & Sharma, M. (2017). Exploiting biohydrogen pathways of cyanobacteria and green algae: an industrial production approach. In *Biohydrogen Production: Sustainability of Current Technology and Future Perspective* (pp. 97–113). Springer.

Khalife, E., Tabatabaei, M., Najafi, B., Mirsalim, S. M., Gharehghani, A., Mohammadi, P., Aghbashlo, M., Ghaffari, A., Khounani, Z., Shojaei, T. R., & Salleh, M. A. M. (2017). A novel emulsion fuel containing aqueous nano cerium oxide additive in diesel–biodiesel blends to improve diesel engine performance and reduce exhaust emissions: Part I–Experimental analysis. *Fuel, 207*, 741–750.

Ko, J. K., Enkh-Amgalan, T., Gong, G., Um, Y., & Lee, S. M. (2020). Improved bioconversion of lignocellulosic biomass by *Saccharomyces cerevisiae* engineered for tolerance to acetic acid. *GCB Bioenergy, 12*(1), 90–100.

Koutra, E., Economou, C. N., Tsafrakidou, P., & Kornaros, M. (2018). Biobased products from microalgae cultivated in digestates. *Trends in Biotechnology, 36*, 819–833. https://doi.org/10.1016/j.tibtech.2018.02.015 (accessed on 5th November 2025).

Kumar, A., & Singh, J. S. (2016). Microalgae and cyanobacteria biofuels: a sustainable alternate to crop-based fuels. In *Microbes and Environmental Management* (Vol. 1, pp. 1–20). Studium Press Pvt. Ltd.

Lacey, J. A., Aston, J. E., Westover, T. L., Cherry, R. S., & Thompson, D. N. (2015). Removal of introduced inorganic content from chipped forest residues via air classification. *Fuel, 160*, 265–273.

Li, L., Li, K., Wang, Y., Chen, C., Xu, Y., Zhang, L., Han, B., Gao, C., Tao, F., & Ma, C. (2015). Metabolic engineering of *Enterobacter cloacae* for high-yield production of enantiopure (2R,3R)-2,3-butanediol from lignocellulose-derived sugars. *Metabolic Engineering, 28*, 19–27.

Li, M., Yoo, C. G., Pu, Y., Biswal, A. K., Tolbert, A. K., Mohnen, D., & Ragauskas, A. J. (2019). Downregulation of pectin biosynthesis gene GAUT4 leads to reduced ferulate and lignin-carbohydrate cross-linking in switchgrass. *Communications Biology, 2*, 22, 8450–8461.

Li, P., Fu, X., Zhang, L., & Li, S. (2019). CRISPR/Cas-based screening of a gene activation library in *Saccharomyces cerevisiae* identifies a crucial role of OLE1 in thermotolerance. *Microbial Biotechnology, 12*(6), 1154.

Lian, J., Chao, R., & Zhao, H. (2014). Metabolic engineering of a *Saccharomyces cerevisiae* strain capable of simultaneously utilizing glucose and galactose to produce enantiopure (2R,3R)-butanediol. *Metabolic Engineering, 23*, 92–99.

Liao, C. J., Mi, L., Pontrelli, S., & Luo, S. (2016). Fueling the future: microbial engineering for the production of sustainable biofuels. *Nature Reviews Microbiology, 14*, 288–304. https://doi.org/10.1038/nrmicro.2016.32 (accessed on 5th November 2025).

Liew, F., Henstra, A. M., Köpke, M., Winzer, K., Simpson, S. D., & Minton, N. P. (2017). Metabolic engineering of *Clostridium autoethanogenum* for selective alcohol production. *Metabolic Engineering, 40*, 104–114.

Liu, R., Zhu, F., Lu, L., Fu, A., Lu, J., Deng, Z., & Liu, T. (2014). Metabolic engineering of fatty acyl-ACP reductase-dependent pathway to improve fatty alcohol production in *Escherichia coli*. *Metabolic Engineering, 22*, 10–21.

Losse, M., & Geissdoerfer, M. (2021). Mapping socially responsible investing: a bibliometric and citation network analysis. *Journal of Cleaner Production, 296*(4), 126376.

Ma, F., Fu, C., Yang, J., & Yang, Q. (2020). Control strategy for adaptive active energy harvesting in sediment microbial fuel cells. *Journal of Energy Engineering, 146*(1), 04019034.

Madvar, M. D., Ahmadi, F., Shirmohammadi, R., & Aslani, A. (2019). Forecasting of wind energy technology domains based on the technology life cycle approach. *Energy Reports, 5*, 1236–1248.

Martín-Pascual, J., Jódar, J., Rodríguez, M. L., & Zamorano, M. (2020). Determination of the optimal operative conditions for the torrefaction of olive waste biomass. *Sustainability, 12*, 6411.

Matsakas, L., Nitsos, C., Raghavendran, V., Yakimenko, O., Persson, G., Olsson, E., Rova, U., Olsson, L., & Christakopoulos, P. (2018). A novel hybrid organosolv: steam explosion method for the efficient fractionation and pretreatment of birch biomass. *Biotechnology for Biofuels, 11*, 160.

Maurya, D. P., Singla, A., & Negi, S. (2015). An overview of key pretreatment processes for biological conversion of lignocellulosic biomass to bioethanol. *3 Biotech, 5*, 597–609. https://doi.org/10.1007/s13205-015-0279-4 (accessed on 5th November 2025).

Mercer, J. (2015). Microbial fuel cells: generating power from waste. *Review of Engineering in Everyday Life, 42*(8), 3053–3058.

Milano, J., Ong, H. C., Masjuki, H., Chong, W., Lam, M. K., Loh, P. K., et al. (2016). Microalgae biofuels as an alternative to fossil fuel for power generation. *Renewable and Sustainable Energy Reviews, 58*, 180–197.

Molinuevo-Salces, B., Mahdy, A., Ballesteros, M., & González-Fernández, C. (2016). From piggery wastewater nutrients to biogas: microalgae biomass revalorization through anaerobic digestion. *Renewable Energy, 96*, 1103–1110.

Muhammad, G., Alam, M. A., Mofijur, M., Jahirul, M. I., Lv, Y., Xiong, W., Ong, H. C., & Xu, J. (2021). Modern developmental aspects in the field of economical harvesting and biodiesel production from microalgae biomass. *Renewable and Sustainable Energy Reviews, 135*, 110209.

Muylaert, K., Vandamme, D., Foubert, I., & Brady, P. V. (2015). Harvesting of microalgae by means of flocculation. In *International Springer Publishing* (pp. 251–273).

Nikolić, S., Pejin, J., & Mojović, L. (2016). Challenges in bioethanol production: utilization of cotton fabrics as a feedstock. *Chemical Industry and Chemical Engineering Quarterly, 22*, 375–390.

Oncel, S., & Kose, A. (2014). Comparison of tubular and panel type photobioreactors for biohydrogen production utilizing *Chlamydomonas reinhardtii* considering mixing time and light intensity. *Bioresource Technology, 151*, 265–270.

Park, J., Naresh, K. A., Cayetano, R. D. A., & Kim, S. H. (2020). Assessment of *Chlorella* sp. as a potential feedstock for biological methane production. *Bioresource Technology, 305*, 123075. https://doi.org/10.1016/j.biortech.2020.123075 (accessed on 5th November 2025).

Parkash, A. (2016). Microbial fuel cells: A source of bioenergy. *Journal of Microbial & Biochemical Technology, 8*, 247–255. https://doi.org/10.4172/1948-5948.1000293 (accessed on 5th November 2025).

Passos, F., Carretero, J., & Ferrer, I. (2015). Comparing pretreatment methods for improving microalgae anaerobic digestion: thermal, hydrothermal, microwave, and ultrasound. *Chemical Engineering Journal, 279*, 667–672.

Prasad, S., Kumar, S., Yadav, K. K., Choudhry, J., Kamyab, H., Bach, Q. V., Sheetal, K. R., Kannojiya, S., & Gupta, N. (2020a). Screening and evaluation of cellulitis fungal strains for saccharification and bioethanol production from rice residue. *Energy, 25*, 116422.

Prasad, S., Singh, A., Korres, N. E., Rathore, D., Sevda, S., & Pant, D. (2020b). Sustainable utilization of crop residues for energy generation: A life cycle assessment (LCA) perspective. *Bioresource Technology, 303*, 122964.

Qin, L., Zhao, X., Li, W. C., Zhu, J. Q., Liu, L., Li, B. Z., & Yuan, Y. J. (2018). Process analysis and optimization of simultaneous saccharification and co-fermentation ethylenediamine-pretreated corn stover for ethanol production. *Biotechnology for Biofuels, 11*, 1–10.

Rashid, N., Nayak, M., Lee, B., & Chang, Y. K. (2019). Efficient microalgae harvesting mediated by polysaccharides interaction with residual calcium and phosphate in the growth medium. *Journal of Cleaner Production, 234*, 150–156.

Raut, M. P., Couto, N., Pham, T. K., Evans, C., Noirel, J., & Wright, P. C. (2016). Quantitative proteomic analysis of the influence of lignin on biofuel production by *Clostridium acetobutylicum* ATCC 824. *Biotechnology for Biofuels, 9*, 113.

Rodionova, M. V., Poudyal, R. S., Tiwari, I., Voloshin, R. A., Zharmukhamedov, S. K., Nam, H. G., Zayadan, B. K., Bruce, B. D., Hou, H. J. M., & Allakhverdiev, S. I. (2017). Biofuel production: Challenges and opportunities. *International Journal of Hydrogen Energy, 42*(12).

Rollin, J. A., del Campo, J. M., Myung, S., Sun, F., You, C., Bakovic, A., & Senger, R. S. (2015). High yield hydrogen production from biomass by *in vitro* metabolic engineering: mixed sugars co-utilization and kinetic modeling. *Proceedings of the National Academy of Sciences of the United States of America, 112*, 4964–4969.

Sahay, S., & Braganza, V. J. (2016). Microalgae-based biodiesel production–Current and future scenario. *Journal of Experimental Sciences, 7*, 31–35.

Schadeweg, V., & Boles, E. (2016). Increasing n-butanol production with *Saccharomyces cerevisiae* by optimizing acetyl-CoA synthesis, NADH levels and trans-2-enoyl-CoA reductase expression. *Biotechnology for Biofuels, 9*(1), 257.

Sekar, M., Mathimani, T., Alagumalai, A., Chi, N. T. L., Duc, P. A., Bhatia, S. K., Brindhadevi, K., & Pugazhendhi, A. (2021). A review on the pyrolysis of algal biomass for biochar and biooil–Bottlenecks and scope. *Fuel, 283*.

Sengmee, D., Cheirsilp, B., Suksaroge, T. T., & Prasertsan, P. (2017). Biophotolysis-based hydrogen and lipid production by oleaginous microalgae using crude glycerol as exogenous carbon source. *International Journal of Hydrogen Energy, 42*, 1970–1976.

Sheldon, R. A. (2018). Enzymatic conversion of first- and second-generation sugars. In *Biomass and Green Chemistry* (pp. 169–189). Springer.

Sheng, L., Kovács, K., Winzer, K., Zhang, Y., & Minton, N. P. (2017). Development and implementation of rapid metabolic engineering tools for chemical and fuel production in *Geobacillus thermoglucosidasius* NCIMB 11955. *Biotechnology for Biofuels, 10*, 5.

Silveira, M. H. L., Morais, A. R. C., Da Costa Lopes, A. M., Olekszyszen, D. N., Bogel-Łukasik, R., Andreaus, J., & Pereira Ramos, L. (2015). Current pretreatment technologies for the development of cellulosic ethanol and biorefineries. *ChemSusChem, 8*(20), 3366–3390.

Singh, A., Sharma, R., Pant, D., & Malaviya, P. (2021). Engineered algal biochar for contaminant remediation and electrochemical applications. *Science of the Total Environment, 774*, 145676.

Singh, R., Shukla, A., Tiwari, S., & Srivastava, M. (2014). A review on delignification of lignocellulosic biomass for enhancement of ethanol production potential. *Renewable and Sustainable Energy Reviews, 32*, 713–728.

Singh, R., Singh, A., & Rathore, D. (2017). Biohydrogen: Global trend and future perspective. In A. Singh & D. Rathore (Eds.), *Biohydrogen Production: Sustainability of Current Technology and Future Perspective* (pp. 291–315). New Delhi: Springer India. http://dx.doi.org/10.1007/978-81-322-3577-4 (accessed on 5th November 2025).

Sivagurunathan, P., Kumar, G., Mudhoo, A., Rene, E. R., Saratale, G. D., Kobayashi, T., et al. (2017). Fermentative hydrogen production using lignocellulose biomass: An overview of pre-treatment methods, inhibitor effects and detoxification experiences. *Renewable and Sustainable Energy Reviews, 77*, 28–42. http://dx.doi.org/10.1016/j.rser.2017.03.091 (accessed on 5th November 2025).

Solé-Bundó, M., Carrère, H., Garfí, M., & Ferrer, I. (2017). Enhancement of microalgae anaerobic digestion by thermo-alkaline pretreatment with lime (CaO). *Algal Research, 24*, 199–206.

Tahvildari, K., Anaraki, Y. N., Fazaeli, R., Mirpanji, S., & Delrish, E. (2015). The study of CaO and MgO heterogenic nano-catalyst coupling transesterification reaction efficacy in the production of biodiesel from recycled cooking oil. *Journal of Environmental Health Science and Engineering, 13*, 73.

Tsegaye, B., Balomajumder, C., & Roy, P. (2018b). Biodegradation of wheat straw by *Ochrobactrum oryzae* BMP03 and *Bacillus* sp. BMP01 bacteria to enhance biofuel production by increasing total reducing sugars yield. *Environmental Science and Pollution Research, 25*(30), 30585–30596. https://doi.org/10.1007/s11356-018-3056-1 (accessed on 5th November 2025).

Vaid, S., Nargotra, P., & Bajaj, B. K. (2018). Consolidated bioprocessing for biofuel-ethanol production from pine needle biomass. *Environmental Progress & Sustainable Energy, 37*, 546–552.

Valdivia, M., Galan, J. L., Laffarga, J., & Ramos, J. L. (2020). A research and technological valuation model for decision analysis in the environmental and renewable energy sectors. *Renewable and Sustainable Energy Reviews, 122*, 109726.

Van Kuijk, S. J., Sonnenberg, A. S., Baars, J. J., Hendriks, W. H., & Cone, J. W. (2015). Fungal treated lignocellulosic biomass as ruminant feed ingredient: A review. *Biotechnology Advances, 33*(1), 191–202. https://doi.org/10.1016/j.biotechadv.2014.10.014 (accessed on 5th November 2025).

Varman, A. M., Xiao, Y., Pakrasi, H. B., & Tang, Y. J. (2013). Metabolic engineering of *Synechocystis* sp. strain PCC 6803 for isobutanol production. *Applied and Environmental Microbiology, 79*(3), 908–914.

Venkata Mohan, S., Hemalatha, M., Chakraborty, D., Chatterjee, S., Ranadheer, P., & Kona, R. (2020). Algal biorefinery models with self-sustainable closed loop approach: Trends and prospective for blue bioeconomy. *Bioresource Technology, 295*, 122128. https://doi.org/10.1016/j.biortech.2019.122128 (accessed on 5th November 2025).

Vohra, M., Manwar, J., Manmode, R., Padgilwar, S., & Patil, S. (2014). Bioethanol production: Feedstock and current technologies. *Journal of Environmental Chemical Engineering, 1*(1), 13. https://doi.org/10.1016/j.jece.2013.10.013 (accessed on 5th November 2025).

Voloshin, R. A., Rodionova, M. V., Zharmukhamedov, S. K., Veziroglu, T. N., & Allakhverdiev, S. I. (2016). Review: Biofuel production from plant and algal biomass. *International Journal of Hydrogen Energy, 41*, 17257–17273.

Vuppaladadiyam, A. K., Yao, J. G., Florin, N., George, A., Wang, X., Labeeuw, L., et al. (2018). Impact of flue gas compounds on microalgae and mechanisms for carbon assimilation and utilization. *ChemSusChem, 11*, 334–355. https://doi.org/10.1002/cssc.201701611 (accessed on 5th November 2025).

Xue, C., Zhao, J., Chen, L., Yang, S. T., & Bai, F. (2017). Recent advances and state-of-the-art strategies in strain and process engineering for biobutanol production by *Clostridium acetobutylicum*. *Biotechnology Advances, 35*, 310–322.

Yang, X., Xu, M., & Yang, S. T. (2015). Metabolic and process engineering of *Clostridium cellulovorans* for biofuel production from cellulose. *Metabolic Engineering, 32*, 39–48.

Yao, L., Qi, F., Tan, X., & Lu, X. (2014). Improved production of fatty alcohols in cyanobacteria by metabolic engineering. *Biotechnology for Biofuels, 7*, 94.

Yeong, T. K., Jiao, K., Zeng, X., Lin, L., Pan, S., & Danquah, M. K. (2018). Microalgae for biobutanol production – Technology evaluation and value proposition. *Algal Research, 31*, 367–376. https://doi.org/10.1016/j.algal.2018.02.029 (accessed on 5th November 2025).

Yu, L., Xu, M., Tang, I. C., & Yang, S. T. (2015). Metabolic engineering of *Clostridium tyrobutyricum* for n-butanol production through co-utilization of glucose and xylose. *Biotechnology and Bioengineering, 112*(10), 2134–2141.

Zhang, H., Liu, C., Ou, Y., Chen, T., Yang, L., & Hu, Z. (2019). Development of a helical coagulation reactor for harvesting microalgae. *Journal of Bioscience and Bioengineering, 127*, 447–450.

Zhang, S., Guo, F., Yan, W., Dai, Z., Zhou, J., Dong, W., Jiang, M., Zhang, W., & Xin, F. (2019). Recent advances of CRISPR-Cas9-based genetic engineering in industrial biology. *Frontiers in Bioengineering and Biotechnology, 7*, 459.

Zhang, Y., Gu, Z., Ren, Y., Wang, L. U., Zhang, J., Liang, C., Tong, S., Wang, Y., Xu, D., Zhang, X., & Ye, N. (2021). Integrating transcriptomics and metabolomics to characterize metabolic regulation to elevated $CO_2$ in *Chlamydomonas reinhardtii*. *Marine Biotechnology, 23*(2), 255–275.

## CHAPTER 3

# Cyanobacterial Cell Factories: An Overview of Polyhydroxyalkanoate Bioplastic Production

PRITI PAL,[1] AKHILESH KUMAR SINGH,[2,*] BRIJESH PANDEY,[2] ANAND PRAKASH,[2] PRAKASH KUMAR SARANGI,[3] SAURABH SINGH RATHORE,[2] RAJESH KUMAR SRIVASTAVA,[4] and RISHI KUMAR SINGH[5]

[1]*Amity Institute of Biotechnology, Amity University Uttar Pradesh, Lucknow Campus, Lucknow, India*

[2]*Department of Biotechnology, School of Life Sciences, Mahatma Gandhi Central University, Motihari, Bihar, India*

[3]*College of Agriculture, Central Agricultural University, Imphal, Manipur, India*

[4]*Department of Biotechnology, School of Core Engineering, GITAM (Deemed to be University), Visakhapatnam, Andhra Pradesh, India*

[5]*School of Biosciences, IMS Institute, University Courses Campus, Ghaziabad, Uttar Pradesh, India*

*Corresponding author

## ABSTRACT

Cyanobacteria are considered a promising feedstock for the sustainable production of polyhydroxyalkanoates (PHA), a biodegradable biopolymer viewed as an alternative to petroleum-based plastics. Compared with other prokaryotes, cyanobacteria produce higher-quality PHA and can

Industrial Biotechnology: Current Progress and Novel Technologies.
Prakash Kumar Sarangi, Akhilesh Kumar Singh, Rajesh Kumar Srivastava, and Brijesh Pandey (Eds.)


DOI: 10.1201/9781779642233-3

accumulate it intracellularly by utilizing $CO_2$ and sunlight, making the process more environmentally friendly and less resource-intensive. However, large-scale PHA production from conventional bacteria remains costly due to the need for sugar-based fermentation. Therefore, improving PHA production in cyanobacteria through optimized strains, efficient cultivation systems, and cost-effective recovery processes is essential. Process optimization, including reactor design and nutrient management, plays a crucial role in enhancing PHA accumulation and reducing production costs. Although many wild-type and genetically modified cyanobacteria show high PHA yields under laboratory conditions, only limited studies have demonstrated successful large-scale production. Advances in genetic engineering further enhance the potential of cyanobacteria by improving metabolic pathways and increasing PHA storage capacity. This chapter provides an overview of cyanobacterial PHA biosynthesis, the influence of nutrient conditions, the role of reactors in upstream processing, and strategies for cost-effective downstream recovery. It also highlights current technical challenges and the importance of process optimization for achieving industrial-scale PHA production using genetically modified cyanobacterial strains.

## 3.1 INTRODUCTION

Polyhydroxyalkanoates (PHA), a group of polyesters produced by cyanobacteria that resemble synthetic plastics chemically, has drawn the attention of researchers since 1966 (Iasimone et al., 2020). PHA is a compound that is known to accumulate as granules in the cytoplasm of cyanobacteria and is derived from a particular type of microalga (Papadopoulos et al., 2021). Despite the development of industrial PHA production from cyanobacteria, widespread use is constrained by lower yields that drive up production costs. Cyanobacteria have also undergone metabolic modification to increase PHA output and decrease operational bottlenecks. PHB is the most typical type of PHA. Due to its intracellular PHA level, the thermophilic cyanobacterium *Synechococcus* sp. MA19 produced 55% of the DW PHA when phosphorus was limited (Shrivastav et al., 2010). Similarly, *Synechocystis* sp. PCC6803 was shown to be unaffected by light intensity or carbon source when it came to PHA synthesis. Numerous cyanobacterial strains have been discovered to contain 1–55% PHA, including *Calothrix* sp., *Oscillatoria* sp., *Microcystis* sp., *Nostoc* sp., *Spirulina* sp., and *Synechocystis* sp. Under nitrogen deprivation conditions, *Oscillatoria okeni* TISTR 8549 naturally produced 42% of the functionally superior poly (3-hydroxybutyrate-co-3-hydroxy valerate) (González-Resendiz et al., 2021). Recently, efforts have been made to improve cyanobacterial traits through genetic engineering, with some degree of success, to enhance PHA synthesis productivity, diversity, and regulation (Amelia et al., 2019). Microbial PHA production for various industrial applications, particularly food packaging, has not yet established a strong presence despite being commercialized (Kourmentzao et al., 2017). However, due to the rise in oil prices and the drive toward a carbon-neutral economy, PHA will soon be produced and commercialized from cyanobacteria. The scaffold for numerous biomolecules is provided by naturally occurring biopolymers called PHA, which are found in the form of esters accumulated within a variety of microbes. PHA is produced by many prokaryotic microorganisms when their nutritional needs are not met, such as when they need to store carbon and energy. PHA has attracted a lot of commercial and academic interest from the eco-friendly polymer market since Lemoine first discovered them in 1926 because of their beneficial qualities, such as high biocompatibility, excellent biodegradability, diverse chemical structure, and production from renewable carbon resources. PHA is a biopolymer with physicochemical characteristics resembling those of commonly used industrial materials polypropylene, polystyrene, and polyethylene. The structural characteristics of PHA are influenced by the carbon precursor, microbial strain, media composition, fermentation process, and recovery methods (Choi et al., 2021). The natural cycle of circulation and renewability is aided by the degradation of PHA-based products into $CO_2$, $H_2O$, and $CH_4$ when they are left in the environment. Additional optically pure building blocks that can be used as synthons for the synthesis of drugs, organic compounds, and fragrances can be produced by hydrolyzing the used PHA (Lan and Wei, 2016). In intracellular inclusions, PHA can make up 80% of a cell's weight and be synthesized to store carbon and energy (Roja et al., 2019). When oxygen, phosphorus, or nitrogen are in short supply, these other essential nutrients are synthesized inside the cell as insoluble cytoplasmic inclusions. Because it does not significantly change the osmotic state of the cell, this polymeric material can be stored there in high concentrations (Wagner et al., 2016). These inclusions typically have spherical shapes and mean diameters between 0.2 and 0.7 m.

They are encased in a 2 nm membrane made up of 0.5% lipids and 2% protein. The granules are surrounded by a phospholipid layer, polymerases, depolymerizes, and unspecific cytosolic proteins. Lipids, proteins, and carbohydrates are the most important components of biobased products, such as bioplastics, biopolymers, and biobased polyurethane, and cyanobacteria are capable of producing large amounts of these substances (Rueda et al., 2020). For several cyanobacteria, including *Synechocystis* sp., *Spirulina* sp., *Nostoc* sp., *Oscillatoria* sp., and *Calothrix* sp., PHA content of 1–10% has been reported (Kamravamanesh et al., 2019). The most widely studied and commercially available short-chain-length PHA (scl-PHA) is P (3HB), which is produced by cyanobacteria most frequently (Oliveira et al., 2019). The cyanobacteria species *Synechococcus* sp., *Aphanothece* sp., *Gloeothece* sp., *Spirulina* sp., and *Calothrix scytonemicola* are known to be capable of producing P (3HB) using $CO_2$ as a carbon source (Kamravamanesh et al., 2019). PHA serves as a compound that most organisms, including cyanobacteria, use to store energy and carbon. When cyanobacteria are exposed to environmental stressors like nutrient-limited cultivation conditions, they frequently exhibit their high potential for the production of PHA. On the other hand, a system for producing photosynthetically could offer a substitute for sustainable PHA production. Cyanobacteria are photosynthetic prokaryotes, and some of them, including *Aulosira fertilissima* and *Synechococcus* sp., are known to produce PHA. *Nostoc muscorum, Calothrix scytonemicola* TISTR 8095, and numerous others. These photosynthetic microorganisms can grow and reproduce in confined spaces without competing with food crops for space (Wang et al., 2020). They also do not need exogenous sugar to grow. The ability of cyanobacteria to use $CO_2$ for growth and their easy genetic tractability are two distinguishing characteristics that make them useful in industry (Koch et al., 2019). Cyanobacteria, which removes excess nitrogen and phosphate from water as well as PHA formation, can grow in wastewater. Aquaculture wastewater can be reused because cyanobacteria can use extra nitrogen and phosphate for growth and PHA accumulation from wastewater (Troschl et al., 2018). In this chapter, an overview of the production of green PHA by cyanobacteria, the impact of different nutrients, as well as the role of reactors in upstream processing are discussed. The emphasis in this chapter is also on genetically altered cyanobacteria that may be able to boost PHA formation as well as improve PHA recovery together with the cost-effective downstream processing. Additionally, it highlights the difficulties of industrial cyanobacterial cultivation/ growth as well as the importance of process optimization for scale-up.

## 3.2 BIOSYNTHETIC PATHWAY OF CYANOBACTERIAL PHA

Numerous experts in this field have provided in-depth explanations of how polyhydroxyalkanoate production occurs during a photoautotrophic bacterial fermentative process. The three fundamental steps of the traditional PHA biosynthetic pathway, which are each catalyzed by a different enzyme, are well-known: phaA-encoded β-ketothiolase catalyzes the condensation of two acetyl-CoA molecules into one acetoacetyl-CoA; phaB-encoded NADPH-dependent acetoacetyl-CoA dehydrogenase reduces acetoacetyl-CoA; and phaC-encoded PHA synthase polymerizes 3-hydroxyacid (3HA) units, or (R)-3 Fatty acid oxidation pathway and the pathway. As is clear, PHA synthase is essential for the biosynthesis of PHA (Jordan et al., 2017). A wide range of substrates, including sugars (glucose, fructose, sucrose, maltose, and lactose), starch, glycerol, FAs and their derivatives, methanol, lignin, and agricultural, industrial, and dairy byproducts, have been reported as potential PHA substrates based on the presence of these enzymes (Park et al., 2021). PHA compositions and content have been seen to increase with the addition of various substrate combinations and precursor substrates, as well as with the adoption of various feeding regimens (Troschl et al., 2017). However, cyanobacteria that can adapt to both photoautotrophic and heterotrophic cultivation share a lot of the same biosynthetic pathways for using the three fundamental steps mentioned above. The majority of the information gleaned comes from studies on *Synechocystis* sp. PCC 6803. Two PhaEC subunits make up the synthase enzyme in this instance. Therefore, the PHA synthase in cyanobacteria is also a type-III PHA synthase. The genes for the PhaA and PhaB enzymes are similar to how the genes for PhaE and PhaC are organized. They are said to be organized into a single operon. Consequently, only SCL-PHAs have been described in cyanobacterial species to date (Wang et al., 2013). In addition to *Synechococcus* sp. strains MA19 and PCC 6715, *Chlorogloeopsis fritschii* PCC 6912, *Anabaena cylindrica* SAG 1403-2, *Cyanothece* sp. strains PCC 7424, PCC 8303, and PCC 8801, and *Gloeocapsa* sp. strain PCC 7428, the presence of a type-III PHA synthase. However, because cyanobacteria are a diverse group, it is unknown whether they contain other varieties of PHA synthase, which soon offers a valuable opportunity (Kamravamanesh et al., 2018). When cyanobacteria were grown autotrophically using $CO_2$, ribulose-1,5-bisphosphate carboxylase/oxygenase was used to fix the carbon source in the Calvin-Benson-Bassham (CBB) cycle (RuBisCO). Around 90% of the carbon found in biomass on Earth is known to be assimilated by RuBisCO, which is also more efficient at absorbing $CO_2$ than $O_2$. Inorganic carbon (Ci) transporters help to move atmospheric $CO_2$ across the wall, assisting in preserving the local RuBisCO carbon concentration. The Calvin cycle's byproduct, glyceraldehyde-3-phosphate, can be changed into 3-phosphoglycerate (PGA), which can then go through one of three pathways for sugar metabolism: the Entner-Doudoroff (ED) pathway, glycolysis, or finally, acetyl-CoA, which is used in the PHA synthesis pathway (Monshupanee et al., 2019). Even though the PHA synthesis pathway and subsequent metabolic engineering studies have been extensively demonstrated in cyanobacteria, the PHA synthesis pathway begins with acetyl coenzyme A. Numerous metabolic processes have acetyl-CoA as a precursor, including the synthesis of fatty acids, and it can be produced from both the degradation of fatty acids and photosynthesis-obtained carbohydrates. Acetyl-CoA flux thus regulates PHA production. The enzyme 3-ketothiolase catalyzes the first step in the synthesis of PHA, which condenses two acetyl-CoA molecules into acetoacetyl-CoA. Acetoacetyl-CoA is converted to 3-hydroxybutyryl-CoA by the NADPH-dependent Acetoacetyl-CoA reductase enzyme, which is encoded by the *PhaB2* gene. PHA synthase, a product of the PhaC gene, catalyzes the joining of R-Hydroxybutyric with the expanding PHB chain to enable the polymerization (Hendry et al., 2020). In addition, cyanobacteria use glycerol and other photoautotrophic carbon sources to produce PHA, and these sources are controlled by different biosynthetic pathways (Ansari and Fatima, 2019). In addition, PHA granules play some regulatory and protective roles in cyanobacteria, strong in the face of osmotic and oxidative stress managed brought on by oxidants, heat, desiccation, and UV radiation (Tarawat et al., 2020).

## 3.3 PHA PRODUCTION BY PHOTOAUTOTROPHIC CYANOBACTERIA

Since cyanobacteria are prokaryotic, they lack the specialized organelles found in eukaryotes and instead have photosynthetic pigments in their cytoplasm (Figure 3.1). Cyanobacteria make up 20–30% of all photosynthetic organisms and carry out the majority of photosynthesis on Earth (Bhati et al., 2010). These organisms can fix atmospheric nitrogen and inorganic carbon using the nitrogenase enzyme. Cyanobacteria have carboxysomes to achieve carbon dioxide concentrating mechanisms, in contrast to the proteinaceous micro-compartments called pyrenoids that are found in algae and contain the enzyme (RuBisCO) (Samantaray et al., 2011). Although cyanobacterial RuBisCOs typically have a low affinity for $CO_2$, carbonic anhydrase allows them to grow rapidly even in the presence of low $CO_2$ levels. Because of its simple structure, it is therefore more effective than algae at fixing carbon from the atmosphere (Balaji et al., 2013). To produce useful chemicals from inorganic carbon fixation, RuBisCO's biomass yield and $CO_2$ affinity can be easily increased in cyanobacteria through genetic engineering (Carpine et al., 2015). As a result of metabolic engineering, cyanobacteria are now much more capable of converting $CO_2$ into ethanol, isobutanol, isoprene, and a wide range of other products (Drosg et al., 2015). Due to their rich amino acid composition, certain cyanobacteria, including *Spirulina* sp. (45–65%), *Arthrospira maxima* (70–75%), and *Synechococcus* sp. (60–65%), have attracted research attention. PHA have a variety of uses and are a more environmentally friendly option than conventional plastics. They were first developed as a result of an in-depth investigation into bio-based and biodegradable polymers (Phalanisong and Plangklang, 2021). There is no evidence of long-chain-length PHA or mcl-PHA in cyanobacteria at this time. The best-known catalyst for PHA production in cyanobacteria is nitrogen limitation (Koller, 2015). The MA19 strain of cyanobacteria, which was later determined to be *Synechococcus* sp., was the first to produce PHA in cyanobacteria. Cyanobacteria of the *Spirulina* species are frequently discovered in freshwater that are very alkaline. It can, however, be grown in any kind of water, including fresh, brackish, and saltwater. It contains anywhere between 46 and 63% protein. *Spirulina* has more advantageous commercial properties for blending than *Chlorella* due to its superior blend properties. *Spirulina*'s high protein content makes it a potentially healthy food. Another blue-green alga, *Scenedesmus almeriensis*, can accumulate PHA and is found in freshwater and brackish waters (Roh et al., 2021). A photoautotrophic freshwater cyanobacterium called *Calothrix Scytonemicola* turns $CO_2$ into the biopolymer PHA (Fedeson et al., 2017). The cyanobacteria *Aulosira fertilissima* synthesizes

PHA in about 10% of the carbon utilization, compared to bacteria (Wagner et al., 2016). This demonstrates that, compared to many other PHA-producing strains, cyanobacteria can reduce the cost of oxygen and carbon supply, which lowers the cost of the entire production process. Many challenges in their biosynthesis may prevent cyanobacteria from being used in industry, even though they appear to have a high potential for producing PHA. When cyanobacteria are exposed to environmental stressors like nutrient-limited cultivation conditions, they frequently produce PHA. Cyanobacteria to increase PHA synthesis, which will also help to improve the viability from an economic standpoint. Numerous studies have demonstrated that cyanobacteria, such as *Spirulina* sp., *Nostoc* sp., *Oscillatoria* sp, *Synechocystis* sp., can convert $CO_2$ to PHA with a content of 10–50% by using sunlight (Roja et al., 2019).

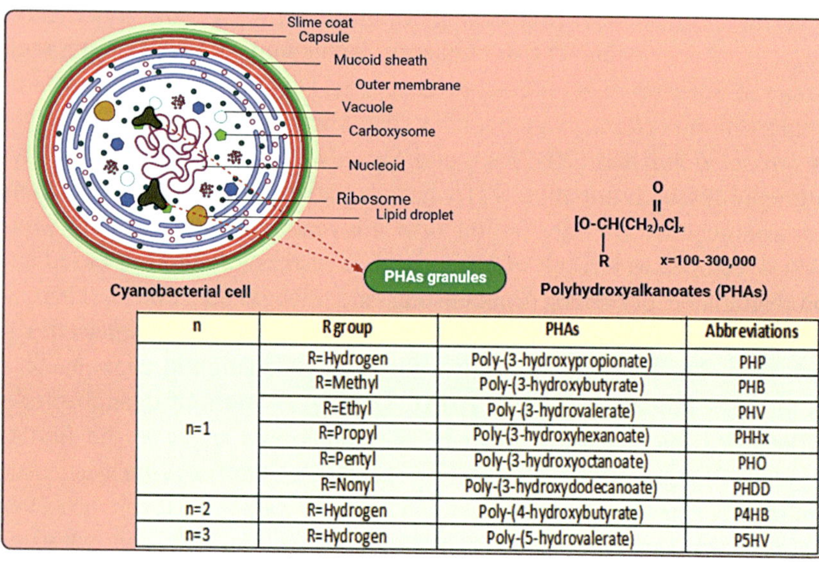


| n | R group | PHAs | Abbreviations |
|---|---|---|---|
| n=1 | R=Hydrogen | Poly-(3-hydroxypropionate) | PHP |
| | R=Methyl | Poly-(3-hydroxybutyrate) | PHB |
| | R=Ethyl | Poly-(3-hydrovalerate) | PHV |
| | R=Propyl | Poly-(3-hydroxyhexanoate) | PHHx |
| | R=Pentyl | Poly-(3-hydroxyoctanoate) | PHO |
| | R=Nonyl | Poly-(3-hydroxydodecanoate) | PHDD |
| n=2 | R=Hydrogen | Poly-(4-hydroxybutyrate) | P4HB |
| n=3 | R=Hydrogen | Poly-(5-hydrovalerate) | P5HV |

**FIGURE 3.1** Chemical composition of PHAs and their derivatives in cyanobacterial cells.

### 3.3.1 PHA ACCUMULATION BY NOSTOC

*Nostoc* is the name given to a group of organisms that can be found near freshwater sources on land and in the water. *Nostoc* is a diverse group of filamentous cyanobacteria that can reach a temperature of about 20°C (86F) at its most active stage. Numerous species have been identified as producing

PHA under phosphate and nitrogen limitation since *Nostoc muscorum* produced 8.6% of dry cell weight (dcw) PHA under photoautotrophic circumstances (Bhati and Mallick, 2016). Under photoautotrophic conditions, PHA content of up to 19.27% with *N. ellipsosporum* and 22% with *N. muscorum* was discovered (Hondo et al., 2015). Utilizing the metabolic inhibitors carbonyl cyanide *m*-chlorophenylhydrazone (CCCP) and dicyclohexylcarbodiimide (DCCD), we were able to redirect the flux toward the PHA production pathway, which caused PHA concentrations to increase from an initial dry weight content of 8.5% to up to 21 and 17%, respectively (Aikawa et al., 2014). It is interesting to note that production of the PHA copolymer poly (3-hydroxybutyric acid-co-3-hydroxyvaleric acid), or P (3HB-co-3HV), has also been reported from *Nostoc*, but only when propionate or valerate are added to the culture medium under mixotrophic or heterotrophic conditions (Gupta et al., 2017). Under nitrogen and phosphate limitation, respectively, the addition of these precursor substrates increased P (3HB-co-3HV) production up to 28.2–31.4% and 58–60% of dcw. Under heterotrophic conditions, this content increased even further, reaching a maximum of 78% of dcw (Kamravamanesh et al., 2018). As a nutrient supplement, poultry litter was added to the culture at a rate of 10 g/L along with glucose, acetate, valerate, and $CO_2$. As a result, a P (3HB-co-3HV) copolymer yield of 774 mg $L^{-1}$ was created (65–70% of dcw) (Gupta et al., 2017). Notably, PHA accumulation in the biomass was observed in the late exponential phase, and the yield of *Nostoc*-produced biomass was typically around 1 g/L.

### 3.3.2 PHA ACCUMULATION BY ARTHROSPIRA

*Arthrospira*, formerly known as *Spirulina,* is a type of filamentous bacteria that can be grown in freshwater and is found in alkaline (salt) lakes. *Arthrospira* is presently primarily grown as a food supplement due to its high protein and vitamin content. It is a strong candidate for use in the production of PHA because of its rapid growth and minimal water needs. According to reports, *Arthrospira* can produce 5000–15,000 tons of dry weight annually (Koller et al., 2017). Because its cultivation requires high alkalinity, the culture is free of other usual contaminants. It is therefore very likely to be used to keep an open pond culture stable and high in biomass. One of the most frequently investigated species for the production of PHA is *Spirulina platensis* (Kumar et al., 2019). Since the first report of PHA production in 1982, which was accomplished at up to 6% dcw, the rate of PHA production under photoautotrophic conditions has not increased significantly. Various strategies have been employed to raise the yield. Acetate supplementation (2.5–3% of dcw), phosphorus limitation (3.5% of dcw) (Kumar et al., 2019), and increased salinity (14.7 percent) all led to an increase in PHA yield (Koller et al., 2017). The highest yields were produced by the *Spirulina* sp. LEB 18, which in 15 days produced 1.48 g/L/d PHA (20.62% of dcw) (Lam et al., 2017). Increasing the yield of PHA production in mixotrophic or heterotrophic cultures is the main issue. The yields have been improved by condition optimization, and they may be further improved.

### 3.3.3 PHA ACCUMULATION BY SYNECHOCYSTIS AND SYNECHOCOCCUS

Both fresh and saltwater contain tiny cyanobacteria from the genera *Synechocystis* and *Synechococcus*. It was discovered that *Synechocystis* can produce PHA, with a yield of 4.1% under nitrogen-starved conditions (Panith et al., 2016). The findings of this study demonstrated that glucose-based mixotrophic cultivation increased biomass but not PHA yield (% of dcw). In this instance, the yield increased from 4.5% of dcw under balanced culture cultivation to 9.5% and 15.2% of dcw under nitrogen restriction and 11.2% under phosphorus depletion (Ray and Kalia, 2017). Samantaray et al. (2011) found that heterotrophic cultivation in the dark with 0.4% acetate could increase the yield to 22% of dry weight. This yield was then increased to 38% of dry weight when the stationary phase culture was subjected to phosphate and gas exchange limitation in the presence of 0.4% acetate and 0.4% fructose (Yao et al., 2016). The most popular strain currently used to produce PHA is *Synechocystis* PCC6803 (Singh et al., 2015). The literature also mentions the production of PHA by the closely related genus *Synechococcus*. In Japan, wet volcanic rock surfaces were home to the thermophilic cyanobacterium *Synechococcus* sp. MA19, which used up to 27% (w/w) of $CO_2$ to produce PHA. The yields from this strain in photoautotrophic cultivation were further increased to 55% (dcw), or 2.4 g/L, under phosphate limitation. The amount of PHA produced by cyanobacteria under photoautotrophic conditions is at its highest level to date (Panith et al., 2016). Furthermore, it was discovered that *S. salina* produced 7.5% PHA, which was then utilized for the hydrothermal liquefaction-based production of bio-oil (Yao et al., 2016). In a different experiment, after 21 days of incubation in a large tubular photobioreactor with medium circulation, pH control via $CO_2$ flow, artificial illumination, and controlled temperature, comparable yields of 4.8–9% of dcw, up to 2.0 g/L, were attained. In this instance, it was discovered that nitrogen restriction and illumination enhanced the production of PHA, while mixotrophy by the addition of acetate did not contribute due to contamination (Wang et al., 2018). Because *Synechococcus* sp. PHA production has not been extensively studied, to increase production, there is a lot of area for experimentation with mixotrophic or heterotrophic cultivation. Along with the genus already mentioned that is primarily used for PHA production, other genera have also been reported to be able to produce PHA. Some of the genera mentioned include *Chlorogloea fritschii, Gloeocapsa* sp., *Oscillatoria limosa, Gloeothece* sp., PCC 6909, *Aulosira* sp., and *Calothrix* (Zhang et al., 2016). While *Chlorogloeopsis fritschii* PCC 6912, a thermophilic cyanobacteria, had PHA of up to 16% of dcw in its dried biomass, *Brevibacillus invocatus* MTCC 9039 had PHB of up to 13% of cdw accumulated in its stationary phase (Bhati and Mallick, 2016). According to Samantaray and Mallick (2012), the $N_2$-fixing cyanobacterium *Aulosira fertilissima* produces PHA while also treating wastewater in a biological recirculation system (Table 3.1). The production of PHA by these bacteria has also been reported to increase to 85% dcw with 0.26 percent citrate, 0.28% acetate, and 5.58 mg/L $K_2HPO_4$ for an incubation period of 5 days when phosphate deficiency is present (Samantaray et al., 2011). When nitrogen was limited, *Calothrix scytonemicola* TISTR 8095 could produce 25% of dcw (356.6 mg/L) PHA in 44 days (Zhang et al., 2016). *Anabaena cylindrica*, a filamentous cyanobacterium, was able to produce 2% of the dcw PHA, and valerate and propionate supplementation resulted in the production of P (3HBco-3HV) (Bhati and Mallick, 2016).

## 3.4 STRATEGIES FOR ENHANCING UPSTREAM PROCESSING

### *3.4.1 MEDIA OPTIMIZATION*

Cyanobacteria have been grown in a variety of culture mediums, including Pringsheim's Medium, BG11 Medium, Fogg's medium, and so on (Zheng et al., 2020). Researchers typically use BG11 and BG110.

**TABLE 3.1** Photoautotrophic PHA Production By Wild-Type Cyanobacterial Strains/Species Under Different Cultivation Conditions

| Wild-Type Cyanobacteria | Cultivation Conditions | Type of PHA | PHA Bioplastic (% or mg/l of Dry Weight) | References |
|---|---|---|---|---|
| *Spirulina subsalsa* | Batch, photoautotrophic, 5% NaCl, nitrogen free | PHA | 7.45% | Shrivastav et al. (2010) |
| *Aulosira fertilissima* | $CO_2$ + wastewater | PHB | 460.3 mg/l | Samantaray et al. (2011) |
| *Aulosira fertilissima* | Heterotrophic (in the flask), P deficiency | PHA | 85% | Samantaray and Mallick (2012) |
| *Synechocystis* | Overexpression of the sigma factor *sigE* Nitrogen limitation | PHA | 25% | Osanai et al. (2013) |
| *Aulosira fertilissima* | Fructose + valerate supplementation/phosphate deficiency | P(3HB-o-3HV) | 62–77% | Samantaray and Mallick (2014) |
| *Nostoc* | Acetate, glucose, valerate + nitrogen limitation | P(3HB-o-3HV) | 78% | Bhati and Mallick (2015) |
| *Calothrix scytonemicola* TISTR 8095 | Nitrogen limitation | PHA | 25.4% | Kaewbai-ngam et al. (2016) |
| *Nostoc muscorum* NCCU-442 | Phosphate deficiency | PHA | 26.4% | Ansari and Fatma (2016) |
| *Chlorogloea fritschii* TISTR 8527 | Two-stage cultivation: Photoautotrophy followed by heterotrophy | PHB | 51% | Monshupanee et al. (2016) |
| *Oscillatoria okeni* TISTR 8549 | Heterotrophic, Nitrogen limitation, acetate supplementation | P(3HB-co-3HV) | 42% | Taepucharoen et al. (2017) |
| *Nostoc muscorum* | Phosphate limitation | PHA | 19.27% | Martins et al. (2017) |
| *Synechocystis salina* CCALA192 | Optimized BG-11 media | PHA | 200 mg/l | Troschl et al. (2017) |
| *Synechocystis* sp. CCALA192 | Two-stage cultivation, N depletion, $CO_2$ as sole C source | PHB | 12.5% | Troschl et al. (2018) |
| *Scytonema geitleri* Bharadwaja | 30 mM acetate supplementation, 14:10 h light cycle | PHA | 7.12% | Singh et al. (2019) |
| *Chlamydomonas reinhardtii* | D-xylose supplementation, *N* limitation | PHB | 206 mg/l | Cassuriaga et al. (2020) |
| *Synechococcus elongatus* UAM–C/ S03 | Nitrogen limitation | PHA | 29.4% | González-Resendiz et al. (2021) |

Nitrate and phosphate restrictions caused *Synechococcus* sp. MA19 to grow photoautotrophically, which increased PHB to 27% and 55% (w/w), respectively. PHA in *Nostoc muscorum* increased in photoautotrophic conditions due to phosphorus restriction and shortage. Nitrogen and phosphorus starvation had a positive effect on PHA accumulation by 9.5% and 11% (w/w) in a study with *Synechocystis* sp. PCC 6803. However, 29% (w/w) PHA was produced when *Synechocystis* was pre-grown in BG11 with 0.1% glucose and 0.4% acetate under phosphate deficiency conditions. *Nostoc muscorum* accumulated 16.4% (w/w) of PHA in phosphate-deficient media that also contained 1% glucose and 1% acetate (Singh and Mallick, 2017). PHA in *Aulosira fertilissima* with phosphate deficiency was 77% (w/w), but PHB increased to 85% (w/w) with the addition of acetate and citrate. The maximum polymer accumulation of 1.59 g/L was reached when the cells were pre-cultured in 1.0% fructose and then grown in the previously optimized conditions. In *Synechocystis* sp. PCC 6803, mixotrophic growth with 0.4% glucose and nitrogen deficiency increased the PHA yield by 13.5% (Surendran et al., 2020). The percentages of PHA in *Aulosira fertilissima* CCC444 increased to 18.7% (w/w) and 17.6% (w/w), respectively, when nickel (1.0 mg/L) and copper (1.5 mg/L) were added to the culture medium. By adjusting media and physicochemical elements like pH, light intensity, photoperiod, salt concentration, and sugar supplementation, PHA production can be quickly increased. *Nostoc muscorum* had a PHA that was 26.37% (w/w) lower in phosphorus than the control, which was six times higher (Sawant et al., 2017). The industrial-scale cultivation of cyanobacteria is quite expensive and impractical because it needs a lot of fresh water. Utilizing specially created wastewater-based cultivation media for cyanobacteria could solve this problem and promote water reuse. Nitrogen and phosphorous, which are necessary nutrients for the cultivation of cyanobacteria, are present in significant amounts in wastewater from livestock, aquaculture, and agricultural runoff. The concentration of nutrients in wastewater can be optimized to promote the accumulation of biomass and polymers. Utilizing agricultural run-off and simultaneous feeding in three photobioreactors (PBRs) with a total capacity of 11.7 m3 is another method for growing cyanobacteria (Price et al., 2020). This study demonstrated PHA accumulation along with the wastewater's effective nutrient removal capability. Similar approaches can potentially lower production costs and provide an efficient treatment for these waters.

### 3.4.2 ROLE OF NUTRIENT LIMITATION

#### 3.4.2.1 NITROGEN AND PHOSPHATE REGULATION

NtcA and PII-signaling protein, two transcription factors, are necessary for cellular adaptation during nitrogen starvation. NtcA increases the expression of genes like sll0783, phaA, phaB, and phaC/E. An excessive NADPH pool, higher enzyme expression, and a mutation of sll0783 in *Synechocystis* sp. PCC 6803 changed the location of PHA synthase and reduced granulation, all contribute to PHA accumulation (Price et al., 2020). Cells produce PHA primarily from glycogen, which is cellular carbon that is stored when there is a lack of nitrogen. A glycogen synthase mutant of *Synechocystis* sp. PCC 6803 was also reported to produce less PHA. Thus, it is clear from this study that PHA accumulation under nitrogen stress and stored glycogen have a relationship (Ong et al., 2018). Lowered ATP during phosphate starvation increases PHA accumulation because of the high NADPH/ATP ratio (Mendhulkar et al., 2017). Additionally, the PHA operon is activated by phosphorus deprivation, which increases the expression of the genes responsible for PHA synthesis (Meixner et al., 2018). Upstream of phaB, an inducible promoter was discovered in a study using *Acinetobacter* species (a gene encoding for acetoacetyl-CoA reductase). This promoter was activated under phosphate deprivation, increasing the amount of acetoacetyl-CoA reductase and favoring PHA synthesis (Li and Strathmann, 2019).

#### 3.4.2.2 ACETATE AND CITRATE SUPPLEMENTATION

Acetate induces PHA production rather than providing cyanobacteria with a direct source of energy. Acetate is taken up by cells and converted to acetyl-CoA, which increases the acetyl-CoA pool. High levels of citrate synthase produce free CoA-SH, which inhibits the PHA pathway's β-ketothiolase (phaA) activity during typical cyanobacterial growth with sufficient nutrient availability (Grigore et al., 2019). The cell's high NADH concentration inhibits citrate synthase activity and restricts the entry of acetyl-CoA into the TCA cycle when nutrients are in short supply. As a result, acetyl-CoA levels rise, and β-ketothiolase then condenses it (Conca et al., 2020). The acetyl CoA flux towards PHA synthesis is determined by the ratios of [acetyl CoA]/[CoA] and [NADH]/[NAD] (Alcântara et al., 2020).

The addition of citrate to the medium has an impact on PHA accumulation. Citrate chelates $Mg^{2+}$ and lowers the activity of phosphofructokinase, which converts fructose-6-phosphate to fructose-1,6-bisphosphate through phosphorylation (Arias et al., 2018). The conversion of accumulated fructose-6-phosphate to its isomer glucose-6-phosphate by isomerase, which then enters the pentose phosphate pathway and favorably affects PHA accumulation, is known to produce excess NADPH, a known cofactor for acetoacetyl-CoA reductase. The addition of citrate prevents the TCA cycle, rerouting the acetyl-CoA pool to the PHA pathway and impeding citrate synthase (Cha et al., 2020).

## 3.5 CYANOBACTERIAL STRAIN IMPROVEMENT FOR PHA PRODUCTION

Photosynthetic prokaryotes can be genetically modified (GM) to produce PHA by altering the genes that make the three enzymes required for PHA synthesis: acetoacetyl-CoA reductase, β-ketothiolase, and PHA synthase. Many wild-type cyanobacterial strains, such as *Nostoc muscorum, Synechocystis* sp. PCC 6803, and *Aulosira fertilissima*, contain a variety of native PHA synthesis pathways, and genetic engineering can further encourage PHA overproduction in these organisms (Yajima et al., 2020). By incorporating specific genes or entire operons from other PHA-producing microorganisms, cyanobacteria can produce more PHA. PHA can boost a recombinant *Synechococcus* species' dry biomass by up to 25%. After transformation with PHA genes from *Ralstonia eutropha*, high levels of acetyl-CoA and PHA are produced along with the overexpression or deletion of a few other genes (Koller et al., 2017). The cellular carbon partitioning can be altered by the deletion of the enzyme ADP-glucose pyrophosphorylase encoding gene (agp gene) in *Synechocystis* sp. PCC 6803. This increases the production of PHA (18.6% PHA) (Troschl et al., 2018). As a result, altering photosynthetic microorganisms to use $CO_2$ as their carbon source opens up new opportunities for producing PHA at a low cost and on a large scale (Bhati and Mallick, 2015). Breaks of PHA depolymerase (phaZ) under nutrient-poor conditions, it uses intracellular PHA to break down PHA polymer to create 3-hydroxybutyrate. Therefore, gene silencing or depolymerase enzyme inhibition through genetic modification could enhance PHA storage within cyanobacteria. In a different investigation, after *Synechococcus* sp. MA19 was given the PHA synthase gene from *R. eutropha*, soluble PHA synthase and PHA granules devoid of any pigment were created (González-Resendiz et al., 2021).

### 3.5.1 GENETICALLY ENGINEERED CYANOBACTERIA FOR PHA PRODUCTION

Prokaryotic cyanobacteria are easier to manipulate because of their relatively simple genetic background. Most cyanobacterial studies on metabolic engineering and PHA biosynthesis have used a small number of model strains, with *Synechocystis* sp. PCC 6803 being the species that has been the subject of the most research. For both PHA production and other cyanobacterial research, PCC6803 is the most well-researched model of cyanobacterium. In addition, *Synechocystis* sp. PCC6803 holds the distinction of being the first photoautotrophic organism to have its entire genome sequenced in 1997 and the first recombinant cyanobacterium used for PHA production (Kamravamanesh et al., 2018a, b). PHA biosynthesis can be enhanced by introducing multiple copies of heterologous PHA synthase genes up to 11% of the dcw (Bhati and Mallick, 2015). After the erythromycin resistance cassette was inserted into the ADP-glucose pyrophosphorylase gene (*agp*), photoautotrophic PHA production under nitrogen depletion increased to 14.6%. This increased to 18.6% under mixotrophic cultivation with acetate (Shrivastav et al., 2010). The sll0783 gene significance in PHA production was revealed by the use of kanamycin/bleomycin resistance cassettes and cultivation under nitrogen depletion (Samantaray and Mallick, 2012). The native *SigE* gene was over-expressed into *Synechocystis* to control modifications in sugar catabolism linked to the glycogen pathway, resulting in 1.4% of dcw phototrophi-cally adapted cells (Osanai et al., 2013). Similar to this, *Synechocystis* overexpressed the PHA biosynthetic operon from *Microcystis aeruginosa* NIES-843 under nitrogen depletion, resulting in 7% of dcw photoauto-trophic PHA production (Bhati and Mallick, 2015). In contrast to the wild types, phaAB overexpression was used to achieve the highest PHA content of 26% of dry weight in a different study, and it increased to 35% under mixotrophic conditions with the addition of 0.4% acetate under nitrogen depletion (Monshupanee et al., 2016). While heterologously expressing the thioesterase gene (*tesB*) from *E. coli* and the *phaAB* gene from *Cupriavidus necator* H16 in a photoautotrophic environment using $CO_2$, Osanai et al. (2013) reported that phaEC-inactivated *Synechocystis* produced 3-hydroxybutyrate despite not being PHA. Under the influence of the light-inducible psbAII promoter, overexpression of the genes for PHA synthase from *Chromobacterium* sp. USM2 (*phaCCs*), acetoacetyl-CoA synthase from *Streptomyces* sp. CL190 (*nphT7Ss*), and *C. necator* acetoacetyl-CoA reductase (phaBCn) (Samantaray and Mallick, 2014). The production of 14% of dcw (232 mg/L) of acetyl-CoA was achieved recently by inducing deletions of the enzymes phosphotransacetylase (Pta) and acetyl-CoA hydrolase (Ach), as well as the expression of a heterologous phosphoketolase (XfpK) from the bacterium *Bifidobacterium breve* (Thinagaran and Sudesh, 2019). The acetyl CoA reductase binding site was optimized with $CO_2$ to produce 1.84 g/L PHA with a productivity of 263 mg/L/d (Yadav et al., 2020). Genetic engineering has also been applied to *Synechococcus* with success. *Synechococcus* sp. PCC7942, which has PHA synthesizing genes from *Alcaligenes eutrophus*, produced 3.01% of dcw PHA under photoautotrophic and nitrogen-starved conditions. When acetate was added, this amount increased to 25.6% of dcw. Recombinant cyanobacteria *Synechococcus* sp. PCC7002 recA null mutation with the *E. coli* recA gene in antibiotic-free cultivation produced 52% of the dcw PHA from carbon dioxide (Van Thuoc et al., 2019). *Synechococcus* PCC7942 with heterologous expression of the *C. necator* PHA operon showed improved PHA accumulation, ranging from 3 to 25% of dcw, and the addition of GABA shunt with $CO_2$ feed produced a PHA yield of 4.5% dcw, according to Ansari and Fatma (2016). In an intriguing study, PHA biosynthetic genes from *Chlorogloeopsis fritschii* PCC 9212 were inserted into copolymer P (3HB-co-4HB), which also contains 4-hydroxybutyrate (4HB) monomer, and the ccmR gene from *Synechococcus* sp. PCC 702 was deleted. This study provided a PHA content of 4.5% of dcw and showed the potential for P (3HBco-4HB) production in cyanobacteria using light and $CO_2$ (Tu et al., 2019a).

### 3.5.2 CRISPR/CAS BASED GENOME EDITING IN CYANOBACTERIA

Cyanobacteria is a promising platform for the synthesis of biofuels and biobased chemicals. However, the metabolic engineering of cyanobacteria poses many challenges (Kamravamanesh et al., 2018a, b). Gene replacement, marker-less point mutations, gene knockouts, and knock-ins are now more efficient methods for modifying the cyanobacterial genome (Behler et al., 2018). PHA and glycogen production have so far been down-regulated by the CRISPRi system to increase fluxes toward succinate and other carbon storage compounds of interest (Sangkharak et al., 2020). The overexpression of PHA biosynthetic genes using CRISPRi-based gene editing, however, has not been documented. While marker-free knockouts and knock-ins can be made using CRISPR-based editing, the developed cyanobacterial strains could be regarded as commercially viable and secure for outdoor cultivation and $CO_2$ sequestration in the future.

## 3.6 DOWNSTREAM PROCESSING FOR PHA RECOVERY

### *3.6.1 BIOMASS HARVESTING*

In order to extract useful products from cyanobacterial mass cultures, biomass harvesting involves concentrating the cultures into thick cakes. Filtration, coagulation/flocculation, sedimentation, and flotation are methods for obtaining cyanobacteria. Large-scale production necessitates cost-effective biomass recovery because cell harvesting accounts for 20–30% of the total cost of biomass production (Mannina et al., 2020).

#### *3.6.1.1 FILTRATION*

A membrane is used in the straightforward technique of filtering to separate pressure drop from biomass. Techniques for extracting cyanobacteria from broth have been used with both ultrafiltration and microfiltration (Singh et al., 2015). When compared to other dewatering techniques like centrifugation, the filtration process uses less energy (Figure 3.2). However, cake formation as filtration proceeds raises resistance and lowers flux, leading to high operational costs. Using tangential flow filtration, fragile cyanobacterial cells were successfully removed without clogging the membrane (Kumar et al., 2019). In order to recover cyanobacteria, hollow fiber and tubular membranes were also employed (Wang et al., 2018). With an estimated energy requirement of 0.3–0.7 kW h $m^{-3}$, this polymeric membrane was able to produce 150 g $L^{-1}$ (dry wt.) of *Nannochloropsis* sp. biomass and a 99% volume reduction (Khatami et al., 2021). *Elliptio complanata,* a freshwater mussel, was used to filter the water at different flow rates, assisting in the removal of the water's numerous cyanobacterial (Microcystis) species (Roja et al.2019).

#### *3.6.1.2 COAGULATION/FLOCCULATION*

Coagulation or flocculation is a harvesting technique that balances charges on the surface of cells using chitosan-like polymers and cationic salts like $AlCl_3$, $Fe_2(SO_4)_3$, or $Al_2(SO_4)_3$ (Yadav et al., 2020). Although it can be harvested, the chemicals alter the cell's biochemical make-up and raise the risk of contamination. By genetically altering cyanobacterial strains, chemicals were avoided. By using magnetic beads coated with protein A, 70% of the biomass was recovered from the *Synechococcus elongatus* PCC 7942 outer envelope with reduced S-protein expression and increased flag tag in surface porın SomA (Fedeson et al., 2017). *Microcystis aeruginosa* 1343 (M1) and 905 (M9) were subjected to magnetic nanoparticle settling using iron oxide nanoparticles coated with polyethyleneimine. This method recovered 93.3% and 97.5% of the biomass, respectively, by neutralizing surface charges and removing extracellular organic matter (Yajima et al., 2020). For cell recovery, bioflocculation is an alternative to chemical flocculants. In contrast, MNXY1, a quinovose-containing bioflocculant from *Klebsiella pneumoniae* strain NY1, flocculated *Synechocystis* UTEX 2470 to 50% of its initial amount. After 1 hour, 95% of the biomass was recovered (Van Thuoc et al., 2019). Effective bioflocculation of *Synechococcus subsalsus* and *Spirulina maxima* with *Aspergillus niger* pellets (1:5 cyanobacterial-to-fungal ratio) achieved a biomass concentration factor of 62.8 and a biomass recovery efficiency of 94% (González-Resendiz et al., 2021). A study on air bubbling and shaking-grown biofilm found that while the decline phase produced a poor recovery, the log phase of growth produced a biomass recovery of 70%. The highest initial biomass concentration (IBC) bubbled system recovered more quickly, demonstrating that the growth phase, type of mixing system, and IBC all influence bioflocculation (Conca et al., 2020).

#### *3.6.1.3 AUTO SEDIMENTATION*

Autosedimentation is the term for the instantaneous settling of cyanobacterial cells caused by cell clumping and cluster formation. *Desmodesmus* sp. F2 and *Chlorella minutissima*, two lipid-rich cyanobacteria, demonstrated this phenomenon and facilitated rapid recovery after cultivation (Singh et al., 2019). This property was demonstrated by the cyanobacterium *Chlorogloea fritschii* TISTR 8527, which recovered 91% of its biomass in one minute (Roh et al., 2021). The settling rate can be changed by modifying the morphology of cyanobacterial cells. FtsZ is a cytoskeletal protein that aids in cell growth, division, and sedimentation. It resembles tubulin. Overexpression of minC and cdv3 in *Synechococcus elongatus* PCC 7942 caused FtsZ dislocation and up to a few millimeters of elongation, which caused natural cell settling (Taepucharoen et al., 2017). Overexpression of bolA, a transcription factor of the actin-like protein MreB, causes elongation up to five folds in the filamentous cyanobacterium *Fremyella diplosiphon* without impairing cell function, and it improves sedimentation (Roh et al., 2021). Therefore, input reuse enables media separation and streamlines the subsequent procedure.

### *3.6.1.4 FLOTATION*

A high flocculation rate is a result of the filamentous structure and mucilage secretion of the heterocystous cyanobacterium *Anabaena* sp. PCC 7120. The autoflotation of cells produced 0.72–1.10 mol $H_2$ per mg of dcw, resulting in the formation of floc, which allowed 91.71% of the biomass to be recovered (Papadopoulos et al., 2021). When cyanobacterial cells were floated in the air at 0.3 mass flow rate with biodegradable methylated ovalbumin (MeOA), 85% of the cells were recovered (Price et al., 2020). Magnesium is a crucial nutrient for the healthy development of cyanobacteria. Around 84% of the biomass was recovered when *M. aeruginosa* was harvested using magnesium chloride as a coagulant at a high pH (> 10) (Hondo et al., 2015). Microbial biomass harvesting is difficult due to the method's reliance on a number of variables, including cell morphology, surface charge and density, culture pH, PBR design, and the desired product. Centrifugation and filtration can harvest delicate microbial cells with intact structures, but the operational cost is increased by filter clogging and high energy requirements for large culture volumes (Figure 3.2). Both flotation and sedimentation are density-based separation techniques, with the latter requiring the addition of surfactant and continuous bubbling at high densities while the former failing at low culture densities. Due to the variety in biomass types and culture conditions, the benefits and drawbacks of recovery techniques indicate that no single strategy can guarantee successful harvesting in all circumstances. When compared to individual recovery methods, the addition of flocculants/coagulants before gravity sedimentation and centrifugation can increase the settling of small-sized cells while also lowering the amount of energy required (Zheng et al., 2020). To recover cyanobacterial biomass with the least amount of energy use and expense, combined harvesting techniques are therefore required. The easiest method for quick cell separation and media re-use is auto-sedimentation because no chemical agents are needed during the procedure. However, cyanobacterial strains only occasionally exhibit this phenomenon. A suitable strain or a multi-factorial process optimization that supports auto-sedimentation is required for industrial-scale cell recovery to achieve cost-effective recovery.

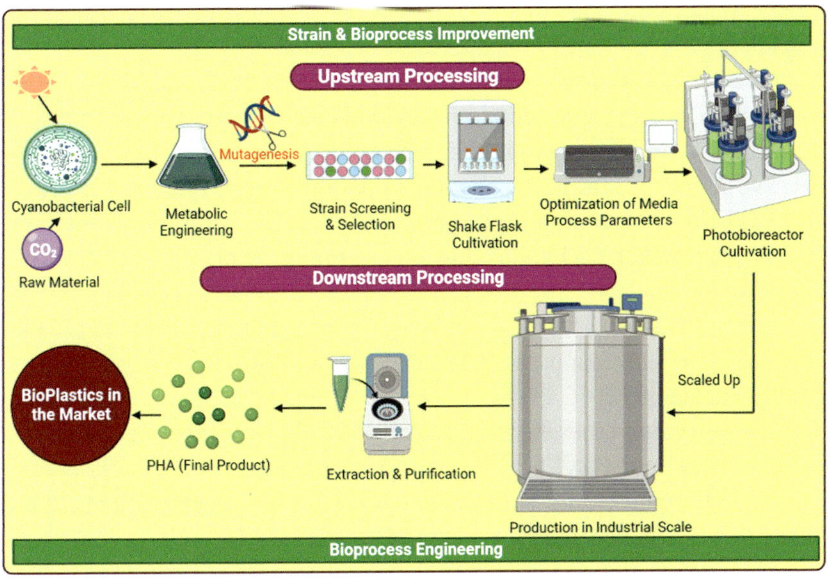


**FIGURE 3.2** Diagrammatic representation of the cyanobacterial PHA production process. The selection and improvement of strains, extensive cultivation in closed and open systems, and biomass harvesting to the final product are steps needed in the industrial-scale production of PHA.

### *3.6.2 PHA RECOVERY*

PHA is kept in the form of intracellular granules, which are visible with a clear and simple stain. Cell walls and cell membranes must be harmed using a variety of methods to extract PHA. Compared to other gram-negative bacteria (6 nm), the cyanobacterial cell wall is more rigid and has a thicker peptidoglycan layer (10 nm) (Bhati and Mallick, 2016). PHA has been extracted from cyanobacterial cells using several different solvent techniques. Intracellular PHA from cyanobacterial biomass can be extracted in a single step using halogenated solvents like hypochlorite, chloroform, and dichloromethane (Cassuriaga et al., 2020). PHA can be purified and extracted from bacterial and cyanobacterial biomass using high sodium hypochlorite solution concentrations (10–13%, v/v), but it requires multiple washings of the pellets and results in low molecular weight polymers (Troschl et al., 2017). Chloroform was used as an extraction solvent to produce high molecular weight PHA (1,700,000 kDa) from the same bacterial biomass without the need for washing (Wagner et al., 2016). When extracted, many cyanobacterial pigments have a negative impact on the properties of PHA. As a result, pigment removal from cyanobacteria is crucial before PHA recovery with the fewest solvents and steps. The food, cosmetics, and pharmaceutical industries may benefit from these cyanobacterial pigments. Soxhlet apparatus: Before extracting PHA with chloroform in the Soxhlet apparatus, pigment can be removed at 4°C using methanol (Carpine et al., 2015). This process yields high-quality PHA, but it is a lengthy and energy-intensive process. Solvents like dichloromethane and chloroform cannot be used on an industrial scale due to their high cost and toxicity. An environmentally friendly solvent called 1,2-propylene carbonate can extract 95% pure PHA from *R. eutropha* at a temperature of 130°C (Wang et al., 2018). PHA recovery has also been investigated using other environmentally friendly solvents like acetic acid, butyl acetate, and ethyl acetate. *Burkholderia cepacia* B27 was used to extract PHA with acetic acid, which resulted in a higher solubility and purity but a lower recovery of only 36%. Because it removes impurities, solvent precipitation using chilled methanol performs better than solvent casting (Singh et al., 2019). The recovery of PHA from cyanobacteria using ionic liquid (IL) as a green solvent. PHA cannot be dissolved in the IL 1-ethyl-3-methylimidazolium methyl phosphonate ([$C_2$mim] [MeO(H)$PO_2$]), but cyanobacterial cell biomass can dissolve in it (Martins et al., 2017). Using this IL, 98% of the PHA recovered from cyanobacteria could be reused. Through the use of methods like alcalase enzyme digestion, SDS, and EDTA surfactant digestion, PHA was extracted without the use of solvents (Taepucharoen et al., 2017). Without crystal formation, the purity of PHA recovered with these methods was greater than 90%. The ball mill and high-pressure homogenizer also demonstrated significant potential for cell disruption for PHA recovery, even though this is an energy-intensive process (Phalanisong and Plangklang, 2021). Extracellular PHA secretion can significantly reduce recovery costs because it can be extracted without the need for cell lysis. The signal peptide HlyA was fused with phasin protein-coated PHA granules to cause genetically altered E to secrete PHA through type I secretion (Cassuriaga et al., 2020). Similar engineering techniques can be used to engineer cyanobacteria to secrete PHA, which reduces the cost of recovery. As a result, it is still challenging to economically recover high purity PHA from harvested biomass while maintaining the quality of the extracted polymer and selecting an environmentally friendly solvent with processes involved.

## 3.7 CHALLENGES ASSOCIATED WITH INDUSTRIAL-SCALE CYANOBACTERIAL PHA PRODUCTION

Cyanobacteria are known to produce respectable amounts of PHA when grown on a lab scale. *A. fertilissima*, a filamentous cyanobacterium, demonstrated that the mutant strain MT a24 of *Synechocystis* sp. PCC 6714 produced 1.16 g of L1 PHA when grown in optimized media (Troschl et al., 2018). Research on mass production has been relatively understudied, although process parameter optimization has received a lot of attention. Many challenges make it difficult to scale up photosynthetic cultures (González-Resendiz et al., 2021). Standardizing factors like light, temperature, mixing, nutrient supply, culture contamination, the development of an algal film that makes the PBR wall opaque, and oxygen buildup are necessary for scale-up. In contrast to open raceway ponds where vertical mixing of the culture is constrained, small reactors enable uniform lighting and nutrient delivery, which reduces cell settling and boosts production. The laminar flow of culture limits light to the cells in the center of tubular PBRs, which affects cell growth. Because productivity may be hindered by shading brought on by high biomass, maintaining optimal growth is essential (Martins et al., 2017). Small-scale jacketed reactors can keep the culture temperature stable, but open ponds and closed PBRs find it difficult or impossible to do so. Because the temperature variations in the outdoor studies reduced productivity, the selection of a robust strain can help to some extent (González-Resendiz et al., 2021). Growth is inhibited by changing the $CO_2$ to $O_2$ ratio, which is brought about by increased RuBisCO oxygenase activity and decreased carbon fixation as a result of oxygen buildup in the tubular PBR. In large-scale production, the cost of the nutrients is crucial, but some strains use inexpensive sources, like urea. Although nitrate needs ATP to be converted to ammonia, adding ammonia directly to the culture can also be toxic because it raises the culture's pH (Kamravamanesh et al., 2018). Better substitutes include varieties of cyanobacteria that can fix atmospheric nitrogen. In a 200 L tubular PBR, *Synechocystis* sp. CCALA192 was grown, producing 0.125 g L1 PHB (Wang et al., 2020). In a 40-liter reactor, the mutant cyanobacterial strain MT a24 of *Synechocystis* sp. PCC 6714 produced 0.356 g L1 of PHA (Yajima et al., 2020). This cyanobacterium produces less PHA in a large reactor system than it does in a lab-scale culture. According to these studies, small-scale production and growth optimizations might need to be redone for industrial-scale production. Along with having the right information to deal with culture contamination and predators, cyanobacteria must be adapted to extensive outdoor studies.

## 3.8 CONCLUSION

Over the next two decades, it is anticipated that there will be a shift toward more recycling of conventional plastics and plastics made from fossil fuels to facilitate the collection, processing, and reuse. Since they are the only microbes capable of producing PHA through photosynthesis, which relies primarily on light and $CO_2$ for energy and requires little in the way of nutrients for growth, cyanobacteria are regarded as a promising source of PHA. Because these cyanobacteria consume $CO_2$, the greenhouse effect brought on by the release of this gas by industry is decreased, benefiting the environment. As a result, PHA made by cyanobacteria decreases carbon dioxide emissions, which has a significant positive impact on the environment in addition to decreasing the use of fossil fuels. The investigation into cyanobacterial stimulation of PHA synthesis is still in its infancy, and the PHA generated is not suitable for commercial use. Regardless, it is evident that cyanobacteria can produce biopolymers at a lower cost while also having a significant impact on the environment. The ability of cyanobacteria to photosynthesize, which functions as a solar cell and lowers $CO_2$ levels in the environment as well as providing the raw materials for the production of cyanobacterial bioplastic, gives them a significant advantage over other microorganisms that produce PHA. Currently, improved strains and recovery techniques are the main areas of focus for international research projects looking at specific cyanobacterial PHA production processes. Although there are many obstacles to increasing cyanobacterial PHA productivity as well as PHA extraction and purification effectiveness, doing so would waste a lot of time and effort and produce sub-optimal results overall. When scaling up and commercializing the production of cyanobacterial PHA, the entire process must be taken into account. It may be possible to achieve an economically viable PHA production point by placing more emphasis on sustainable and viable upstream processing. Apart from emphasizing the optimized media and cultivation conditions on PHA productivity, there is also a need to develop commercial processes that are viable and sustainable and can be applied in non-sterile settings using waste streams and open systems. The focus of the research should be to create strains that are more resistant to alterations in the cultivation environment, including pH, temperature, salinity, and media composition, similar to mixed cultures derived from wastewater. Besides, the time-spaced yield of the resilient strains will be improved, whose PHA production is linked to biomass growth.

## KEYWORDS

- **nanoagrochemicals**
- **nanofertilizers**
- **nanohormones**
- **nanoparticles**
- **nanopesticides**
- **nano-scale**
- **nanotechnology**
- **plasmodesmata**

## REFERENCES


Aikawa, S., Nishida, A., Ho, S. H., Chang, J. S., Hasunuma, T., & Kondo, A. (2014). Glycogen production for biofuels by the euryhaline cyanobacteria *Synechococcus* sp. strain PCC 7002 from an oceanic environment. *Biotechnology for Biofuels, 7*(1), 88. https://doi.org/10.1186/1754-6834-7-88 (accessed on 5th November 2025).

Alcântara, M. G., Distante, F., Storti, G., Moscatelli, D., Morbidelli, M., & Sponchioni, M. (2020). Current trends in the production of biodegradable bioplastics: The case of polyhydroxyalkanoates. *Biotechnology Advances, 42*, 107582.

Amelia, T. S. M., Govindasam, S., Tamothran, A. M., Vigneswari, S., & Bhubalan, K. (2019). Applications of PHA in agriculture. In Kalia, V. C. (Ed.), *Biotechnological Applications of Polyhydroxyalkanoates* (pp. 347–361). Springer, Singapore.

Ansari, S., & Fatima, T. (2016). Cyanobacterial polyhydroxybutyrate (PHB): Screening, optimization and characterization. *PLoS One, 11*(6), e0158168. https://doi.org/10.1371/journal.pone.0158168 (accessed on 5th November 2025).

Ansari, S., & Fatima, T. (2019). Cyanobacterial polyhydroxybutyrate (PHB): Screening, optimization and characterization. *PLoS One, 11*, e0158168. https://doi.org/10.1371/journal.pone.0158168 (accessed on 5th November 2025).

Arias, D. M., Uggetti, E., García-Galán, M. J., & García, J. (2018). Production of polyhydroxybutyrate's and carbohydrates in a mixed cyanobacterial culture: Effect of nutrients limitation and photoperiods. *New Biotechnology, 42*, 1–11.

Balaji, S., Gopi, K., & Muthuvelan, B. (2013). A review on production of poly β hydroxybutyrates from cyanobacteria for the production of bio plastics. *Algal Research, 2*, 278–285.

Behler, J., Vijay, D., Hess, W. R., & Akhtar, M. K. (2018). CRISPR-based technologies for metabolic engineering in cyanobacteria. *Trends in Biotechnology, 36*, 996–1010.

Bhati, R., & Mallick, N. (2015). Poly (3-hydroxybutyrate-co-3-hydroxyvalerate) copolymer production by the diazotrophic cyanobacterium *Nostoc muscorum* Agardh: Process optimization and polymer characterization. *Algal Research, 7*, 78–85. https://doi.org/10.1016/j.algal.2014.12.003 (accessed on 5th November 2025).

Bhati, R., & Mallick, N. (2016). Carbon dioxide and poultry waste utilization for production of polyhydroxyalkanoate biopolymers by *Nostoc muscorum* Agardh: A sustainable approach. *Journal of Applied Phycology, 28*, 161–168.

Bhati, R., Samantaray, S., Sharma, L., & Mallick, N. (2010). Poly-β-hydroxybutyrate accumulation in cyanobacteria under photoautotroph. *Biotechnology Journal, 5*, 1181–1185.

Carpine, R., Olivieri, G., Hellingwerf, K., Pollio, A., & Marzocchella, A. (2015). The cyanobacterial route to produce poly-β-hydroxybutyrate. *Chemical Engineering Transactions, 43*, 289–294.

Cassuriaga, A. P. A., Moraes, L., Morais, M. G., & Costa, J. A. V. (2020). Polyhydroxybutyrate production and increased macromolecule content in *Chlamydomonas reinhardtii* cultivated with xylose and reduced nitrogen levels. *International Journal of Biological Macromolecules, 158*. https://doi.org/10.1016/j.ijbiomac.2020.04.273 (accessed on 5th November 2025).

Cha, D., Ha, H. S., & Lee, S. K. (2020). Metabolic engineering of *Pseudomonas putida* for the production of various types of short-chain-length polyhydroxyalkanoates from levulinic acid. *Bioresource Technology, 309*, 123332.

Choi, S. Y., Oh, J., Jung, J., Park, Y., & Lee, S. Y. (2021). Three-dimensional label-free visualization and quantification of polyhydroxyalkanoates in individual bacterial cell in its native state. *Proceedings of the National Academy of Sciences, 118*(31), e2103956118.

Conca, V., da Ros, C., Valentino, F., Eusebi, A. L., Frison, N., & Fatone, F. (2020). Long-term validation of polyhydroxyalkanoates production potential from the side stream of customizing polyhydroxyalkanoates. *Indian Journal of Microbiology, 55*, 235–249.

Drosg, B., Fritz, I., Gattermayr, F., & Silvestrini, L. (2015). Photo-autotrophic production of poly (hydroxyalkanoates) in cyanobacteria. *Chemical and Biochemical Engineering Quarterly, 29*, 145–156. https://doi.org/10.15255/cabeq.2014.2254 (accessed on 5th November 2025).

Fedeson, D. T., & Ducat, D. C. (2017). Cyanobacterial surface display system mediates engineered interspecies and abiotic binding. *ACS Synthetic Biology, 6*(2), 367–374.

González-Resendiz, L., Sánchez-García, L., Hernández-Martínez, I., et al. (2021). Photoautotrophic poly(3-hydroxybutyrate) production by a wild-type *Synechococcus elongatus* isolated from an extreme environment. *Bioresource Technology, 337*(6), 125508. https://doi.org/10.1016/j.biortech.2021.125508 (accessed on 5th November 2025).

Grigore, M. E., Grigorescu, R. M., Iancu, L., Ion, R. M., Zaharia, C., & Andrei, E. R. (2019). Methods of synthesis, properties and biomedical applications of polyhydroxyalkanoates: A review. *Journal of Biomaterials Science, 30*, 695–712.

Gupta, A., Kumar, M., & Thakur, I. S. (2017). Analysis and optimization of process parameters for production of polyhydroxyalkanoates along with wastewater treatment by *Serratia* sp. ISTVKR1. *Bioresource Technology, 242*, 55–59.

Hauf, W., Watzer, B., Roos, N., Klotz, A., & Forchhammer, K. (2015). Photoautotrophic polyhydroxybutyrate granule formation is regulated by cyanobacterial phasin PhaP in *Synechocystis* sp. strain PCC 6803. *Applied and Environmental Microbiology, 81*(13), 4411. https://doi.org/10.1128/AEM.00604-15 (accessed on 5th November 2025).

Hendry, J. I., Bandyopadhyay, A., Srinivasan, S., Pakrasi, H. B., & Maranas, C. D. (2020). Metabolic model guided strain design of cyanobacteria. *Current Opinion in Biotechnology, 64*, 17–23. https://doi.org/10.1016/j.copbio.2019.08.011 (accessed on 5th November 2025).

Hondo, S., Takahashi, M., Osanai, T., Matsuda, M., Hasunuma, T., Tazuke, A., et al. (2015). Genetic engineering and metabolite profiling for overproduction of polyhydroxybutyrate in cyanobacteria. *Journal of Bioscience and Bioengineering, 120*, 510–517. https://doi.org/10.1016/j.jbiosc.2015.03.004 (accessed on 5th November 2025).

Iasimone, F., Seira, J., Desmond-Le Quéméner, A., Panico, E., De Felice, V., Pirozzi, F., & Steyer, J. P. (2020). Bio flocculation and settling studies of native wastewater filamentous cyanobacteria using different cultivation systems for a low-cost and easy to control harvesting process. *Journal of Environmental Management, 256*, 109957.

Jordan, A., Chandler, J., MacCready, J. S., Huang, J., Osteryoung, K. W., & Ducat, D. C. (2017). Engineering cyanobacterial cell morphology for enhanced recovery and processing of biomass. *Applied and Environmental Microbiology, 83*(9), e00053-17.

Kaewbai-ngam, A., Incharoensakdi, A., & Monshupanee, T. (2016). Increased accumulation of polyhydroxybutyrate in divergent cyanobacteria under nutrient-deprived photoautotroph: An efficient conversion of solar energy and carbon dioxide to polyhydroxybutyrate by *Calothrix scytonemicola* TISTR 8095. *Bioresource Technology, 212*. https://doi.org/10.1016/j.biortech.2016.04.035 (accessed on 5th November 2025).

Kamravamanesh, D., Kovacs, T., Pflugl, S., Druzhinina, I., Kroll, P., Lackner, M., & Herwig, C. (2018). Increased poly-β-hydroxybutyrate production from carbon dioxide in randomly mutated cells of cyanobacterial strain *Synechocystis* sp. PCC 6714: Mutant generation and characterization. *Bioresource Technology, 266*, 34–44. https://doi.org/10.1016/j.biortech.2018.06.057 (accessed on 5th November 2025).

Kamravamanesh, D., Lackner, M., & Herwig, C. (2018b). Bioprocess engineering aspects of sustainable polyhydroxyalkanoate production in cyanobacteria. *Bioengineering, 5*, 111. https://doi.org/10.3390/bioengineering5040111 (accessed on 5th November 2025).

Kamravamanesh, D., Slouka, C., Limbeck, A., Lackner, M., & Herwig, C. (2019). Increased carbohydrate production from carbon dioxide in randomly mutated cells of cyanobacterial strain *Synechocystis* sp. PCC 6714: Bioprocess understanding and evaluation of productivities. *Bioresource Technology, 273*, 277–287.

Khatami, K., Perez-Zabaleta, M., Owusu-Agyeman, I., & Cetecioglu, Z. (2021). Waste to bioplastics: How close are we to sustainable polyhydroxyalkanoates production? *Waste Management, 119*, 374–388.

Koch, M., Doello, S., Gutekunst, K., & Forchhammer, K. (2019). PHB is produced from glycogen turnover during nitrogen starvation in *Synechocystis* sp. PCC 6803. *International Journal of Molecular Sciences, 20*(8), 1942.

Koller, M. (2015). Cyanobacterial polyhydroxyalkanoate production: Status quo and quo Vadis? *Current Biotechnology, 4*(999), 1–1. https://doi.org/10.2174/2211550104666150917010849 (accessed on 5th November 2025).

Koller, M., Khosravi-Darani, K., & Braunegg, G. (2017). Advanced photobioreactor systems for the efficient cultivation of cyanobacteria. In Tsang, Y. F. (Ed.), *Photobioreactors: Advancements, Applications and Research* (pp. 35–90). Nova Science Publishers: New York, NY, USA.

Kourmentza, C., Plácido, J., Venetsaneas, N., Burniol-Figols, A., Varrone, C., Gavala, H. N., & Reis, M. A. M. (2017). Recent advances and challenges towards sustainable polyhydroxyalkanoate (PHA) production. *Bioengineering, 4*, 55.

Kumar, P., & Kim, B. S. (2018). Valorization of polyhydroxyalkanoates production process by C. Zhang, et al. co-synthesis of value-added products. *Bioresource Technology, 269*, 544–556. https://doi.org/10.1016/j.biortech.2018.08.120 (accessed on 5th November 2025).

Lam, W., Wang, Y., Chan, P. L., Chan, S. W., Tsang, Y. F., Chua, H., & Yu, P. H. F. (2017). Production of polyhydroxyalkanoates (PHA) using sludge from different wastewater treatment processes and the potential for medical and pharmaceutical applications. *Environmental Technology, 38*, 1779–1791.

Lan, E. I., & Wei, C. T. (2016). Metabolic engineering of cyanobacteria for the photosynthetic production of succinate. *Metabolic Engineering, 38*, 483–493. https://doi.org/10.1016/j.ymben.2016.10.014 (accessed on 5th November 2025).

Li, Y., & Strathmann, T. J. (2019). Kinetics and mechanism for hydrothermal conversion of polyhydroxybutyrate (PHB) for wastewater valorization. *Green Chemistry, 21*(20), 5586–5597.

Mannina, G., Presti, D., Montiel-Jarillo, G., & Suárez-Ojeda, M. E. (2020). Recovery of polyhydroxyalkanoates (PHAs) from wastewater: A review. *Bioresource Technology, 297*, 122478.

Martins, R. G., Gonçalves, I. S., Morais, M. G. D., & Costa, J. A. V. (2017). New technologies from the bioworld: Selection of biopolymer-producing microalgae. *Polímeros, 27*, 285–289. https://doi.org/10.1590/0104-1428.2375 (accessed on 5th November 2025).

Meixner, K., Kovalcik, A., Sykacek, E., Gruber-Brunhumer, M., Zeilinger, W., Markl, K., Haas, C., Fritz, I., Mundigler, N., Stelzer, F., et al. (2018). Cyanobacteria biorefinery production of poly(3-hydroxybutyrate) with *Synechocystis salina* and utilization of residual biomass. *Journal of Biotechnology, 265*, 46–53.

Mendhulkar, V. D., & Laukik, A. S. (2017). Synthesis of biodegradable polymer polyhydroxyalkanoate (PHA) in cyanobacteria *Synechococcus elongatus* under mixotrophic nitrogen- and phosphate-mediated stress conditions. *Industrial Biotechnology, 13*, 85–93.

Monshupanee, T., Chairattanawat, C., & Incharoensakdi, A. (2019). Disruption of cyanobacterial γ-aminobutyric acid shunt pathway reduces metabolite levels in tricarboxylic acid cycle, but enhances pyruvate and poly(3-hydroxybutyrate) accumulation. *Scientific Reports, 9*(1). https://doi.org/10.1038/s41598-019-44729-8 (accessed on 5th November 2025).

Monshupanee, T., Nimdach, P., & Incharoensakdi, A. (2016). Two-stage (photoautotroph and heterotrophy) cultivation enables efficient production of bioplastic poly-3-hydroxybutyrate in auto-sedimenting cyanobacterium. *Scientific Reports, 6*(1), 37121. https://doi.org/10.1038/srep37121 (accessed on 5th November 2025).

Oliveira, H. R., Bassin, I. D., & Cammarota, M. C. (2019). Bio flocculation of cyanobacteria with pellets of *Aspergillus niger*: Effects of carbon supplementation, pellet diameter, and other factors in biomass densification. *Bioresource Technology, 294*, 122167.

Ong, S. Y., Kho, H. P., Riedel, S. L., Kim, S. W., Gan, C. Y., Taylor, T. D., & Sudesh, K. (2018). An integrative study on biologically recovered polyhydroxyalkanoates (PHAs) and simultaneous assessment of gut microbiome in yellow mealworm. *Journal of Biotechnology, 265*, 31–39.

Osanai, T., Numata, K., Oikawa, A., Kuwahara, A., Iijima, H., Doi, Y., et al. (2013). Increased bioplastic production with an RNA polymerase sigma factor SigE during nitrogen starvation in *Synechocystis* sp. PCC 6803. *DNA Research, 20*, 525–535. https://doi.org/10.1093/dnares/dst028 (accessed on 5th November 2025).

Panith, N., Assavanig, A., Lertsiri, S., Bergkvist, M., Surarit, R., & Niamsiri, N. (2016). Development of tunable biodegradable polyhydroxyalkanoates microspheres for controlled delivery of tetracycline for treating periodontal disease. *Journal of Applied Polymer Science, 133*, 44128–44141.

Papadopoulos, K. P., Economou, C. N., Tekerlekopoulou, A. G., & Vayenas, D. V. (2021). A cyanobacteria-based biofilm system for advanced brewery wastewater treatment. *Applied Sciences, 11*(1), 174.

Park, S. H., Alammar, A., Fulop, Z., Pulido, B. A., Nunes, S. P., & Szekely, G. (2021). Hydrophobic thin film composite nanofiltration membranes derived solely from sustainable sources. *Green Chemistry, 23*(3).

Phalanisong, P., & Plangklang, P. R. A. (2021). Photoautotrophic and mixotrophic cultivation of polyhydroxyalkanoate-accumulating microalgae consortia selected under nitrogen and phosphate limitation. *Molecules, 26*, 7613. https://doi.org/10.3390/molecules26247613 (accessed on 5th November 2025).

Price, S., Kuzhiumparambil, U., Pernice, M., & Ralph, P. J. (2020). Cyanobacterial polyhydroxybutyrate for sustainable bioplastic production: Critical review and Lamperspectives. *Journal of Environmental Chemical Engineering, 8*, 104007.

Ray, S., & Kalia, V. C. (2017). Co-metabolism of substrates by *Bacillus thuringiensis* regulates polyhydroxyalkanoate co-polymer composition. *Bioresource Technology, 224*, 743–747.

Roh, H., Lee, J. S., Il, C. H., Kim, J., Lee, J., & Park, S. (2021). Improved $CO_2$-derived polyhydroxybutyrate (PHB) production by engineering fast-growing cyanobacterium *Synechococcus elongatus* UTEX 2973 for potential utilization of flue gas. *Bioresource Technology, 327*(3), 124789. https://doi.org/10.1016/j.biortech.2021.124789 (accessed on 5th November 2025).

Roja, K., Ruben Sudhakar, D., Anto, S., & Mathimani, T. (2019). Extraction and characterization of polyhydroxyalkanoates from marine green alga and cyanobacteria. *Biocatalysis and Agricultural Biotechnology, 22*, 101358.

Rueda, E., García-Galán, M., Ortiz, A., Uggetti, E., Carretero, J., García, J., & Díez-Montero, R. (2020). Bioremediation of agricultural runoff and biopolymers production from cyanobacteria cultured in demonstrative full-scale photobioreactor. *Process Safety and Environmental Protection, 139*, 241–250.

Samantaray, S., & Mallick, N. (2012). Production and characterization of poly-β-hydroxybutyrate (PHB) polymer from *Aulosira fertilissima. Journal of Applied Phycology, 24*, 803–814. https://doi.org/10.1007/s10811-011-9699-7 (accessed on 5th November 2025).

Samantaray, S., & Mallick, N. (2014). Production of poly(3-hydroxybutyrate-co-3-hydroxyvalerate) co-polymer by the diazotrophic cyanobacterium *Aulosira fertilissima* CCC 444. *Journal of Applied Phycology, 26*, 237–245. https://doi.org/10.1007/s10811-013-0073-9 (accessed on 5th November 2025).

Samantaray, S., Nayak, J. K., & Mallick, N. (2011). Wastewater utilization for poly-β-hydroxybutyrate production by the cyanobacterium *Aulosira fertilissima* in a recirculatory aquaculture system. *Applied and Environmental Microbiology, 77*, 8735–8743. https://doi.org/10.1128/aem.05275-11 (accessed on 5th November 2025).

Sangkharak, K., Paichid, N., Yunu, T., & Prasertsan, P. (2020). Enhancing the degradation of mixed polycyclic aromatic hydrocarbon and medium-chain-length polyhydroxyalkanoate production by mixed bacterial cultures using modified repeated batch fermentation. *Journal of Applied Microbiology, 129*, 554–564.

Sawant, S., Kiet, T., Bipinchandra, T., Salunke, K., & Kim, B. S. (2017). Potential of *Saccharophagus degradans* for production of polyhydroxyalkanoates using cellulose. *Process Biochemistry, 57*, 50–56.

Shrivastav, A., Mishra, S. K., & Mishra, S. (2010). Polyhydroxyalkanoate (PHA) synthesis by *Spirulina subsalsa* from Gujarat coast of India. *International Journal of Biological*

*Macromolecules, 46*(2), 255–260. https://doi.org/10.1016/j.ijbiomac.2010.01.001 (accessed on 5th November 2025).

Singh, A. K., & Mallick, N. (2017). Advances in cyanobacterial polyhydroxyalkanoates production. *FEMS Microbiology Letters, 364*(20). https://doi.org/10.1093/femsle/fnx189 (accessed on 5th November 2025).

Singh, M. K., Rai, P. K., Rai, A., Singh, V. K., Srivastava, A., & Mishra, S. (2019). Poly-β-hydroxybutyrate production by the cyanobacterium *Scytonema geitleri* Bharadwaja under varying environmental conditions. *Biomolecules, 9*(5), 198. https://doi.org/10.3390/biom9050198 (accessed on 5th November 2025).

Singh, M., Kumar, P., Ray, S., & Kalia, V. C. (2015). Challenges and Opportunities for Customizing Polyhydroxyalkanoates. *Indian J Microbiol. 55*(3), 235–249. doi: 10.1007/s12088-015-0528-6.

Sruamsiri, D., Thayanukul, P., & Suwannasilp, B. B. (2020). *In situ* identification of polyhydroxyalkanoate (PHA)-accumulating microorganisms in mixed microbial cultures under feast/famine conditions. *Scientific Reports, 10*, 3752. https://doi.org/10.1038/s41598-020-60609-4 (accessed on 5th November 2025).

Surendran, A., Lakshmanan, M., Chee, J. Y., Sulaiman, A. M., Thuoc, D. V., & Sudesh, K. (2020). Can polyhydroxyalkanoates be produced efficiently from waste plant and animal oils? *Frontiers in Bioengineering and Biotechnology, 8*, 169. https://doi.org/10.3389/fbioe.2020.00169 (accessed on 5th November 2025).

Taepucharoen, K., Tarawat, S., Puangcharoen, M., Kanjanamaneesathian, M., & Kittikun, A. H. (2017). Production of poly(3-hydroxybutyrate-co-3-hydroxyvalerate) under photoautotrophy and heterotrophy by non-heterocystous $N_2$-fixing cyanobacterium. *Bioresource Technology, 239*. https://doi.org/10.1016/j.biortech.2017.05.029 (accessed on 5th November 2025).

Tarawat, S., Incharoensakdi, A., & Monshupanee, T. (2020). Cyanobacterial production of poly(3-hydroxybutyrate-co-3-hydroxyvalerate) from carbon dioxide or a single organic substrate: Improved polymer elongation with an extremely high 3-hydroxyvalerate mole proportion. *Journal of Applied Phycology, 32*, 1095–1102.

Thinagaran, L., & Sudesh, K. (2019). Evaluation of sludge palm oil as feedstock and development of efficient method for its utilization to produce polyhydroxyalkanoate. *Waste and Biomass Valorization, 10*, 709–720.

Troschl, C., Meixner, K., & Drosg, B. (2017). Cyanobacterial PHA production—Review of recent advances and a summary of three years' working experience running a pilot plant. *Bioengineering, 4*, 26. https://doi.org/10.3390/bioengineering4020026 (accessed on 5th November 2025).

Troschl, C., Meixner, K., Fritz, I., Paulik, C., Stelzer, F., & Drosg, B. (2018). Pilot-scale production of poly-β-hydroxybutyrate with the cyanobacterium *Synechocytis* sp. CCALA192 in a non-sterile tubular photobioreactor. *Algal Research, 34*, 116–125. https://doi.org/10.1016/j.algal.2018.07.011 (accessed on 5th November 2025).

Tu, W., Zhang, D., & Wang, H. (2019a). Polyhydroxyalkanoates (PHA) production from fermented thermal-hydrolyzed sludge by mixed microbial cultures: The link between phosphorus and PHA yields. *Waste Management, 96*, 149–157.

Van Thuoc, D., My, D. N., Loan, T. T., & Sudesh, K. (2019). Utilization of waste fish oil and glycerol as carbon sources for polyhydroxyalkanoate production by *Salinivibrio* sp. M318. *International Journal of Biological Macromolecules, 141*, 885–892.

Wagner, J., Bransgrove, R., Beacham, T. A., Allen, M. J., Meixner, K., Drosg, B., et al. (2016). Co-production of bio-oil and propylene through the hydrothermal liquefaction of polyhydroxybutyrate producing cyanobacteria. *Bioresource Technology, 207*, 166–174. https://doi.org/10.1016/j.biortech.2016.01.114 (accessed on 5th November 2025).

Wang, B., Pugh, S., Nielsen, D. R., et al. (2013). Engineering cyanobacteria for photosynthetic production of 3-hydroxybutyrate directly from $CO_2$. *Metabolic Engineering, 21*, 1. https://doi.org/10.1016/j.ymben.2013.01.001 (accessed on 5th November 2025).

Wang, B., Xiong, W., Yu, J., Maness, P. C., & Meldrum, D. R. (2018). Unlocking the photobiological conversion of $CO_2$ to (R)-3-hydroxybutyrate in cyanobacteria. *Green Chemistry, 20*, 3772–3782.

Wang, C., Yang, Y., Hou, J., Wang, P., Miao, L., Wang, X., & Guo, L. (2020). Optimization of cyanobacterial harvesting and extracellular organic matter removal utilizing magnetic nanoparticles and response surface methodology: A comparative study. *Algal Research, 45*, 101756.

Yadav, B., Pandey, A., Kumar, L. R., & Tyagi, R. D. (2020). Bioconversion of waste (water)/ residues to bioplastics – A circular bioeconomy approach. *Bioresource Technology, 298*, 122584.

Yajima, T., Nagatomo, M., Wakabayashi, A., Sato, M., Taguchi, S., & Maeda, M. (2020). Bioconversion of biphenyl to a polyhydroxyalkanoate copolymer by *Alcaligenes denitrificans* A41. *AMB Express, 10*, 155.

Yao, L., Cengic, I., Anfelt, J., & Hudson, E. P. (2016). Multiple gene repression in cyanobacteria using CRISPRi. *ACS Synthetic Biology, 5*, 207–212.

Zhang, S., Qian, X., Chang, S., Dismukes, G. C., & Bryant, D. A. (2016). Natural and synthetic variants of the tricarboxylic acid cycle in cyanobacteria: Introduction of the GABA shunt into *Synechococcus* sp. PCC 7002. *Frontiers in Microbiology, 7*, 1972. https://doi.org/10.3389/fmicb.2016.01972 (accessed on 5th November 2025).

Zheng, Y., Chen, J. C., Ma, Y. M., & Chen, G. Q. (2020). Engineering biosynthesis of polyhydroxyalkanoates (PHA) for diversity and cost reduction. *Metabolic Engineering, 58*, 82–93.

## CHAPTER 4

# Microbial Polysaccharides

PRADEEP KUMAR and VIRENDRA KUMAR*

*Department of NMR and MRI Facility, All India Institute of Medical Sciences, New Delhi, Delhi, India*

*Corresponding author

## ABSTRACT

Polyhydroxyalkanoates (PHA) offer the dual benefits of being biobased and fully biodegradable, making them attractive alternatives to petroleum-derived plastics. Polysaccharides, another major class of biopolymers, consist of monosaccharide units and are broadly classified as homopolysaccharides, containing a single type of monosaccharide, or heteropolysaccharides, composed of multiple types. Examples of homopolysaccharides include glucans and mannans, derived from glucose and mannose. Polysaccharides also contain monosaccharide derivatives such as sugar acids (e.g., glucuronic and iduronic acids), amino sugars (e.g., galactosamine), and modified sugars like N-acetylmuramic and N-acetylneuraminic acids. Microorganisms such as bacteria, fungi, and microalgae produce a wide variety of structurally diverse polysaccharides. Many bacterial polysaccharides are located in or near the cell wall and include well-characterized types such as teichoic acids, exopolysaccharides, peptidoglycans, lipopolysaccharides, and capsular polysaccharides. Fungal cell walls primarily consist of glucans, mannans, and chitin, while most microalgal polysaccharides are heteropolysaccharides often associated with sulfate groups. Common microbial polysaccharides include cellulose, alginate, chitin, curdlan, dextran, xanthan, pullulan, and scleroglucan. These biopolymers have extensive applications across food, medicine, wound healing, tissue

Industrial Biotechnology: Current Progress and Novel Technologies.
Prakash Kumar Sarangi, Akhilesh Kumar Singh, Rajesh Kumar Srivastava, and Brijesh Pandey (Eds.)


DOI: 10.1201/9781779642233-4

engineering, drug delivery, cosmetics, textiles, and environmental fields such as wastewater treatment and bioremediation.

## 4.1 INTRODUCTION

Microbial polysaccharides are extremely hydrated macromolecules composed of a repetition of single units of monosaccharide bonded by glycosidic linkages (Mahmoud et al., 2021; Mohd Nadzir et al., 2021). They can be homo- and hetero-polysaccharides and may be associated with organic and inorganic biomolecules. A diverse range of microbial polysaccharides arises not only from the type of monosaccharide units and their derivatives but also from how these moieties are linked together (Mahmoud et al., 2021; Mohd Nadzir et al., 2021). Therefore, a range of polysaccharides exists due to changes in the building block unit of sugar and sugar-derived compounds, anomeric configuration, glycosidic linkage, non-sugar ornamentation of the monosaccharide, shape, and molecular weight. Consequently, polysaccharides depict a rich base of structurally different biomolecules, many of which may have specific physical and chemical properties (Chaisuwan et al., 2021). The polysaccharides establish the main antigens in the most harmful bacteria by being present at the outer surface membrane of the bacterium. They serve as building blocks, compounds for protection, and storage materials. Several polysaccharides play numerous roles or perform activities and functions which remain to be understood (Limoli et al., 2015). Bacteria frequently have the potential to generate polysaccharides with a variety of biological roles. The production of polysaccharides involves a highly controlled process that utilizes complex interactions for energy conservation, biopolymer modification and biosynthesis, and external ecological activities. Bacteria may make use of a wide range of carbon and nitrogen sources along with other nutrients to produce polysaccharides, from the simple basic to the most complicated (Freitas et al., 2015; Mohammed et al., 2021).

Bacteria produce polysaccharides, which include peptidoglycan, lipopolysaccharides, capsule polysaccharides, and exo-polysaccharides (EPS) (Ullah et al., 2019). These macromolecules serve a variety of metabolic and structural functions, from allowing the bacterium to survive in harsh environments to acting as structural components of the cell wall (Ullah et al., 2019). The knowledge of functions performed by microbial polysaccharides offers unique advantages towards creating newer applications of polysaccharides, such as medicines, vaccines, and other commercial uses (Costa et al., 2018; Schmid et al., 2015). The extensive value of microbial polysaccharides in food, medicine, and pharmaceuticals is due to their excessive diversity in structural and functional features (Mahmoud et al., 2021; Osemwegie et al., 2020). Further, utilizing methods of genetic engineering provides new opportunities for economically viable manufacturing while also increasing the output of microbial polysaccharides (Mahmoud et al., 2021). These bio-polymeric sugar macromolecules are distinguished by their enormous bio-molecular weight because they include a significant number of monosaccharides, particularly fewer than 10 moieties and oligosaccharides, larger than or equal to 10 moieties connected together by glycosidic connections (Mahmoud et al., 2021). Protein and polysaccharide biosynthesis, in a divergence from nucleic acids (DNA and RNA), is not a template-driven process; instead, configuration is largely influenced by the complement of polysaccharide modification proteins or enzymes present in an organism (Mahmoud et al., 2021). The present chapter describes some of the important bacterial polysaccharides, which have potential applications. Fungal polysaccharides such as pullulan, galactosaminogalactan, chitin, scleroglucan, botryosphaeran, pestan, and microalgae/cyanobacteria, their polysaccharides, and their applications are also discussed (Chaisuwan et al., 2021; Mahapatra et al., 2013; Mahmoud et al., 2021).

## 4.2 BACTERIAL CELL WALLS, STRUCTURE AND COMPONENTS

The categorization of bacteria as Gram-negative or Gram-positive is based on the composition of their outer membranes (Salton et al., 1996; Silhavy et al., 2010). Gram-positive bacteria have thick cell walls that include numerous layers of protective polysaccharide conjugates with peptidoglycans and peptides, as well as their complex forms (Silhavy et al., 2010). Gram-negative bacteria have significantly thinner cell walls compared to Gram-positive bacteria, and there is only one layer of peptidoglycan in their inner and outer lipid bilayers. The most commonly used definitions of bacterial polysaccharides include capsular polysaccharides (CPS), extracellular or EPS, lipopolysaccharides (LPS), teichoic acids (TA), and peptidoglycans (Kornberg et al., 1999; Morrissey et al., 2012). Lipopolysaccharides, generally known as LPS, cover the surface of Gram-negative bacteria. Both EPS and CPS are produced by bacteria (Salton et al., 1996; Silhavy et al., 2010). Other biomolecules like TA originate only in certain Gram-positive bacteria like *Bacillus*, *staphylococci*, *streptococci*, and *lactobacilli* species (Silhavy et al., 2010) (Figure 4.1).

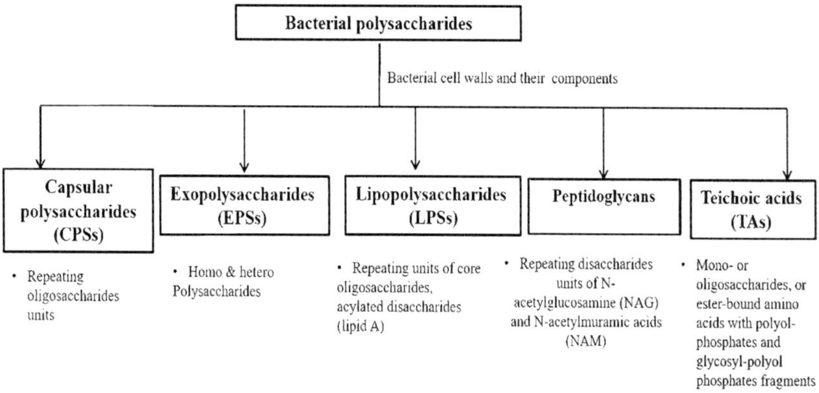


**FIGURE 4.1** Bacterial cell wall and extracellular polysaccharides and their components.

### *4.2.1 EXO-POLYSACCHARIDES (EPS)*

EPS are polysaccharides made and released by bacteria that accumulate outside of the cell membrane (Nwodo et al., 2012). EPS from bacteria continue to be a complicated class of biopolymers with a variety of mono-saccharides and various substituents (Figure 4.2) (Angelin et al., 2020). They are primarily linear strands, and many of them have side chains with mono- and oligosaccharides that are present at regular intervals (Angelin et al., 2020). The majority of these EPS may be made of repeated units of 2–6 monosaccharide moiety that membrane-associated enzymes bring together from glycosyl donors onto a polyisoprene phosphate carrier (Nwodo et al., 2012). The EPS of various microorganisms, such as bacterial and fungal origins, demonstrate a great range of structural combinations and unique capabilities despite the monomeric configuration (Angelin et al., 2020). Bacterial EPS may be produced from easily accessible, renewable, and apparently non-hazardous sources. EPS generated by lactic acid bacteria is crucial in the production of dairy products such drinking yogurt, cheese, and cream, as well as fermented milk-based sweets (Angelin et al., 2020; Mohd Nadzir et al., 2021; Moscovici, 2015).

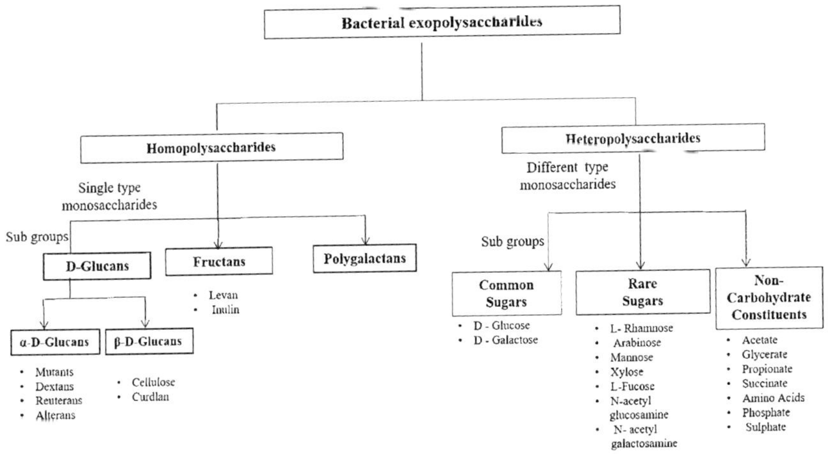


**FIGURE 4.2** Bacterial exopolysaccharide classification and division into subgroups based on homo and hetero monomer units.

## 4.2.2 *LIPOPOLYSACCHARIDES (LPS)*

LPS is the main surface membrane component existing in nearly all Gram-negative bacteria, and it is important to both the form and function of the outer bacterial membrane (Bertani et al., 2018). It is present in *E. coli*, *Pseudomonas* species, and other non-capsulated bacterial strains. Bacterial strains such as *Klebsiella pneumoniae* and *Haemophilus influenzae* are encapsulated; however, LPS is found on their cell surfaces (Farhana et al., 2022). The inner bacterial membrane encloses the cytoplasm; the outside bacterial membrane is exposed to the surrounding environment. Instead of having a double membrane made of phospholipids, the gram-negative bacterial cell membrane is made up of an asymmetric double membrane with phospholipids on the inside and LPS on the outside. The distinguishing structural properties of LPS are central to the protective barrier properties of the bacterial outer membrane (Bertani et al., 2018). Huge glycoconjugates connected to amphipathic are characterized by the presence of a lipid or hydrophobic domain in the core oligosaccharide and polysaccharide. Because they include both lipid and sugar molecules, these biomolecules are often referred to as lipoglycans. LPS is made up of lipid A (an endotoxin and virulence factor), O-antigen (hydrophilic distal oligosaccharide), and the hydrophilic core polysaccharide (Bertani et al., 2018). Innately linked gram-negative bacteria get veracity from LPS, which also serves as a method for the bacterium's contact with other surfaces (Bertani et al., 2018). The majority of LPS biomolecules are thermostable and provoke an inflammatory response in hosts' immune systems (Farhana et al., 2022). Distinct gram-negative bacteria have different types of LPS, and LPS is used to serotype gram-negative bacteria. Additionally, different bacterial species' LPS have remarkably variable sizes and arrangements (Farhana et al., 2022). Similarly, LPS plays a crucial part in host-pathogen interaction, making it one or more recognized biomarkers. There are many applications for LPS in research and medicine development (Bertani et al., 2018). Immune cells may be stimulated, and the innate immune response may be investigated using it (Farhana et al., 2022). Lipid A and other structurally modified LPS formulas have been employed as adjuvants in vaccine development.

### 4.2.3 PEPTIDOGLYCAN

Peptidoglycan, commonly known as murein, is typically present in the bacterial cell wall. It is made up of polysaccharide chains cross-linked by unique peptides comprising D-amino acids. Bacterial cell walls differ from those of fungi and plants (Esko et al., 2009). This rigid peptidoglycan structure is a unique characteristic of bacteria cell walls. In some Gram-positive bacteria, they may make up 95% of the cell wall; however, in Gram-negative bacteria, it may be 5–10%. Peptidoglycan is made of disaccharides (glycan) that are bonded together by short chains of homologous amino acid monomer units (peptides). The N-acetylglucosamine (NAG) and N-acetylmuramic acid (NAM) derivatives of glucose make up the backbone of the peptidoglycan biomolecule, with pentapeptides arising from NAM, with some variations. NAG and NAM strands are synthesized in the cytoplasm of the bacterial cell and then transported through the cytosolic membrane by a carrier molecule, bactoprenol (Navarre et al., 1999).

### 4.2.4 TEICHOIC ACIDS

TA are anionic phosphodiester-linked glycopolymers (glycerol phosphate or ribitol phosphate with carbohydrates) found in the cell wall of many Gram-positive bacteria. The TAs, along with their substituents, contribute charge and hydrophobicity to the bacterial cell surface (Swoboda et al., 2010). Most Gram-positive bacteria, including species from the genera

*Staphylococcus*, *Streptococcus*, *Bacillus*, *Clostridium*, *Corynebacterium*, and *Listeria*, generate TAs within their cell walls (Brown et al., 2013).

## 4.3 BIOSYNTHETIC ROUTES FOR MICROBIAL POLYSACCHARIDES

Bacterial cells may uptake different substrates using different mechanisms; however, they undergo phosphorylation either intracellularly or periplasmically. Intracellular phosphorylation is the most common in bacteria compared to the periplasmic oxidative pathway (Green et al., 2016; Mahmoud et al., 2021). In the cytoplasm, first, the substrate is catabolized via glycolysis. Phosphorylated sugars like nucleoside diphosphate sugars (NDP-sugars) are used to generate precursors for polysaccharide biosynthesis (Schmid et al., 2015). One of the two methods has been identified in gram-negative bacteria (Wang et al., 2011; Wiseman et al., 2021). Wzx flippase, Wzy polymerase, and Wzz chain-length controller proteins of the integral inner membrane have been reported to play a key role in the mechanism (Green et al., 2016; Mahmoud et al., 2021). The biopolymer repeat composite is generally constructed and polymerized on the inner surface of the cytoplasmic membrane, which is found in the periplasm (Wiseman et al., 2021).

EPS synthesis during microbial fermentation may benefit from molecular genetic techniques. An outstanding example has been reported by Wang et al., carried out on the synthesis of the capsular K5 polysaccharides of *Escherichia coli* (K5 EPS) (Wang et al., 2011). The fermentation method has been optimized to increase heparosan output and production. By converting uridine diphosphate glucose (UDP glucose) into UDP glucuronic acid via UDP glucose dehydrogenase and UDP-N-Acetyl-glucosamine, a regulated supply of nucleotide sugars for both cell wall production and heparosan biosynthesis was established (Ahmed et al., 2022; Ates et al., 2031; Soumya et al., 2021).

## 4.4 DIFFERENT TYPES OF MICROBIAL POLYSACCHARIDES: SPECIAL EMPHASIS ON BACTERIA

There are more than a 100 different types of monosaccharide units, including pyruvate, pentoses, hexoses, hexuronic acids, and deoxyhexoses

(De et al., 2010; Kornberg et al., 1999; Morrissey et al., 2012). The majority of CPSs are heteropolysaccharides, made up of oligosaccharide units. There are many different forms of TAs, but frequent fragments include polyolphosphates, glycosylpolyolphosphates, polyolphosphate-glycosylphosphates, and polyolphosphate-glycosylpolyolphosphates. Linear disaccharide polysaccharide repeating units are cross-linked with oligopeptide fragments to form peptidoglycans (De et al., 2010; Kornberg et al., 1999; Morrissey et al., 2012).

## 4.4.1 *HOMOPOLYSACCHARIDES*

### *4.4.1.1 DEXTRAN*

It is a branched bacterial polysaccharide made up of α (1→6) linked d–glucose residues that have some degree of branching across α (1→3) connections (Sarwat et al., 2008). Dextran's obtained from different sources have different molecular weights and degrees of branching and accordingly show physicochemical characteristics. Dextran is have found uses in many applications mainly because of their affordability and presence of hydroxyl functionality (Nwodo et al., 2012; Schmid et al., 2015).

### *4.4.1.2 CELLULOSE*

*Gluconacetobacter xylinus* is a bacterium that can make cellulose. Bacterial cellulose (BC) possesses unique qualities like compatibility, a high capacity to hold water, high crystallinity, a fine network of fibers, and a high tensile strength in the wet condition. *In situ* moldability is a benefit in addition to its affordable and reasonably simple production (Choi et al., 2022; He et al., 2020).

## 4.4.2 *HETEROPOLYSACCHARIDES*

### *4.4.2.1 GELLAN GUM*

It is a bacterial EPS made up of repeating units of tetra saccharide, D-glucose (β1 → 4)D-glucuronic acid (β1 → 4)D-glucose (β1 → 4)L-rhamnose (α1 → 3). It is an anionic polysaccharide produced by the bacterium *Sphingomonas elodea*. In its high acyl form, D-acetate and D-glycerate are present on the same glucose residue (Mohd Nadzir et al., 2021).

The high acyl form produces translucent, soft, elastic, flexible gels that are resistant to heat and acid, whereas the low acyl form produces rigid, nonelastic, brittle gels. Gellan gum has found applications in the food and cosmetic industry. It has potential biomedical applications due to the presence of glucuronic repeating units (Nwodo et al., 2012; Schmid et al., 2015).

#### *4.4.2.2 XANTHAN GUM*

The bacterium *Xanthomonas campestris* ferments glucose to generate xanthan gum. It is made up of pentasaccharide (comprising glucose, mannose, and glucuronic acid) as repeating units. D-Glucose units (β-1,4-linked) form the backbone of the molecule. The alternate glucose units of the backbone have a trisaccharide side chain of D-mannose (β1 → 4) D-glucuronic acid (β1 → 2)D-mannose (β1 → 4). However, there may be substituents present in side chains like pyruvate on the terminal mannose unit, and the mannose attached to the glucose backbone may be acetylated. It can be used to produce hydrogels, and due to its high viscosity imparting properties, it has found many applications in the food and cosmetic industry (Nwodo et al., 2012; Schmid et al., 2015). In addition, Table 4.1 shows applications, monomeric units, and bacterial species, including curdlan, alginate, hyaluronic acid/hyaluronan, colonic acid, glucuronan, succinoglycan, welan, and levan (Barcelos et al., 2020; He et al., 2020; Moscovici, 2015; Nwodo et al., 2012; Schmid et al., 2015).

## 4.5 FUNGAL POLYSACCHARIDES

Fungal polysaccharides may be categorized based on the structure and composition of polysaccharides, and location in the cell, for example, EPS (Chaisuwan et al., 2021). The Fungi produce a variety of polysaccharides including glucans, chitin, and various heteropolysaccharides (Mahapatra et al., 2013; Roca et al., 2015). For the past 20 years, fungus EPS have been acknowledged as high-value biomolecules. Galactosaminogalactan, N-acetylglucosamine (GlcNAc) pullulan, scleroglucan, and botryosphaeran are examples of some of the polysaccharides that have potential applications in pharmaceutical, medical, food, and biotechnology industry (Osemwegie et al., 2020; Osiska et al., 2015). Figure 4.3 summarizes some of the steps in production and harvesting of microbial polysaccharides and

**TABLE 4.1** Basic Biochemistry and Application of the Most Important Bacterial Exopolysaccharides

| Bacterial Polysaccharides | Monosaccharide Units | Bacteria | Application |
|---|---|---|---|
| Cellulose | Glucose | *Acetobacters* spp. | Foods (Fiber), Biomedical (wound healing), domestic, agricultural, and industrial sectors, and so forth [Choi et al. (2022); He et al. (2021); Moscovici et al. (2015)] |
| Curdlan | Glucose | *A. radiobacter* and *R. meliloti* | Heavy metal removal, foods, and medicines [Barcelos et al. (2020); Moscovici et al. (2015); Roca et al. (2015); Schmid et al. (2015)] |
| Dextran | Glucose | *Leuconostoc mesenteroides* | Regulating wound shock and blood plasma volume expansion [Barcelos et al. (2020); Moscovici et al. (2015); Roca et al. (2015); Schmid et al. (2015)] |
| Xantham | Mannose, glucuronic acid, acetate, pyruvate, glucose, and others | *Xanthomonas campestris* | Ion stabilizer and thickener for medicinal creams and suspensions carrier with the controlled release [Barcelos et al. (2020); Moscovici et al. (2015); Roca et al. (2015); Schmid et al. (2015)] |
| Alginate | Mannuronic acid, guluronic cacid, acetate | *Azotobacter vinelandii, Pseudomonas aeruginosa* | Tablet disintegrating agents, pharmaceutical solution thickeners and stabilizers, dental emulsions, antiacid (anti-reflux) imprints, stomach protectors, microspheres for medication administration, and fibers in wound hemostatic dressing and bandages [Barcelos et al. (2020); Moscovici et al. (2015); Roca et al. (2015); Schmid et al. (2015)] |
| Gellan | Glucose, rhamnose, glucuronic acid, glycerate and acetate | *Sphingomonas paucimobilis (formerly Pseudomonaselodea)* | Excipients are used in oral, ophthalmic, and nasal medication formulations for sustained/controlled release of tablets [Barcelos et al. (2020); Moscovici et al. (2015); Roca et al. (2015); Schmid et al. (2015)]. |
| Hyaluronic acid/ hyaluronan | N-acetyl glucosamine and glucuronic acid | *Bacillus subtilis; Streptococcus equisimilis/zooepidemicus (recomb. Str. equisimilis)* | Chronic wounds with slow wound healing, intra-articular injections for osteoarthritis, and vitreous replacement surgery for eyes [Barcelos et al. (2020); Moscovici et al. (2015); Roca et al. (2015); Schmid et al. (2015)] |
| Colonic acid | Glucose, fucose, galactose and glucoronate | *Salmonella spp., E. coli, Enterobacter* spp. *and Shigella spp.* | Individual care products and Cosmetics [Barcelos et al. (2020); Roca et al. (2015); Schmid et al. (2015)] |

**TABLE 4.1** *(Continued)*

| Bacterial Polysaccharides | Monosaccharide Units | Bacteria | Application |
|---|---|---|---|
| Glucuronan | Glucuronic acid | *G. hansenii S. and meliloti* M5N1CS | Cosmetics products and foods [Barcelos et al. (2020); Moscovici et al. (2015); Roca et al. (2015); Schmid et al. (2015)] |
| Succinoglycan | Glucose and galactose | *Agrobacterium radiobacter Agrobacterium tumefaciens, Rhizobium meliloti,* *A. faecalis var. myxogenes* 10C3 | Oil recovery and food [Barcelos et al. (2020); Moscovici et al. (2015); Roca et al. (2015); Schmid et al. (2015)] |
| Welan | Mannose, glucose, and glucuronic acid | *Sphingomonas* sp. | Chemistry Construction [Barcelos et al. (2020); Moscovici et al. (2015); Roca et al. (2015); Schmid et al. (2015)] |
| Levan | Glucose and fructose | *Azotobacter, Bacillus, Pseudomonas, Gluconobacter, Acetobacter, Mycobacterium, Streptococcus, Corynebacterium, Aerobacter, Erwinia, and Zymomonas* | Medicines, Industry, Glue, Feed and Food, and so forth [Barcelos et al. (2020); Moscovici et al. (2015); Roca et al. (2015); Schmid et al. (2015)] |

Figure 4.4 summarizes some of application of microbial polysaccharides in various industries. Table 4.2 describes some of the polysaccharides of fungal origin and their application.

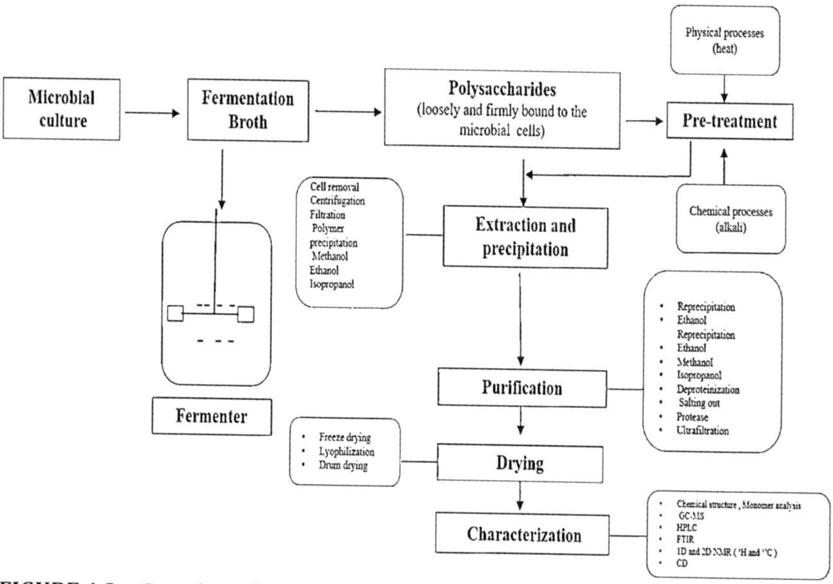


**FIGURE 4.3** Overview of production and harvesting of microbial polysaccharides.

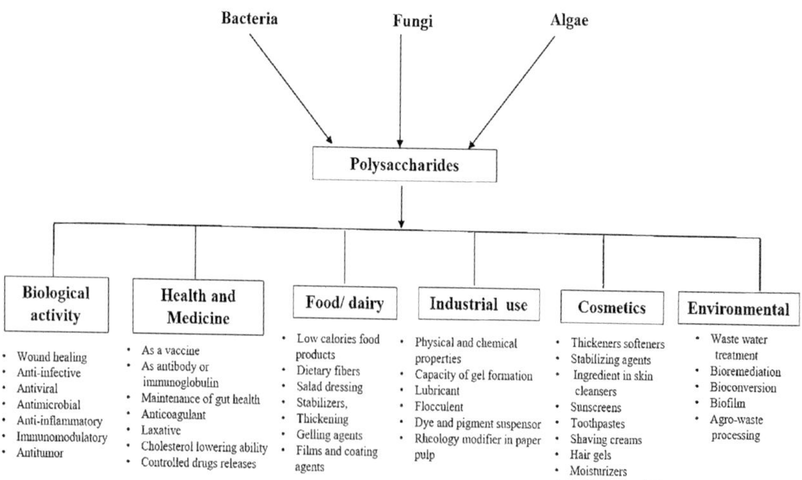


**FIGURE 4.4** Application of microbial polysaccharides (bacterial, fungal, and microalgal/ cyanobacteria).

**TABLE 4.2** Fungal Sources, Monomers Unit of Exopolysaccharides, and Their Application

| Fungal Polysaccharides | Monosaccharide Units | Fungi | Application | References |
|---|---|---|---|---|
| Pullulan | Maltotriose | *Aureobasidium pullulans* | Products for tablet coating, granulation, and oral, wound, and oxygen-impermeable film-forming, non-animal capsules | Cheng et al. (2011); Moscovici (2015) |
| Galactosaminogalactan | Galactose and N-acetyl galactosamine (GalNAc) | *Aspergillus fumigatus* | Adhesin, host immune response regulation, and signaling route | Briard et al. (2016); Fontaine et al. (2011) |
| Chitin | N acetylglucosamine (GlcNAc) | *Candida albicans* | Diet supplements for cartilage and bones. | Chen et al. (2010) |
| Scleroglucan | Glucose (Glucan) | *Sclerotium glucanicum* | Oil recovery, adhesives, watercolors, printing inks, animal feed composition, and cosmetics. | Mahapatra et al. (2013) |
| Botryosphaeran | Glucose (Glucan) | *Botryosphaeria rhodina* | Toxicologically accepted and potent immunomodulator | Mahapatra et al. (2013) |
| Pestan | Glucose (Glucan) | *Pestalotiopsis* sp. | Wastewater treatment like bio sorbent of lead and zinc. | Mahapatra et al. (2013) |

### 4.5.1 PULLULAN

Pullulan is a repeating unit of maltotriose that is α (1 → 4) linked and united by α (1 → 6) linkages. It is an EPS fungal homopolysaccharide of glucose that is synthesized from starch by fermentation. Pullulan is produced from starch by the fungus *Aureobasidium pullulans*. The non-toxicity and absence of immunogenicity of pullulan are some of its benefits. Pullulan appears to be the only EPS of fungal origin that is commercially produced (Moscovici et al., 2013; Valverde et al., 2015). Its current uses as a medicinal component are based on its unique film- and binding-forming abilities, as well as its great oxygen impermeability. Due to these qualities, it is excellent for coating and granulating tablets, creating non-animal capsules, and creating oral and wound care products. Other fungal exopolysaccharides like galactosaminogalactan (Cheng et al., 2011; Fontaine et al., 2011), chitin (Briard et al., 2016), scleroglucan (Osińska et al., 2015), botryosphaeran (Osińska et al., 2015), pestan (Osińska et al., 2015), their applications, fungal species, and monomeric unit are shown in Table 4.2.

## 4.6 MICROALGAE / CYANOBACTERIA POLYSACCHARIDES

Photosynthetic microorganisms like microalgae and cyanobacteria have received a lot of interest due to their adaptability in producing biomass. Solar energy and wastewater (and other waste material) can be used as nutrient sources, making them ecosystem friendly (Chen et al., 2010). The generation of polysaccharides in the species of *Porphyridium, Chlorella, Spirulina,* and *Nostoc* has been reported (Chen et al., 2010). Most microalgal polysaccharides are heteropolysaccharides, which are typically linked to sulphates. The generation of microalgal polysaccharides may depend on the microalgae strain and factors such as available nutrients, salinity, and temperature. In addition to polysaccharides, microalgae have a high concentration of other bioactive compounds such as phycocyanin, peptides, polyunsaturated fatty acids (PUFA), and carotenoids (Dolganyuk et al., 2020). However, different species of microalgae and cyanobacteria may contain a significant amount of fructose, fucose, galactose, glucose, mannose, rhamnose, ribose, xylose, and so forth.

Microalgal and cyanobacterial polysaccharides may have antiviral, antibacterial, and antioxidant properties. Exopolysaccharides production by growing microalgae is a physiological process which is typical under stressful conditions (Dolganyuk et al., 2020). Application of nitrogen restriction during microalgae culture will increase exopolysaccharide accumulation. Microalgae/cyanobacteria sources like *Anabaena* species, *Arthrospira platensis, Chlorella pyrenoidosa, Chlorella vulgaris, Dixoniella grisea, Gloeocapsa* species, *Graesiella* species, *Neochloris oleoabundans*, *Nostoc carneum*, *Porphyridium aerugineum*, and *Spirulina* species (Ahmed et al., 2014; Barboríková et al., 2019; Bhunia et al., 2018; De Jesus et al., 2018; Hussein et al., 2015; Li et al., 2020; Naggar et al., 2020; Netanel Liberman et al., 2020; Rossi et al., 2012; Trabelsi et al., 2016; Wan et al., 2020), monomers unit of exopolysaccharides and their application are shown in Table 4.3.

## 4.7 MICROBIAL POLYSACCHARIDE PRODUCTION

Microbial polysaccharides may be located inside a section of the cytoplasmic membrane, as a cell wall component, and attached to the outer layer of the cell wall (as a capsule or as slime). Polysaccharides, which are located inside the cytoplasm or are present in the cell wall, are difficult to harvest (Chen et al., 2010). Exopolysaccharides from bacteria, fungi, and microalgae/cyanobacteria are isolated by combining physical techniques (like sonication, centrifugation, heating) and chemical techniques (like cationic exchange resin, glutaraldehyde, NaOH, ethylenediaminetetraacetic acid-EDTA, and formaldehyde). Despite the obvious industrial advantages of microbial exopolysaccharides, their production is highly limited. Costs are frequently associated with the substrate required for microbial growth and the fermenters used to cultivate (Osemwegie et al., 2020) (Figure 4.3).

### *4.7.1 FERMENTER*

Numerous fermentation techniques have been reported to produce bacterial and fungal exopolysaccharides (as well as other compounds). Fermentation in anaerobic conditions employs microbial metabolism to bio-transform composite materials. Normal fermentation by-products

**TABLE 4.3** Microalgae/Cyanobacteria Sources, Monomers Unit of Exopolysaccharides, and Their Application

| Microalgae/Cyanobacteria | Monosaccharide Units | Application | References |
|---|---|---|---|
| *Anabaena species* | Glucose, xylose, rhamnose, and uranic Acids | Heavy metals from wastewater removed | Bhunia et al. (2018) |
| *Arthrospira platensis* | Fructose, glucose, mannose, fucose, galactose, rhamnose, ribose, xylose, and uranic Acids | Bio-stimulant | Ahmed et al. (2014) |
| *Chlorella pyrenoidosa* | Glucose, mannose, fucose, xylose, rhamnose, arabinose, and uranic Acids | Antioxidant activities | Wan et al. (2020) |
| *Chlorella Vulgaris* | Glucose, maltose, Fructose, lactose, arabinose, rhamnose, uranic Acids sulphates, and amino acids | Anti-obesity agents prevent chronic airway inflammation | Barboríková et al. (2019); Naggar et al. (2020) |
| *Dixoniella grisea* | Xylose, rhamnose Uranic Acids Sulphates Methylated Sugars | Unique rheological properties and bioactivities | Netanel Liberman et al. (2020) |
| *Gloeocapsa species* | Glucose, fructose, fucose, galactose, ribose, rhamnose, arabinose, mannose, xylose, | Phototrophic biofilms | Rossi et al. (2012) |
| *Graesiella species* | Glucose, fucose, arabinose, galactose, rhamnose, xylose, ribose, mannose, uranic Acids, sulphates, and amino acids | Antioxidant and antiproliferative activities | Trabelsi et al. (2016) |
| *Neochloris oleoabundans* | Galactose, glucose, mannose, ribose, arabinose, xylose, rhamnose, uranic Acids, and amino acids | (immunomodulatory activity) | Li et al. (2020) |
| *Nostoc carneum* | Xylose, glucose Uranic Acids Sulphates | antioxidant activity | Hussein et al. (2015) |
| *Porphyridium aerugineum* | Xylose, glucose, galactose Uranic Acids Sulphates Methylenated sugars | Unique rheological properties and bioactivities | Netanel Liberman et al. (2020) |
| *Spirulina species* | Glucose, fructose, galactose Uranic Acids, and amino acids | anti-obesity agent's bio flocculant and food industries | De Jesus et al. (2018) |

include alcohol and carbon dioxide, and monomers are polymerized to create microbial polysaccharides (Osemwegie et al., 2020). Exopolysaccharide extraction has mostly employed two types of fermentation: submerged fermentation and solid-state fermentation (SSF). Different species produce different chemicals throughout the fermentation process, and the present environmental conditions have a big influence on those molecules.

## 4.8 ISOLATION AND EXTRACTION METHODS OF MICROBIAL POLYSACCHARIDES

Microbial polysaccharides can be isolated and purified using a variety of techniques. The main consideration when choosing a method for isolating microbial polysaccharides is to maintain the inherent features of these compounds throughout the isolation and purification processes. The bulk of polysaccharides in bacteria, fungi, and microalgae/cyanobacteria are found as a component of the cell wall (Mahmoud et al., 2021). Therefore, the initial stage in the extraction of polysaccharides is crushing materials from bacteria, fungi, and microalgae/cyanobacteria. By rupturing the cell walls of bacteria, fungi, and microalgae/cyanobacteria, ultrasonic gas flow crushing technology has recently been used in addition to conventional crushing techniques to considerably increase the efficiency of polysaccharide extraction. Mechanical crushing must be followed by lipid removal since the cell walls of bacteria, fungus, and microalgae/cyanobacteria are predominantly coated by lipid. Ethanol reflux employing a Soxhlet extractor is a typical technique for extracting fat. The raw material can be used to extract polysaccharides once the lipids have been removed (Mahmoud et al., 2021).

### *4.8.1 EXTRACTION WITH HOT WATER METHOD*

This is one of the most widely used methods for microbial polysaccharide extraction because the majority of the polysaccharides are soluble in hot water, and hot water does not cause any noticeable change in the polysaccharides. The polysaccharide of interest from the solution can be extracted by filtration or centrifugation as deemed suitable (Mahmoud et al., 2021).

### 4.8.2 METHOD OF EXTRACTING DILUTED ALKALI-WATER SOLUTION

Some polysaccharides show low solubility in hot water, especially acidic ones, or those with a high molecular weight. For such polysaccharides, a dilute alkali solution generally works to dissolve them. NaOH or $NaCO_3$ solutions are frequently utilized for this purpose. However, polysaccharides are susceptible to breakdown at temperatures over 10°C when employing a dilute alkali solution. Polysaccharides are often extracted with hot water as a first step, and then residual polysaccharides are next extracted with a diluted alkali solution (Mahmoud et al., 2021).

### 4.8.3 OTHER APPROACHES

Hot water or dilute alkali extraction methods are the two most commonly used methods for polysaccharide extraction; however, in a few cases, other methods like dimethyl sulfoxide (DMSO), 2-methoxy ethanol-LiCl, or acidic aqueous solution may be preferred (Mahmoud et al., 2021).

### 4.8.4 EXCLUSION OF IMPURITIES IN MICROBIAL POLYSACCHARIDE EXTRACTS

The extracted solutions of polysaccharides often contain other compounds as contaminants with a range of impurities, which may include inorganic salts, monosaccharides, oligosaccharides, low molecular weight non-polar substances, and high molecular weight organic impurities like proteins and lignin. These contaminants can be eliminated using the dialysis process. Since various dialysis bags have varying criteria for molecular weight cut-off, therefore, the first step is to select an appropriate dialysis bag for dialysis (Mahmoud et al., 2021). Dialysis bags must be pre-treated before use. They are frequently boiled for a few hours in boiling water to remove contaminants before use. Dialysis bags may be re-used after thoroughly washing them, treated with a preservative (such as benzoic acid), and kept refrigerated till further use. The pH of the extract solution of polysaccharides should be adjusted to pH 5–9 first before dialysis since dialysis bags are typically stable in the pH range of 5 to 9. It should be noted that although dialysis bags have a specific molecular weight exclusion range, some polysaccharide molecules are linear and may occasionally pass through the dialysis bag despite being larger than the exclusion range. Additionally, inorganic salts like charged anions and cations are removed using ion exchange resins. Salts may be eliminated on a large industrial scale using ion exchange resin mixed beds (Mahmoud et al., 2021).

#### 4.8.4.1 ENZYMATIC METHOD

Proteins or peptides are digested using appropriate protease. As enzymes work at a particular pH, the extract solution's pH is adjusted to 7–8, and then enzyme pronase is added, allowing it to digest proteins for 2–4 hours at 37°C. After the required digestion, the process is stopped by boiling it for 5 minutes (Mahmoud et al., 2021).

#### 4.8.4.2 SEVAG TECHNIQUE

Chloroform is added to the polysaccharide aqueous solution (pH 4–5) to denature the proteins, followed by addition of n-butanol. When this mixture is shaken vigorously, denatured proteins will form a jelly at the interface between polar and solvent. Therefore, denatured proteins may then be eliminated by centrifugation. However, this method has low efficiency. These steps are repeated a few times to remove proteins efficiently (Mahmoud et al., 2021).

### 4.8.5 PURIFICATION OF POLYSACCHARIDES

It may be difficult to describe isolation and purification separately and may employ a combination of methods. The actual method or combination of methods used may depend on the location of the polysaccharide in the cell. For instance, polysaccharides are first extracted with water and then with an alkaline solution. Additional contaminant extraction for purification may be carried out using column chromatography (Mahmoud et al., 2021). Figure 4.3 summarizes the different separation and purification procedures used for microbial polysaccharides. Colorimetric techniques can be used to visualize polysaccharide content during microbial growth on agar plates. Various monosaccharides interact with dyes, and this phenomenon may be used to quickly and simply determine the presence of EPS (Fontaine et al., 2011).

#### 4.8.5.1 ELECTROPHORESIS

The technique for detecting the presence of ionic polysaccharides and monitoring the purification process during the various phases is electrophoresis on polyacrylamide gels (SDS – or DOC-PAGE). In fact, this method may be used to evaluate charged polysaccharides, proteoglycans, and lipopolysaccharides (LPSs). Alcian Blue and silver staining can be applied (Fontaine et al., 2011; Jackson et al., 1990).

#### 4.8.5.2 CHROMATOGRAPHIC METHODS

Microbial polysaccharides are often purified and fractionated using chromatographic techniques such as ion-exchange chromatography, size exclusion chromatography, and affinity chromatography. Ion exchange chromatography is based on separation by differences in charge characteristics among biomolecules. Higher selectivity can be attained by adjusting the pH to affect the net surface charge of charged molecules. To separate microbial polysaccharides with various molecular weights or sizes, size exclusion chromatography might be utilized (Fontaine et al., 2011). Targeted affinity is used in affinity chromatography to fix the target and particular biomolecule charged by the mobile phase to the immobilized ligand on the stationary phase. These biomolecules can be recovered once additional washing and elution processes have been completed. The kind of applications and the state of the polysaccharide's purity determine the best technique for microbiological purification. For instance, chromatographic procedures offer a high purity of polysaccharides, trying to make them relevant for research and other fields (Dolganyuk et al., 2020; Fontaine et al., 2011).

## 4.9 ANALYTICAL METHODS FOR CHARACTERIZATION OF MICROBIAL POLYSACCHARIDES

### 4.9.1 NUCLEAR MAGNETIC RESONANCE (NMR) SPECTROSCOPY

Spectroscopy methods in combination with chemical methods such as compositional analyses, partial degradation, and methylation analysis may be used determine the structure of bacterial polysaccharides.

Particularly mass spectrometry (MS) and nuclear magnetic resonance (NMR) spectroscopy provide crucial information for structural elucidation of bacterial polysaccharides. The polysaccharides are often subjected to chemical or enzymatic de-polymerization to yield oligosaccharides that are readily amenable to structural analysis. Quantitative NMR has some advantages as little or no sample preparation is required. One dimensional (1D) and two-dimensional (2D) NMR techniques allow structure elucidation and quantification of microbial polysaccharides (Ren et al., 2019).

1D 1H-NMR may be used to determine the number of sugar residues and their anomeric structure. The number and kind of methyl groups are also determined. The relationship between the nuclei of a single residue as well as between the nuclei of other residues may be found using 2D NMR. 2D NMR experiments such as COSY, TOCSY, HSQC-DEPT, HSQC-TOCSY, HMBC, and NOESY investigations, are used. Homonuclear COSY and TOCSY spectra allow assignment of particular monosaccharide. Each signal in a heteronuclear spectrum, like HSQC-DEPT, denotes a specific connection between a proton and a carbon (Moscovici, 2015). The DEPT experiment permits the separation of CH and CH3 protons (positive signals) from $CH_2$ protons (negative signals). Circular dichroism, small-angle neutron scattering (SANS), and measuring NMR NOEs in combination with molecular dynamics simulations are further methods for detecting secondary structure (Larsen et al., 2020).

### *4.9.2 MASS SPECTROMETRY*

Gas chromatography-mass spectrometry (GC-MS), matrix-assisted laser desorption/ionization time-of-flight mass spectrometry (MALDI-TOF MS), rapid atom bombardment mass spectrometry (FAB-MS), and electrospray ionization ion trap mass spectrometry (ESI-ITMS) are used to identify and characterize polysaccharides. EI mass spectra and GC retention times are used in GC-MS to identify volatile substances (Han et al., 2013; Larsen et al., 2020). EI can be substituted with moderate desorption and ionization techniques such MALDI-TOF MS, FAB-MS, and ESI-ITMS. With detection limits ranging from picomolar to femtomolar, they enable the analysis of polysaccharides, oligosaccharides, and monosaccharides. Alditol acetates, partially methylated alditol acetates, and pertrimethylsilylated (+)- or (-)-2-butyl glycosides, which are evaluated using GC-MS, have all been used to create the monosaccharide composition (Han et al., 2013).

## 4.10 MICROBIAL POLYSACCHARIDE MODIFICATION

The formation of polysaccharides is significantly influenced by a variety of environmental factors, such as pH and temperature, carbon and nitrogen source, ion source, oxygen, and aeration rate, as well as dilution rate (Ahmed et al., 2022). In addition, physical and chemical cross-linking reactions result in changes in microbial polysaccharides. In the pharmaceutical industry, cross-linked polysaccharides operate as a coating or an embedding agent for the drug's active ingredient. Physical cross-linking occurs regardless of the presence of the cross-linking agent, in contrast to chemical cross-linking. Chemical cross-linking results in either intra- or intermolecular linkages that are covalently connected to other polymer chains. Chemical cross-linking involves two important variables: the concentration of the cross-linking agents and the length of the cross-linking process (Ahmed et al., 2022).

## 4.11 APPLICATIONS OF MICROBIAL POLYSACCHARIDES

Microbial polysaccharides are considered safe compared to synthetic polymers. Therefore, microbial polysaccharides are receiving increased interest in the food industry, pharmacological, biomedical, and cosmetic applications due to their new properties and physicochemical makeup.

### *4.11.1 HEALTH AND MEDICINE AND BIOLOGICAL ACTIVITIES*

Polysaccharides have qualities like increased solubility, biodegradability, biocompatibility, and non-immunogenicity for potential biomedical applications. For instance, biological applications such as wound treatment, regenerative medicine, and controlling medication delivery have made substantial use of polysaccharides derived from algae. Heparin-loaded hydrogels, for example, have been effectively employed to distribute bone morphogenetic proteins (BMP). The polysaccharide has been shown to increase mechanical qualities, which helps compensate for synthetic polymer's low biological performance.

Exopolysaccharides are particularly finding potential applications in biomedical applications (Angelin et al., 2020; Patel et al., 2012). The survival rate of encapsulated bacterial probiotics has been improved by using polysaccharides for micro-encapsulation. Additionally, the majority of the properties of polysaccharides, such as enteric dissolution, ion-induced gelation, and electrostatic activity, are perfect for creating micro-capsules. Alginates (negatively charged) and chitosan (positively charged) interact to create a semi-permeable membrane system, resulting in capsules with a sturdy texture and less permeability to water-soluble biomolecules. In particular, the single-layer chitosan-coated alginate beads may be coated repeatedly by putting them into such an alginate or chitosan solution, increasing the potential of the probiotic bacteria (Angelin et al., 2020; Patel et al., 2012).

EPSs have significant antiviral, antioxidant, antitumor, and immunomodulatory properties. Atherosclerosis, Parkinson's disease, rheumatoid arthritis, and cancer are just a few of the diseases brought on by reactive oxygen species (ROS) like nitric oxide ($NO^-$), hydroxyl ($OH^-$), superoxide ($O^-$), and so forth, and others. Exopolysaccharides have been shown to possess antioxidant and free radical-scavenging properties. EPSs, which are produced by probiotic bacteria, have anti-ulcer properties. Using ethanol-induced erosion models and acetic acid-induced stomach ulcers in rats, researchers examined the anti-ulcer properties of *Lactobacilli*, *Bifidobacteria*, and *Streptococci*. EPSs with rhamnose content of over 60% were more effective at treating stomach ulcers. EPSs have been reported to demonstrate immune system-stimulating and anti-cancer properties (Kurutas et al., 2016; Pizzino et al., 2017).

For vaccination to provide long-lasting protection against microbial invasion, particular antibodies must be present. A wide variety of type-specific capsular and exopolysaccharide structures are shown by pathogenic bacteria such as *E. coli*, *Klebsiella pneumoniae*, *Streptococcus* species (including *Pneumococcus*), *Haemophilus influenza*, *Neisseria meningitides*, and *Salmonella typhi*. A very intricate interaction of many cells and chemical components makes up the immune response to infections with harmful bacteria, with the goal of eradicating the invading organism (Cress et al., 2014; Mostowy et al., 2018).

Superparamagnetic iron oxide nanoparticles with cross-linked dextran coating or large series of multifunctional imaging agents have been developed as a complete platform for magnetic resonance imaging (MRI), positron emission tomography (PET) imaging, and fluorescence molecular tomography (FMT). As a result of magnetic field-induced hyperthermia, acetylated pullulan-coated magnetic nanoparticles exerted a theragnostic effect, killing tumor cells. Recurrent dose delivery is required for the theragnostic use of such diagnostics, and it mostly depends on how iron particles are metabolized and eliminated (Nikolova et al., 2020).

Antitumor properties are present in several microbial polysaccharides. Tumors are a major health concern and the number one cause of death globally. Numerous polysaccharides, including schizophyllan, have been shown to be potent anticancer agents (Mohammed et al., 2021). Polysaccharide-protein conjugates have been shown to have anticancer action and can boost the effectiveness of standard chemotherapy medicines. Recent studies have demonstrated the immunosuppressive properties of polysaccharides in preventing tumor development. Despite the diversity in their chemical structures and conjugated sections, mushrooms have long been utilized as food and medicine because they are rich suppliers of various therapeutic substances (Chen et al., 2019; Ren et al., 2012; Zong et al., 2012).

It is known that polysaccharides generated from mushrooms have undergone substantial research to determine their potential for use in pharmacological and anticancer treatments. Ganoderma lucidum, which demonstrated *in vitro* immune activation and anticancer action on the breast cancer cells, and Lentinus edodes, which had a notable antitumor impact against subcutaneously transplanted sarcoma, are two examples of polysaccharides from fungi such as mushrooms (Pandya et al., 2019; Schepetkin et al., 2006). Mushroom-derived polysaccharides have been shown to have anticancer effects via immune system stimulation, suppression of tumorigenesis, and stimulatory in tumor cells directly through tumor-inhibitory actions.

Algal polysaccharides are also particularly significant due to their wide range of pharmacological properties, which include anticancer properties (Costa et al., 2010; Meng et al., 2016). The expression of cytokines like TNF-$\alpha$, IFN-$\gamma$, and $IL^{-1}$ by effector cells like macrophages, T lymphocytes, B lymphocytes, cytotoxic T lymphocytes, and natural killer cells is induced by polysaccharides. Cytokines always have antiproliferative activity, lead to tumor cell apoptosis and differentiation, and also secrete products like reactive nitrogen, oxygen intermediates, and interleukin. Saccharide-coated nanoparticles have a longer circulatory circulation lifespan. They also significantly build up in tumor tissues (Jiao et al., 2011). In order to control inflammatory diseases, microbial polysaccharides are frequently utilized in nanomaterials, and their anti-inflammatory capabilities have been experimentally evaluated. For instance, the anti-inflammatory activity of TCM polysaccharides is primarily attributed to the inhibition of chemotactic factors and adherence control variables as well as the activities of key enzymes involved in the inflammation process. Sulfated polysaccharides made from algae show their anti-inflammatory effect by obstructing the migration of leukocytes to inflammatory sites, in comparison to other polysaccharides that have an inhibitory effect on inflammatory-related mediators like cytokines (IL-1b, IL-6, TNF-α), and NO and decreased the infiltration of inflammatory cells (Mohammed et al., 2021).

### *4.11.2 FOOD AND DAIRY PRODUCT INDUSTRY*

Microbial polysaccharides act as thickeners, stabilizers, texturizers, and gelling agents to improve the food's quality, texture, and flavor (Nwodo et al., 2012; Oner, 2013). Utilizing polysaccharides in food items causes water's rheological characteristics to change, which consequently affects the product's texture. The mouthfeel, which is challenging to characterize but connected to the physical characteristics of polysaccharides, is another easily quantifiable characteristic of polysaccharide additions (Khan et al., 2007; Ramalingam et al., 2014). Mouth feel is correlated with viscosity, particularly with the polysaccharide's non-Newtonian activity. This is related to viscosity because of how it reduces the strength of food flavors. The evaluation of the initial sensation on the palate of the first bite via mastication and swallowing is connected to the mouth-feel characteristics of polysaccharides. Microbial polysaccharides also affect how cooked meals taste, look, and color (Xu et al., 2009; Yang et al., 2013).

Polysaccharides also help fermented milk products have better rheology, texture, stability, and mouthfeel (Ahmed et al., 2005). Microbial polysaccharides can be used to address issues that typically arise during the production of yogurts, such as poor viscosity, gel fracture, or excessive syneresis (whey separation). A texture profile investigation of cheese produced by fermentation using EPS-producing *Streptococcus thermophilus* and *Lactobacillus delbrueckii* species revealed that the cheese's hardness, consistency, adhesiveness, chewiness, relaxation, and modulus were much reduced (Patel et al., 2012; Torino et al., 2015). The industries manufactured using the EPS-producing cultures becomes smooth, creamy, moist, and soft, whereas the one made without the EPS-producing strains turns dry and granular. It has been established that EPS-producing cultures enhance consumer acceptability (Salazar et al., 2016). Numerous polysaccharide molecules create an ordered polysaccharide conformation structure, or the gel structure, as a result of hydrogen bonding and ionic interactions.

The EPS generated by microorganisms is mostly used to replace plant and marine algal gums in various applications. Due to their unique and diverse macromolecular structures, they have particular rheological characteristics such as gelling, emulsifying, or thickening agents, for example, xanthan, gellant, and curdlan (Ates, 2015; Osemwegie et al., 2020). Due to its ability to thicken liquids, cellulose is anticipated to be used in a variety of culinary applications. Numerous culinary products, including cheese spreads, ice creams, puddings, and other sweets, employ xanthan. The use of xanthan could assist milk products to have better textures, which would raise their quality (Ates, 2015; Osemwegie et al., 2020). Many food applications can benefit from dextran, including enhancing the qualities of dough products. Additionally, it is used to improve the viscoelastic qualities of frozen meals. In order to improve oxygen delivery, dextran hemoglobin molecules are used as blood supplements and plasma expanders.

### *4.11.3 WASTEWATER TREATMENTS, BIOFILM AND BIOREMEDIATION*

Polysaccharides have demonstrated outstanding removal capability for a variety of contaminants, such as aromatic compounds, dyes, and heavy metal ions. The microbial polysaccharides used to make the sorbent material are very selective, have a high rate of adsorption, and have a high capacity for detoxifying (Mahmoud et al., 2021). Insoluble beads, gels, sponges, capsules, films, membranes, and fibers may all be made using them. Recently, the development of sorbents based on natural polysaccharides has received interest, with the majority of the focus being on the use of chitin, starch, and their derivatives. The capacity of many microbial polysaccharides to bind metals has also been demonstrated, and they have been proposed as prospective replacements for the extensively used traditional sorbents (Mahmoud et al., 2021). Bacteria like *Enterobacter* and *Pseudomonas* can break down or absorb harmful heavy metals when bioremediation procedures are used (Banerjee et al., 2021; Mahapatra et al., 2013; Osemwegie et al., 2020).

### 4.11.4 COSMETICS AND OTHER INDUSTRIAL USE

Bacterial polysaccharides have physicochemical characteristics that make them acceptable for usage as cosmetic components. They are biocompatible, biodegradable, and typically nontoxic natural biopolymers (Mahmoud et al., 2021). Hyaluronic acid (HA), BC, and levan are three of them that are employed as active ingredients in cosmetic formulations because of their biological features that include skin regeneration and protection. Other bacterial polysaccharides, such as xanthan gum and gellant gum, are utilized in cosmetic vehicles like emulsions, gels, and suspensions and are primarily employed as viscosity controllers and psych-sensorial agents. Levan is a blending ingredient in cosmetics and has been demonstrated to have great cell-proliferating, skin hydrating, and skin irritation-alleviating benefits. Due to pectin's great performance in the cosmetics industry, specifically for personal care product compositions, pectin has recently broadened its number of possible uses (Mzoughi et al., 2018). It has shown excellent activity as a skin anti-aging ingredient and as a stabilizer for shampoos and lotions. Another significant substance that is extensively used in the food and cosmetics sectors is starch derivatives made from native polysaccharides that have undergone chemical or physical alteration.

### 4.11.5 OTHER APPLICATIONS OF FUNGAL POLYSACCHARIDES

There are several uses for fungal EPSs in the food and pharmaceutical industries. Pullulan, scleroglucan, and botryosphaeran are a few of the several fungal EPSs (Briard et al., 2016; Cheng et al., 2011; Fontaine et al., 2011; Mahapatra et al., 2013; Moscovici, 2015). Pullulan, an EPS of *A. pullulans*, may be made into non-toxic, biodegradable, and edible plastics as well as utilized as a thickener and viscosity stabilizer in the food sector. EPS scleroglucan is developed in the oil industry for enhanced oil recovery. The commercial, bacterial polysaccharide known as xanthan gum is used to prepare drilling fluids (water-based muds) with minimal mud toxicity. Scleroglucan is often referred to as schizophyllan. This EPS was used in the manufacturing of adhesives, watercolors, printing inks, and animal feed composition, among other things. As a bio-sorbent for lead and zinc, the pestan, a fungal polysaccharide EPS produced by *Pestalotiopsis* species, has uses in waste-water treatment.

### *4.11.6 OTHER APPLICATIONS OF MICROALGAE/CYANOBACTERIA POLYSACCHARIDES*

A variety of polysaccharides with intriguing physicochemical characteristics and antioxidants may be produced by microalgae. Wan et al. isolated and purified polysaccharides from *Chlorella pyrenoidosa* microalga and assessed their impact on extending *Caenorhabditis* worms' lifespan (Wan et al., 2020). Due to an increase in the activity of an antioxidant enzyme like superoxide dismutase (SOD), they reported a reduction in ROS and lipid peroxidation. These microalgal polysaccharides may be able to slow down the ageing process and disorders linked to oxidative stress (Wan et al., 2020). Li et al. showed that Nostoc (Nostoglycan) polysaccharides can decrease ROS, prevent lipid peroxidation, and limit the growth of cancer cells (Li et al., 2020). Furthermore, due to properties like bioactivity and membrane permeability capacity, as well as effects on key plant mechanisms like photosynthesis, which also causes an increase in carotenoids and proteins, polysaccharides from microalgae and cyanobacteria have been studied for applications as plant bio-stimulants. Polysaccharides might thus be used to lessen the need for pesticides and support the development of sustainably farmed crops (Ahmed et al., 2014; Barborková et al., 2019; Bhunia et al., 2018; Naggar et al., 2020; Netanel Liberman et al., 2020; Wan et al., 2020).

The bio-remediation of various wastewater toxins has recently attracted the attention of researchers who are searching for ecologically acceptable alternatives. Extracellular polymeric components from *Cyanothece* species are used in this context to remove nano- and microplastics from water. Due to the high production costs, the diagnostic stage of EPS from microalgae, and the numerous existing proposals for its uses in a variety of fields, its use is often restricted to expensive products like food and nutraceuticals, cosmetics, and pharmaceuticals (De Jesus et al., 2018; Hussein et al., 2015; Li et al., 2020; Rossi et al., 2012; Trabelsi et al., 2016).

## 4.12 CONCLUSION

In conclusion, microbial polysaccharides are an important class of biopolymers with unique properties, which have found a potential role in biomedicine, the food industry, the cosmetics industry, and environmental applications. They require further research and exploration for better methods of not only production and purification but also applications. They offer safer alternatives to chemical synthetic polymers and compounds, especially in the healthcare, pharmaceutical, and food industry.

## KEYWORDS

- **capsular polysaccharides**
- **exopolysaccharides**
- **lipopolysaccharides**
- **microbial polysaccharides**
- **peptidoglycans**
- **teichoic acids**

## REFERENCES

Ahmed, M., Moerdijk-Poortvliet, T. C. W., Wijnholds, A., Stal, L. J., & Hasnain, S. (2014). Isolation, characterization and localization of extracellular polymeric substances from the cyanobacterium *Arthrospira platensis* strain MMG-9. *European Journal of Phycology, 49*, 143–150.

Ahmed, N. H., El Soda, M., Hassan, A. N., & Frank, J. (2005). Improving the textural properties of an acid-coagulated (Karish) cheese using exopolysaccharide producing cultures. *LWT–Food Science and Technology, 38*, 843–847.

Angelin, J., & Kavitha, M. (2020). Exopolysaccharides from probiotic bacteria and their health potential. *International Journal of Biological Macromolecules, 162*, 853–865.

Ates, O., Arga, K. Y., & Oner, E. T. (2013). The stimulatory effect of mannitol on Levan biosynthesis: Lessons from metabolic systems analysis of *Halomonas smyrnensis* AAD6(T). *Biotechnology Progress, 29*(6), 1386–1397.

Banerjee, A., Sarkar, S., Govil, T., González-Faune, P., Cabrera-Barjas, G., Bandopadhyay, R., Salem, D. R., & Sani, R. K. (2021). Extremophilic exopolysaccharides: Biotechnologies and wastewater remediation. *Frontiers in Microbiology, 12*, 721365.

Barboríková, J., Šutovská, M., Kazimierová, I., Jošková, M., Fraňová, S., Kopecký, J., & Capek, P. (2019). Extracellular polysaccharide produced by *Chlorella vulgaris*–Chemical characterization and anti-asthmatic profile. *International Journal of Biological Macromolecules, 135*, 1–11.

Barcelos, M. C. S., Vespermann, K. A. C., Pelissari, F. M., & Molina, G. (2020). Current status of biotechnological production and applications of microbial exopolysaccharides. *Critical Reviews in Food Science and Nutrition, 60*, 1475–1495.

Bertani, B., & Ruiz, N. (2018). Function and biogenesis of lipopolysaccharides. *EcoSal Plus, 8*, 10.

Bhunia, B., Prasad Uday, U. S., Oinam, G., Mondal, A., Bandyopadhyay, T. K., & Tiwari, O. N. (2018). Characterization, genetic regulation and production of cyanobacterial exopolysaccharides and its applicability for heavy metal removal. *Carbohydrate Polymers, 179*, 228–243.

Briard, B., Muszkieta, L., Latgé, J. P., & Fontaine, T. (2016). Galactosaminogalactan of *Aspergillus fumigatus*, a bioactive fungal polymer. *Mycologic, 108*, 572–580.

Brown, S., Santa Maria, J. P., Jr., & Walker, S. (2013). Wall teichoic acids of gram-positive bacteria. *Annual Review of Microbiology, 67*, 313–336.

Chaisuwan, W., Phimolsiripol, Y., Chaiyaso, T., Techapun, C., Leksawasdi, N., Jantanasakulwong, K., Rachtanapun, P., Wangtueai, S., Sommano, S. R., You, S., Regenstein, J. M., Barba, F. J., & Seesuriyachan, P. (2021). The antiviral activity of bacterial, fungal, and algal polysaccharides as bioactive ingredients: Potential uses for enhancing immune systems and preventing viruses. *Frontiers in Nutrition, 8*, 772033.

Chen, J. K., Shen, C. R., & Liu, C. L. (2010). N-acetylglucosamine: Production and applications. *Marine Drugs, 8*, 2493–2516.

Chen, L., Ge, M. D., & Zhu, Y. J. (2019). Structure, bioactivity and applications of natural hyperbranched polysaccharides. *Carbohydrate Polymers, 223*, 115076.

Cheng, K. C., Demirci, A., & Catchmark, J. M. (2011). Pullulan: Biosynthesis, production, and applications. *Applied Microbiology and Biotechnology, 92*, 29–44.

Choi, S. M., Rao, K. M., Zo, S. M., Shin, E. J., & Han, S. S. (2022). Bacterial cellulose and its applications. *Polymers (Basel), 14*, 1080.

Costa, J. A. V., Lucas, B. F., Alvarenga, A. G. P., Moreira, J. B., & De Morais, M. G. (2021). Microalgae polysaccharides: An overview of production, characterization, and potential applications. *Polysaccharides, 2*, 759–772.

Costa, L. S., Fidelis, G. P., & Cordeiro, S. L. (2010). Biological activities of sulfated polysaccharides from tropical seaweeds. *Biomedicine & Pharmacotherapy, 64*, 21–28.

Costa, O. Y. A., Raaijmakers, J. M., & Kuramae, E. E. (2018). Microbial extracellular polymeric substances: Ecological function and impact on soil aggregation. *Frontiers in Microbiology, 9*, 1636.

Cress, B. F., Englaender, J. A., He, W., Kasper, D., Linhardt, R. J., & Koffas, M. A. (2014). Masquerading microbial pathogens: Capsular polysaccharides mimic host-tissue molecules. *FEMS Microbiology Reviews, 38*, 660–697.

De Castro, C., Parrilli, M., Holst, O., & Molinaro, A. (2010). Microbe-associated molecular patterns in innate immunity: Extraction and chemical analysis of gram-negative bacterial lipopolysaccharides. *Methods in Enzymology, 480*, 89–115.

De Jesus, C. S., De Jesus Assis, D., Rodriguez, M. B., Menezes Filho, J. A., Costa, J. A. V., De Souza Ferreira, E., & Druzian, J. I. (2019). Pilot-scale isolation and characterization of extracellular polymeric substances (EPS) from cell-free medium of *Spirulina* sp. LEB-18 cultures under outdoor conditions. *International Journal of Biological Macromolecules, 124*, 1106–1114.

Dolganyuk, V., Belova, D., Babich, O., Prosekov, A., Ivanova, S., Katserov, D., Patyukov, N., & Sukhikh, S. (2020). Microalgae: A promising source of valuable bioproducts. *Biomolecules, 10*, 1153.

El-Naggar, N. E., Hussein, M. H., Shaaban-Dessuuki, S. A., & Dalal, S. R. (2020). Production, extraction and characterization of *Chlorella vulgaris* soluble polysaccharides and their applications in AgNPs biosynthesis and bio stimulation of plant growth. *Scientific Reports, 10*, 3011.

Farhana, A., & Khan, Y. S. (2022). *Biochemistry, Lipopolysaccharide*. In StatPearls [Internet]. Treasure Island (FL): Stat Pearls Publishing. https://www.ncbi.nlm.nih.gov/books/NBK526012/ (accessed on 5th November 2025).

Fontaine, T., Delangle, A., Simenel, C., Coddeville, B., Van Vliet, S. J., Van Kooyk, Y., Bozza, S., Moretti, S., Schwarz, F., Trichot, C., Aebi, M., Delepierre, M., Elbim, C., Romani, L., & Latgé, J. P. (2011). Galactosaminogalactan, a new immunosuppressive polysaccharide of *Aspergillus fumigatus*. *PLoS Pathogens, 7*, e1002372. https://doi.org/10.1371/journal.ppat.1002372 (accessed on 5th November 2025).

Freitas, F., Alves, V. D., & Reis, M. A. M. (2015). Bacterial polysaccharides: Production and applications in cosmetic industry. In *Polysaccharides* (pp. 2017–2043). Springer. https://doi.org/10.1007/978-3-319-16298-0_45 (accessed on 5th November 2025).

Green, E. R., & Mecsas, J. (2016). Bacterial secretion systems: An overview. *Microbiology Spectrum, 4*, 10.

Gupta, A., Sharma, V., Sharma, K., Kumar, V., Choudhary, S., Mankotia, P., Kumar, B., Mishra, H., Moulick, A., Ekielski, A., & Mishra, P. K. (2021). A review of adsorbents for heavy metal decontamination: Growing approach to wastewater treatment. *Materials (Basel), 14*, 4702.

Han, L., & Costello, C. E. (2013). Mass spectrometry of glycans. *Biochemistry (Moscow), 78*, 710–720.

He, W., Wu, J., Xu, J., Mosselhy, D. A., Zheng, Y., & Yang, S. (2021). Bacterial cellulose: Functional modification and wound healing applications. *Advances in Wound Care (New Rochelle), 10*, 623–640.

Hussein, M., Abou-ElWafa, G. S., Shaaban-Dessuuki, S. A., & Hassan, N. I. (2015). Characterization and antioxidant activity of exopolysaccharide secreted by *Nostoc carneum*. *International Journal of Pharmacy, 11*, 432–439.

Jackson, P. (1990). The use of polyacrylamide-gel electrophoresis for the high-resolution separation of reducing saccharides labelled with the fluorophore 8-aminonaphthalene-1,3,6-trisulphonic acid. Detection of picomolar quantities by an imaging system based on a cooled charge-coupled device. *Biochemical Journal, 270*, 705–713.

Jiao, G., Yu, G., Zhang, J., & Ewart, H. S. (2011). Chemical structures and bioactivities of sulfated polysaccharides from marine algae. *Marine Drugs, 9*, 196–223.

Jin, T., Mohammad, M., Pullerits, R., & Ali, A. (2021). Bacteria and host interplay in *Staphylococcus aureus* septic arthritis and sepsis. *Pathogens, 10*, 158.

Kamerling, J. P., & Gerwig, G. J. (2007). Strategies for the structural analysis of carbohydrates. In *Comprehensive Glycoscience: From Chemistry to Systems Biology, 2*, 1–68.

Khan, T., Park, J. K., & Kwon, J. H. (2007). Functional biopolymers produced by biochemical technology considering applications in food engineering. *Korean Journal of Chemical Engineering, 24*, 816–826.

Kornberg, A., Rao, N. N., & Ault-Riché, D. (1999). Inorganic polyphosphate: a molecule of many functions. *Annual Review of Biochemistry, 68*, 89–125.

Kurutas, E. B. (2016). The importance of antioxidants which play the role in cellular response against oxidative/nitrosative stress: current state. *Nutrition Journal, 15*, 71.

Larsen, A. H., Wang, Y., Bottaro, S., Grudinin, S., Arleth, L., & Lindorff-Larsen, K. (2020). Combining molecular dynamics simulations with small-angle X-ray and neutron scattering data to study multi-domain proteins in solution. *PLoS Computational Biology, 16*, e1007870.

Li, Y., Wang, C., Liu, H., Su, J., Lan, C. Q., Zhong, M., & Hu, X. (2020). Production, isolation and bioactive estimation of extracellular polysaccharides of green microalga *Neochloris oleoabundans*. *Algal Research, 48*, 101883.

Liberman, G. N., Ochbaum, G., Mejubovsky-Mikhelis, M., Bitton, R., & Malis Arad, S. (2020). Physic-chemical characteristics of the sulfated polysaccharides of the red microalgae *Dixoniella grisea* and *Porphyridium aerugineum*. *International Journal of Biological Macromolecules, 145*, 1171–1179.

Limoli, D. H., Jones, C. J., & Wozniak, D. J. (2015). Bacterial extracellular polysaccharides in biofilm formation and function. *Microbiology Spectrum, 3*, 10.

Mahapatra, S., & Banerjee, D. (2013). Fungal exopolysaccharide: production, composition and applications. *Microbiology Insights, 6*, 1–16.

Mahmoud, Y. A., El-Naggar, M. E., Abdel-Megeed, A., & El-Newehy, M. (2021). Recent advancements in microbial polysaccharides: synthesis and applications. *Polymers (Basel), 13*, 4136.

Meng, X., Liang, H., & Luo, L. (2016). Antitumor polysaccharides from mushrooms: a review on the structural characteristics, antitumor mechanisms and immunomodulating activities. *Carbohydrate Research, 424*, 30–41.

Mohammed, A. S. A., Naveed, M., & Jost, N. (2021). Polysaccharides; classification, chemical properties, and future perspective applications in fields of pharmacology and biological medicine (a review of current applications and upcoming potentialities). *Journal of Polymers and the Environment, 29*, 2359–2371.

Mohd Nadzir, M., Nurhayati, R. W., Idris, F. N., & Nguyen, M. H. (2021). Biomedical applications of bacterial exopolysaccharides: a review. *Polymers (Basel), 13*, 530.

Morrissey, J. H., Choi, S. H., & Smith, S. A. (2012). Polyphosphate: an ancient molecule that links platelets, coagulation, and inflammation. *Blood, 119*, 5972–5979.

Moscovici, M. (2015). Present and future medical applications of microbial exopolysaccharides. *Frontiers in Microbiology, 6*, 1012.

Mostowy, R. J., & Holt, K. E. (2018). Diversity-generating machines: genetics of bacterial sugar-coating. *Trends in Microbiology, 26*, 1008–1021.

Mzoughi, Z., Abdelhamid, A., Rihouey, C., Le Cerf, D., Bouraoui, A., & Majdoub, H. (2018). Optimized extraction of pectin-like polysaccharide from *Suaeda fruticosa* leaves: characterization, antioxidant, anti-inflammatory and analgesic activities. *Carbohydrate Polymers, 185*, 127–137.

Navarre, W. W., & Schneewind, O. (1999). Surface proteins of gram-positive bacteria and mechanisms of their targeting to the cell wall envelope. *Microbiology and Molecular Biology Reviews, 63*, 174–229.

Nikolova, M. P., & Chavali, M. S. (2020). Metal oxide nanoparticles as biomedical materials. *Biomimetics (Basel), 5*, 27.

Nwodo, U. U., Green, E., & Okoh, A. I. (2012). Bacterial exopolysaccharides: functionality and prospects. *International Journal of Molecular Sciences, 13*, 14002–14015.

Oner, E. T. (2013). Microbial production of extracellular polysaccharides from biomass. In Z. Fang (Ed.), *Pretreatment Techniques for Biofuel and Biorefineries* (pp. 35–56). Springer-Verlag Berlin Germany.

Osemwegie, O. O., Adetunji, C. O., Ayeni, E. A., Adejobi, O. I., Arise, R. O., Nwonuma, C. O., & Oghenekaro, A. O. (2020). Exopolysaccharides from bacteria and fungi: current status and perspectives in Africa. *Helion, 6*, e04205.

Osińska-Jaroszuk, M., Jarosz-Wilkołazka, A., Jaroszuk-Ściseł, J., Szałapata, K., Nowak, A., Jaszek, M., Ozimek, E., & Majewska, M. (2015). Extracellular polysaccharides from Ascomycota and Basidiomycota: production conditions, biochemical characteristics, and biological properties. *World Journal of Microbiology and Biotechnology, 31*, 1823–1844.

Pandya, U., Dhuldhaj, U., & Sahay, N. S. (2019). Bioactive mushroom polysaccharides as antitumor: an overview. *Natural Product Research, 33*, 2668–2680.

Patel, S., Majumder, A., & Goyal, A. (2012). Potentials of exopolysaccharides from lactic acid bacteria. *Indian Journal of Microbiology, 52*, 3–12.

Ramalingam, C., Jhanu, P., & Shraddha, M. (2014). Applications of microbial polysaccharides in food industry. *International Journal of Pharmaceutical Sciences Review and Research, 27*, 322–324.

Ren, L., Perera, C., & Hemar, Y. (2012). Antitumor activity of mushroom polysaccharides: a review. *Food & Function, 3*, 1118–1130.

Ren, Y., Bai, Y., Zhang, Z., Cai, W., & Del Rio Flores, A. (2019). The preparation and structure analysis methods of natural polysaccharides of plants and fungi: A review of recent development. *Molecules, 24*, 3122.

Roca, C., Alves, V. D., Freitas, F., & Reis, M. A. (2015). Exopolysaccharides enriched in rare sugars: bacterial sources, production, and applications. *Frontiers in Microbiology, 6*, 288.

Rossi, F., Micheletti, E., Bruno, L., Adhikary, S. P., Albertano, P., & Philippis, R. D. (2012). Characteristics and role of the exocellular polysaccharides produced by five cyanobacteria isolated from phototrophic biofilms growing on stone monuments. *Biofouling, 28*, 215–224.

Salazar, N., Gueimonde, M., Reyes-Gavilan, C. G. D. L., & Madiedo, P. R. (2016). Exopolysaccharides produced by lactic acid bacteria and bifidobacteria as fermentable substrates by the intestinal microbiota. *Critical Reviews in Food Science and Nutrition, 56*, 1440–1453.

Salton, M., & Kim, K. S. (1996). Structure. In S. Baron (Ed.), *Medical Microbiology* (4th ed.). University of Texas Medical Branch at Galveston.

Sarwat, F., Ul Qader, S. A., Aman, A., & Ahmed, N. (2008). Production & characterization of a unique dextran from an indigenous *Leuconostoc mesenteroides* CMG713. *International Journal of Biological Sciences, 4*, 379–386.

Schepetkin, I. A., & Quinn, M. T. (2006). Botanical polysaccharides: macrophage immunomodulation and therapeutic potential. *International Immunopharmacology, 6*, 317–333.

Schmid, J., Sieber, V., & Rehm, B. (2015). Bacterial exopolysaccharides: biosynthesis pathways and engineering strategies. *Frontiers in Microbiology, 6*, 496.

Silhavy, T. J., Kahne, D., & Walker, S. (2010). The bacterial cell envelope. *Cold Spring Harbor Perspectives in Biology, 2*, a000414.

Soumya, M. P., & Nampoothiri, K. M. (2021). An overview of functional genomics and relevance of glycosyltransferases in exopolysaccharide production by lactic acid bacteria. *International Journal of Biological Macromolecules, 184*, 1014–1025.

Swoboda, J. G., Campbell, J., Meredith, T. C., & Walker, S. (2010). Wall teichoic acid function, biosynthesis, and inhibition. *Chembiochem, 11*, 35–45.

Torino, M. I., Valdez, G. F. D., & Mozzi, F. (2015). Biopolymers from lactic acid bacteria: novel applications in foods and beverages. *Frontiers in Microbiology, 6*, 834.

Trabelsi, L., Chaieb, O., Mnari, A., Abid-Essafi, S., & Aleya, L. (2016). Partial characterization and antioxidant and antiproliferative activities of the aqueous extracellular polysaccharides from the thermophilic microalgae *Graesiella* sp. *BMC Complementary and Alternative Medicine, 16*, 210.

Ullah, S., Khalil, A. A., Shaukat, F., & Song, Y. (2019). Sources, extraction and biomedical properties of polysaccharides. *Foods, 8*, 304.

Valverde, M. E., Hernández-Pérez, T., & Paredes-López, O. (2015). Edible mushrooms: improving human health and promoting quality life. *International Journal of Microbiology, 2015*, 376387.

Wan, X. Z., Ai, C., Chen, Y. H., Gao, X. X., Zhong, R. T., Liu, B., Chen, X. H., & Zhao, C. (2020). Physicochemical characterization of a polysaccharide from green microalga *Chlorella pyrenoidosa* and its hypolipidemic activity via gut microbiota regulation in rats. *Journal of Agricultural and Food Chemistry, 68*, 1186–1197.

Wang, Z., Dordick, J. S., & Linhardt, R. J. (2011). *Escherichia coli* K5 heparosan fermentation and improvement by genetic engineering. *Bioengineered Bugs, 2*, 63–67.

Wiseman, B., Nitharwal, R. G., Widmalm, G., & Högbom, M. (2021). Structure of a full-length bacterial polysaccharide co-polymerase. *Nature Communications, 12*, 369.

Xu, C., Willför, S., Holmlund, P., & Holmbom, B. (2009). Rheological properties of water-soluble spruce O-acetyl galactoglucomannans. *Carbohydrate Polymers, 75*, 498–504.

Yadav, P., Yadav, H., Shah, V. G., Shah, G., & Dhaka, G. (2015). Biomedical biopolymers, their origin and evolution in biomedical sciences: A systematic review. *Journal of Clinical and Diagnostic Research, 9*, ZE21–ZE25.

Yang, K., Wang, Z., Nakajima, T., Nishinari, K., & Brenner, T. (2013). The effect of degradation on κ-carrageenan/locust bean gum/konjac glucomannan gels at acidic pH. *Carbohydrate Polymers, 98*, 744–749.

Yu, M. K., Park, J., & Jon, S. (2012). Targeting strategies for multifunctional nanoparticles in cancer imaging and therapy. *Theragnostic, 2*, 3–44.

Zayed, A., Mansour, M. K., Sedeek, M. S., Habib, M. H., Ulber, R., & Farag, M. (2022). Rediscovering bacterial exopolysaccharides of terrestrial and marine origins: novel insights on their distribution, biosynthesis, biotechnological production, and future perspectives. *Critical Reviews in Biotechnology, 42*, 597–617.

Zong, A., Cao, H., & Wang, F. (2012). Anticancer polysaccharides from natural resources: a review of recent research. *Carbohydrate Polymers, 90*, 1395–1410.

CHAPTER 5

# From Microbial World to Industry: Role of Enzymes

HARISH CHANDRA,[1] ARCHANA YADAV,[2,*] KALPANA SAGAR,[1,*] VIRENDRA KUMAR,[3] NITIN BHARDWAJ,[4] KARTIKEY KUMAR GUPTA,[1] and SWINDER JEET SINGH KALRA[5]

[1]*Department of Botany and Microbiology, Gurukula Kangri (Deemed to be University), Haridwar, Uttarakhand, India*

[2]*Department of Microbiology, Institute of Biosciences and Biotechnology, C.S.J.M. University, Kanpur, Uttar Pradesh, India*

[3]*Department of NMR, All India Institute of Medical Sciences, New Delhi, Delhi, India*

[4]*Department of Zoology and Environmental Sciences, Gurukula Kangri (Deemed to be University), Haridwar, Uttarakhand, India*

[5]*Department of Chemistry, DAV College, Kanpur, Uttar Pradesh, India*

*Corresponding author

## ABSTRACT

Natural resources such as herbs, minerals, and animal products are important sources of raw materials in the pharmaceutical industry. Due to the increasing population and the development of lifestyle-related diseases such as high blood pressure, gastrointestinal disturbances, diabetes, and other ailments, immense pressure is put on pharmaceutical industries to meet the demand. Therefore, the exploitation of these natural resources for producing medicines has increased, resulting in the scarcity of raw materials or the cost of the product. Microorganisms, particularly fungi

Industrial Biotechnology: Current Progress and Novel Technologies.
Prakash Kumar Sarangi, Akhilesh Kumar Singh, Rajesh Kumar Srivastava, and Brijesh Pandey (Eds.)


DOI: 10.1201/9781779642233-5

and bacteria, are good sources of primary and secondary metabolites, and these metabolites are important sources of enzymes, which can be easily exploited to produce industrially important products. This chapter focused on the important microbial enzymes, which can be exploited for the production of pharmaceutical products.

## 5.1 INTRODUCTION

The microbial source is another important aspect of industrial applications, and it has been exploited since time immemorial. In ancient literature, the making of curd and alcoholic beverages was well documented. Most of the pharmaceutical and liquor industries are dependent on industrially important microbes, that is, bacteria and fungi. Since the discovery of Penicillin, antibiotic researchers have been in continuous search of new active metabolites from microbes that have an industrially important attribute. Microbial enzymes do not always have a beneficial effect; they often have deleterious effects as well.

The market for microbial enzymes was estimated to be 9.9 billion USD in 2019 and is expected to grow at a CAGR of 7.1% between 2020 and 2027 (Enzymes Market Size, Share, and Trends Analysis Report by Application, 2020). The reasons behind the burgeoning interest in microbes as a source of microbial enzymes for therapeutic agents are that they are easy to cultivate in medium and can be exploited for mass production, the cost of production is low or economical, and they can be easily purified (Vachher et al., 2021). Microbes are troves of various metabolites or biocatalysts for carrying out various biochemical reactions. Further, the interest in enzymes is due to their vast application in the food industry, pharmaceuticals, cosmetics, diagnostics, therapeutics, beverages, paper, and pulp industries, for the production of animal feed, detergent industries, and so on (Mehta and Sehgal, 2019) (Figure 5.1). The sources of enzymes can be animals, plants, or microorganisms. The ease of handling, modification, increased effectiveness, and stability of microbial enzymes, however, make them favored over other sources because they can be produced in large numbers quickly via fermentation on a variety of cheap, widely available, and very diversified carbon and nitrogen sources. They are thought to be potentially promising candidates for industrial uses.

The isolation and characterization of industrially important microbes from different sources such as soil, water, and air can be proven beneficial, but microorganisms from extreme environments such as cold environments, hot springs, marine environments, and harsh environments can be important and novel sources of enzymes and other metabolites which are less explored. These places are not much explored or investigated by researchers from different countries. Diseases such as Dengue, SARS, MERS, Japanese Encephalitis, Cancer, and the recent SARS-CoV-2 pandemic pose challenges to scientific communities in their efforts to develop a treatment for this potentially fatal entity. The recent SARS CoV2 pandemic brought most developed or developing countries to their knees in terms of economy and medical facilities; medical facilities during the first and second waves of COVID-19 became inappropriate, and millions of deaths were recorded worldwide due to a lack of sufficient oxygen cylinders or life-saving drugs (Bhardwaj and Chandra, 2021). In search of treatment, people use all their scientific skills to find an efficient treatment, but still no effective treatment or process has been devised. Nowadays, scientific communities are exploring microbial enzymes that show some promising attributes against pathogenic bacteria, viruses, fungi, and cancer. The present chapter focuses on some of the important properties and activities of industrially important microbial enzymes.

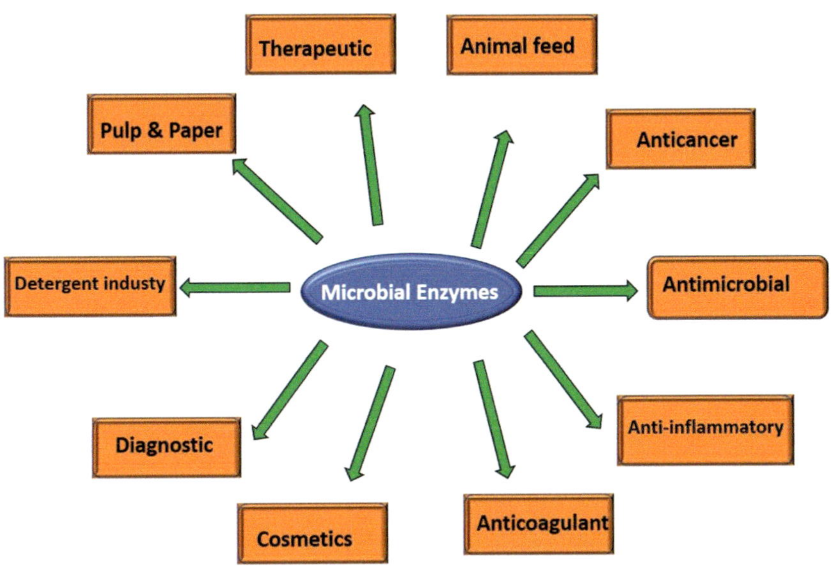


**FIGURE 5.1** Application of microbial enzyme in different fields.

## 5.2 MICROBIAL ENZYMES USED IN DETERGENT INDUSTRIES

The detergent sector, which accounts for 30–40% of all industrial enzymes, is the largest sector and is growing at a faster rate day by day. The stability of enzymes is an important factor for the detergent industry because detergent enzymes should act in the presence of bleaching agents, surfactants, builders, and other enzymes. Alkaline proteases are widely used and more suitable for basic washing conditions as they are used in the formulation of detergents for the degradation of stains such as food, blood, and body secretions (Jain et al., 2012).

Children and adults frequently get food stains on their clothing while eating, and these stains are most likely made of starch, protein, or lipids. These stains can be eliminated by vigorously combining detergents with hot water at high temperatures. However, this procedure is expensive since it involves boiling the water and time-consuming because it involves mixing or beating, which reduces the lifespan of clothing. Utilizing microbial enzymes enables lower temperatures and shorter agitation times. Microbial enzyme detergents remove stains from clothes more effectively than non-enzymatic detergents. Cellulases promote the loosening of the fibers, which helps to remove the stain easily, and during washing, they digest fine fibers to provide a final touch. Proteases, amylases, cellulases, and lipases are the most popular types of enzymes utilized in the detergent industry (Table 5.1). For the manufacture of detergent, only a very small quantity of these enzymes—approximately 0.4–0.8% crude enzyme by weight (around 1% in terms of cost) is used. These enzymes are also active at low temperatures and at alkaline pH.

**TABLE 5.1** Microbial Enzymes Used in Detergent Industries

| Sl. No. | Enzyme | Function | Microorganisms | References |
|---|---|---|---|---|
| 1. | Amylase | Carbohydrate stain removal | *Bacillus subtilis*, *Aspergillus* sp. | Yassin et al. (2021) |
| 2. | Cellulase | Color clarification | *Aspergillus niger*, *Bacillus* sp. | Kim et al. (2012); Sulyman et al. (2020) |
| 3. | Cutinase | Triglyceride removal | *Fusarium solani f.* sp. *pisi* | Egmond et al. (2002) |
| 4. | Lipase | Fat stain elimination | *A. flavus*, *Aspergillus oryzae* | Kareem et al. (2017); Li et al. (2021) |
| 5. | Mannanase | Mannan spot removal | *Bacillus sp.* | Liu et al. (2021) |
| 6. | Protease | Protein stain removal | *Aspergillus oryzae*, *Bacillus subtilis* | Gao et al. (2019); Mahmoud et al. (2021) |

## 5.3 MICROBIAL ENZYMES USED IN THE PAPER AND PULP INDUSTRIES

Food preparation using microorganisms is an age-old process (Raveendran et al., 2018). In the food industry, microorganisms like fungi, yeast, and bacteria are frequently used not only to improve taste and quality but also to provide significant economic benefits. Advanced technology such as strain improvement has also improved the activity and specificity of microbial enzymes, resulting in their use at a wide range of physiological parameters such as pH and temperature for various applications. The fermentation technology using microorganisms has been used since ancient times and is still applied in the food industry. Using microbial enzymes reduces the cost, time as well as space (Gurung et al., 2013). Enzymes are used in a variety of applications in the food industry, including starch hydrolysis, the brewing industry, the beverages industry, the baking industry, the juice industry, and the dairy industry.

Cellulases are microbial enzymes that are used to deink cellulose fibers during recycling. Amylases are employed specifically to modify starch when creating paper, which improves the paper's stiffness, strength, and erasability. The viscosity of the starch suspension is achieved by the addition of the amylase enzyme. The pitch in the paper and pulp industry is composed of lipids which are mainly present in softwoods. Pitch causes problems for the paper machine due to lipid content. Therefore, lipases are used to remove the pitch (Table 5.2).

**TABLE 5.2** Microbial Enzymes Used in Paper and Pulp Industries

| Sl. No. | Enzyme | Function | Microorganisms | References |
|---|---|---|---|---|
| 1. | Amylase | Deinking, drainage improvement | *Bacillus licheniformis* | Hmidet et al. (2008) |
| 2. | Cellulase | Deinking, drainage improvement | *Aspergillus niger*, *Bacillus* sp. | Li et al. (2018); Ncube et al. (2012) |
| 3. | Lipase | Pitch control | *Candida antarctica* | Carniel et al. (2017) |
| 4. | Laccase | Non-chlorine bleaching, delignification | *Bacillus subtilis* | Gangola et al. (2018) |
| 5. | Protease | Biofilm removal | *Bacillus subtilis* | Pant et al. (2015) |
| 6. | Xylanase | Bleach boosting | *Trichoderma reesei*, *Thermomyces lanuginosus*, *Aureobasidium pullulans* | Gauterio et al. (2021); Jampala et al. (2017); Shrivastava et al. (2011) |

## 5.4 MICROBIAL ENZYMES IN FOOD INDUSTRY

The starch-degrading enzyme in the food business was the first microbial enzyme to be used extensively. Two enzymes, alpha-amylase and glucoamylase, convert starch into glucose throughout this process (Pandey et al., 2008). Pullulans and a few other debranching enzymes are also utilized to increase the glucose output. The enzyme beta-amylase, which is made from barley grains, produces the disaccharide maltose (Selvakumar et al., 1996). The enzyme transglutaminase is a texturing agent and is also used for the processing of noodles, yogurt, and sausages. Bacterial and fungal alpha-amylases are widely used for the improvement of bread quality and also to increase shelf life. Both fungal and bacterial amylases are used. Xylanases are used to provide more stable dough by decreasing the water absorption in baking industries and, therefore, reducing the amount of water required in baking. Proteinases are used to improve the properties of dough-handling, while glucose oxidase is used to replace chemical oxidants. The enzyme lipase is used to strengthen gluten to provide better bread quality. Galactosidase is used to break down lactose from milk into glucose and galactose, and chymosin is added to the cheese-making process to help milk proteins coagulate. Consumers who are lactose intolerant use these modified milk products. Fruit juice production makes better use of pectinase, xylanase, and cellulase to better separate the juice from the pulp. Pectinases and amylases are the enzymes utilized in the clearing of juice. Wine production also makes extensive use of pectinases to achieve greater extraction and a high yield (Table 5.3).

Dairy enzymes are another component of the food business, utilized to improve the yields of milk-based products as well as to produce and enhance organoleptic qualities including scent, flavor, and color. For the mass manufacture of cheese and the coagulation of milk into curds, Rennet, a mixture of pepsin and chymosin, is employed. To improve the quality and shelf life of dairy products, such as cheese, yogurt, and milk products, enzymes such aminopeptidase, catalase, esterases, lipases, lactase, lysozyme, proteases, and transglutaminase are utilized (Kuraishi et al., 2001). Microbial enzymes are widely used in the beverage industry in breweries to digest the cell walls of plant material to provide color, aroma, and clearer products and also to produce good yields and high-quality products (Karlund et al., 2014).

**TABLE 5.3** Microbial Enzymes Used in Food Industry

| Sl. No. | Enzyme | Function | Microorganisms | References |
|---|---|---|---|---|
| 1. | Amylase | Starch hydrolysis, bread softness | *Aspergillus* sp., *Bacillus* sp. | Kubrak et al. (2010); Suganthi et al. (2011) |
| 2. | Maltogenic alpha-amylase | lengthen the loaves' shelf lives | *Bacillus stearothermophilus* | Straksys et al. (2016) |
| 3. | Aminopeptidase | rapid ripening of cheese | *Lactobacillus* sp. | Stressler et al. (2016) |
| 4. | Lipase | rapid ripening of cheese, flavor customized cheese, dough stability, and conditioning | *Aspergillus niger, A. oryzae* | Helal et al. (2021); Nema et al. (2019) |
| 5. | Lactase (Beta-galactosidase) | Lactose reduced milk and whey products | *Escherichia coli, Kluyveromyces* sp. | Alves et al. (2019); Duan et al. (2017) |
| 6. | Acid proteinase | Milk coagulation | *Aspergillus* sp. | Shivakumar et al. (2012) |
| 7. | Glucose oxidase | Dough strengthening | *Aspergillus niger, Penicillium chrysogenum* | Konishi et al. (2013); Leskovac et al. (2005) |
| 8. | Neutral proteinase | Faster cheese ripening, debittering | *Bacillus subtilis, A. oryzae* | Ao et al. (2018); Padmapriya et al. (2012) |
| 9. | Catalase | Cheese processing | *Aspergillus niger* | Eberhardt et al. (2004) |
| 10. | Transglutaminase | Protein cross linking, laminated dough strength | *Streptomyces* sp., *Streptoverticillium* sp. | Ceresino et al. (2018); Lin et al. (2004) |
| 11. | Xylanase | Dough conditioning | *Aspergillus niger* | Uday et al. (2017) |
| 12. | Protease | Restrict haze formation | *Aspergillus niger* | Purushothaman et al. (2019) |
| 13. | Pullulanase | Starch saccharification | *Bacillus* sp., *Klebsiella* sp. | Francetic and Pugsley (2005); Kunamneni et al. (2006) |
| 14. | Cellulase | Fruit liquefaction | *Aspergillus niger, Trichoderma atroviride* | Fang et al. (2018); Ncube et al. (2012) |

## 5.5 MICROBIAL ENZYMES AS ANIMAL FEED

As helpful additives, enzymes are crucial to the animal feed business. Endogenous enzymes are those produced by the animal itself or by the microorganisms that live naturally in the animal's stomach and are used by animals to digest food (Table 5.4). About 25% of the feed used by pigs and poultry is indigestible because it contains components that are difficult for animals to digest. Animal feed enzymes can be added to the diet formulation process to help break down toxic or nutritionally inert indigestible feed components. The microbial enzymes utilized in industries decrease viscosity, improve nutrient absorption, and encourage nutrient release either by hydrolysis of non-degradable fibers or by releasing nutrients obstructed by these fibers. Animal feed industries use four different categories of enzymes based on their requirements: (1) Phytate-targeting enzymes; (2) Enzymes that target viscous cereals (for example, barley); (3) non-viscous cereal enzymes (e.g., maize, jowar); and (4) Noncereal and legume enzymes (e.g., linseed meal).

In the production of animal feed, microbial enzymes are included at high temperatures (80–90°C). Therefore, during the production of feed, these enzymes must be thermally stable. The addition of β-glucans to the feed encourages the weight gain of animals by lowering viscosity, which is caused by the presence of β-glucan in animal feed derived from barley. Phosphodiesterase, or Phytase, is added to plant-based feed components to release the phosphate from the phytic acid. Phytase reduces the amount of phosphorous in animal feces, which reduces environmental pollution (Selle et al., 2009). Phytase also minimizes the requirement to add phosphorus to the feed. Phytases isolated from fungal sources are potent feed enzymes (Pandey et al., 2011). The use of another important enzyme, xylanase, in wheat-based feed increases metabolizable energy by 7–10%. The preparation of multienzyme cocktails using guanase's, xylanases, proteinases, and amylases for animal feed is very effective in the animal feed industry (Adeola et al., 2011).

**TABLE 5.4** Microbial Enzymes Used as Animal Feed

| Sl. No. | Enzyme | Function | Microorganisms | References |
|---|---|---|---|---|
| 1. | Phytase | Breakdown of phytic acid to liberate phosphorous | *Aspergillus niger* | Monteiro et al. (2015) |
| 2. | Beta-glucanase | Digestive aid | *Aspergillus niger* | Heidary et al. (2021) |
| 3. | Xylanase | Improved digestibility of starch | *Aspergillus* sp., *Bacillus* sp. | Irfan et al. (2016); Thomas et al. (2016) |

## 5.6 MICROBIAL ENZYMES IN DISEASE DIAGNOSTIC

Diagnosis is an important aspect of medical science. Without a diagnosis, it is not possible to get treatment specifically for any disease. The medical practitioner prescribed some of the enzyme-based diagnoses such as ELISA, PCR, RT-PCR, and other enzyme-based tests, which are proving to be important diagnostic tools in the medical field. It helps the medical practitioner detect the disease in its early stages so that the patient will get treatment on time. The advantages of microbial enzymes over other options include their economic viability, high yields, consistency, ease of product modification and optimization, lack of seasonal fluctuations in supply, rapid microbial growth on low-cost media, stability, and increased catalytic activity (Gurung et al., 2013). The presence of elevated levels of microbial enzymes in the bodies of human beings is indicative of infection and can be a useful indicator for the diagnosis of certain diseases.

## 5.7 MICROBIAL ENZYME AS THERAPEUTICS

### *5.7.1 ANTICANCER ACTIVITY*

Cancer is one of the leading diseases and causes the death of many people in India as well as in other countries. The leading causes of cancer are environmental factors, genetic factors, and a sedentary lifestyle. Environmental factors include the emission of poisonous gases from industry, smoking, chewing tobacco, and irrational use of pesticides for increasing the productivity of crops. Medical sciences somehow manage the disease, but at the ground level, the treatment is expensive and does not have a patient-friendly approach; most deaths are reported during chemotherapy and radiotherapy. During treatment, there are drastic changes that appear in the blood profile. All the components of the blood profile decrease, but to save life, the treatment should be continued until the patient is cured. However, medical researchers are in continuous search of new alternatives, and hope is seen in microbial-based enzymes (Table 5.5) such as L-Asparaginase, L-Glutaminase, L-Tyrosinase, and Galactosidase. L-Asparaginases isolated from *Bacillus licheniformis* from the Red Sea showed anticancer activity against HepG-2 cells, MCF-7, and HCT-116 cells (Alrumman et al., 2019). The colorectal adenocarcinoma cells LS 174 T and HCT 116 were extensively damaged by the enzyme's (L-Glutaminase) anticancer efficiency (IC50: 7.0 g/mL and 13.2 g/mL, respectively) (Mostafa et al., 2021). The effectiveness of L-glutaminase as an anticancer agent was also evaluated using the *in vitro* MTT assay against five different types of human cancer cell lines (Table 5.5). L-glutaminase has little effect on the proliferation of MCF-7 cells but is quite effective against Hep-G2 and HeLa cells (IC50, 6.8 and 8.3 g/mL, respectively). On RAW 264.7 and HCT-116 cells, L-glutaminase had a modest cytotoxic effect (IC50: 59.3 g/mL and 64.7 g/mL, respectively) (Reda et al., 2015). Further, the mechanism of action of microbial enzymes produced by the bacteria may be due to the bacterial endotoxin's indirect killing of cancer cells, causing hemorrhagic necrosis, which in turn causes circulatory stasis and ischemia in the tumor. Tumor Necrosis Factor (TNF) facilitates endotoxin-induced tumor necrosis and may be the cause of altered cells being suppressed by activated macrophages (Carswell et al., 1975).

**TABLE 5.5** Microbial Enzymes as Anticancer Agents

| Sl. No. | Name of Microorganism | Anticancer Molecule | Cell Line | References |
|---|---|---|---|---|
| 1. | *Bacillus licheniformis* | L-Asparaginases | HepG-2 cells, MCF-7 and HCT-116 | Alrumman et al. (2019) |
| 2. | *Halomonas meridian* | L-Glutaminase | LS 174T, HCT 116 | Mostafa et al. (1963) |
| 3. | *Streptomyces canarius* | L-Glutaminase | Hep-G2 cell, HeLa cells, HCT-116 cell, RAW 264.7 | Reda et al. (2015) |
| 4. | *Idiomarina sediminum* | L-Glutaminase | Hep-G2 cell lines | Unissa et al. (2018) |
| 5. | *Thermus thermophilus* | L-Asparaginase | K562, MCF7 and BT20 | Pritsa et al. (2001) |
| 6. | *Streptococcus erysipelas* and *Bacillus prodigiosus*). | Mixed Toxin (Coley toxin) | Sarcoma | Coley et al. (1910) |

## 5.7.2 MICROBIAL ENZYMES AS ANTI-COAGULATING AGENTS

When anybody encounters any kind of accident or wound, the immune system is activated and causes vasodilation, and increases the flow of blood to the site of injury. The process includes the migration of phagocytes, neutrophils, and other factors. After these consequences, finally, there is the sealing of the cut or damaged tissue so that no more blood oozes from the site of infection. The sealing of a wound is done by coagulation of blood; if the coagulation of blood does not occur within the stipulated time, then the patient will lose a huge amount of blood, which may result in the death of a person. In most of the accidental cases, death is due to blood loss (Gitto et al., 2019). Thrombosis, or blood clots, can develop in the veins or arteries. According to Boos and Lip (2006), the accumulation of platelets, fibrin, and thrombin causes arterial thrombosis, which is the primary factor in the majority of heart attacks (myocardial infarction) (Mackman, 2008). To counter this problem, there should be an immediate need for blood anticoagulant, and the most effective anticoagulant used is the streptokinase enzyme produced by *Streptococcus*. Proteases called fibrinolytic enzymes break down fibrin into the thrombus. Two categories of fibrinolytic enzymes can be distinguished based on their mechanisms: Both plasminogen activators and fibrinolytic enzymes, such as tissue-type plasminogen activator (t-PA) and urokinase, have the ability to hydrolyze plasminogen into plasmin (Table 5.6).

**TABLE 5.6** Microbial Enzymes Used as Anticoagulant

| Sl. No. | Name of Microorganism | Enzyme produced | Mechanism of action | References |
|---|---|---|---|---|
| 1. | *Bacillus velezensis* Z01 | Velefibrinase | Anti-aggregation of platelets, and improvement in blood coagulation | Liang (2022); Zhou et al. (2022) |
| 2. | *Bacillus flexus* | Fibrinolytic | Fibrin degradation | Al Farraj et al. (2020) |
| 3. | *Serratia rubidaea* KUAS001 | Fibrinolytic | Fibrin degradation | Anusree et al., 2020 |
| 4. | *Staphylococcus aureus* GH38 | Staphylokinase | Activate plasminogen to form plasmin, which digest fibrin clot than cause thrombosis clot | Noori and Aziz (2020) |
| 5. | *Bacillus subtilis* D21–8 | Fibrinolytic | Fibrin degradation | Pan et al. (2019) |

### *5.7.3 MICROBIAL ENZYMES AS ANTIMICROBIAL AGENT*

The medical practitioner faces challenges such as irrational antibiotic use and the transfer of resistance in bacteria (Chandra et al., 2017). The problems are burgeoning day by day due to the emergence of MDR (Multiple Drug Resistance) and XDR (Extreme Drug Resistance). Since the first antibiotic, that is, Penicillin, was discovered, there have been so many antibiotics discovered till date, but in the past few years, there have been several reports suggesting that there are many microorganisms like *Acinetobacter baumannii*, *Pseudomonas aeruginosa*, *Klebsiella pneumoniae*, *Streptococcus pneumoniae*, and *Staphylococcus aureus* (Hawkey, 2008). Therefore, there is now a need to develop some strategy to combat drug resistance, but most of the strategies seem inefficient. The microbial enzymes and antimicrobial peptides from microorganisms are now being explored against pathogenic bacteria for treatment (Table 5.7). The known antimicrobial enzymes, which have the potential to control bacterial infections caused by pathogenic bacteria, are: (a) subtilisin; (b) lysostaphin; (c) bacteriophage lysins; and (d) glucose oxidase. These microbial enzymes control pathogenic bacteria through different mechanisms, such as (1) hydrolysis of adhesins required for adherence to the host body; (2) breakdown of the cell wall; and (3) disruption of the cell membrane.

**TABLE 5.7** Microbial Enzymes Used as Antimicrobial Agent

| S. No. | Name of Microorganism | Enzyme Produced | Mechanism of Action | References |
|---|---|---|---|---|
| 1. | *Bacillus* sp. | Subtilisin's | Serine proteases hydrolyse adhesin | Molobela et al. (2010) |
| 2. | *Staphylococcus simulans* | Lysostaphin | It causes the hydrolysis of the cell wall of Staphylococcus aureus resulting in disruption of the cell wall. | Recsei et al. (1987) |
| 3. | Bacteriophage | Bacteriophage lysins | Lysis of bacterial cell wall | Borysowski et al. (2006) |
| 4 | *Aspergillus niger* | Glucose oxidase | Bacterial cells are killed by hydrogen peroxide by oxygen oxidation, peroxidation, and rupture of cell membranes. | Alt et al. (1999) |
| 5. | *Actinobacillus actinomycetemcomitans* | Dispersin B (DspB) | It breaks down 1,6-N-acetylglucosamine, which is necessary for biofilm attachment to surfaces. | Chaignon et al. (2007) |
| 6. | *Streptococcus equis* sp. *zooepidemicus* 4881 | Zoocin A | Endopeptidase activity against *Streptococcus mutans* and *S. pyogenes* | Akesson et al. (2007) |

### 5.7.4 ANTI-INFLAMMATORY ACTIVITY

Inflammation is a common immunological reaction to an aggressor, which could be a disease, foreign substance, or thorn. Infections are brought on by pathogens, which include bacteria, viruses, and other creatures.

The breakdown of tissue proteins and the release of lysosomal enzymes are what cause its distinctive symptoms of pain, redness, swelling, and heat. As a result, protein denaturation inhibition and lysosomal membrane stabilization may postpone the onset of inflammation. Enzymatic anti-inflammatory medications are more widely used today than traditional non-steroidal anti-inflammatory medications (NSAIDs). Due to its growing popularity, enzymatic treatment reduces the negative side effects of NSAIDs and offers benefits like specificity and high efficiency (Tiwari, 2017). By reducing inflammatory cytokines and adhesion molecules, SEPD regulates the migration of inflammatory cells to the site of inflammation. As it reduces the appearance of cytokines, enzymes, and several transcription factors involved in the onset and progression of the inflammatory response, the peptide SET-M33D containing D amino acids exhibits potent anti-inflammatory effect (Brunetti et al., 2020). Additionally, the pathophysiology and progression of complications, severity, and mortality in COVID-19 are significantly impacted by the high levels of inflammatory cytokines, such as interleukin (IL)-6 (Wang et al., 2020). The substantial rise in IL-6 levels especially induced by acute respiratory distress has been linked to the severity of the disease, prognosis, and death. According to Jaiswal and Mishra (2018), serratiopeptidase (SEPD) has a potent IL-6 inhibitory effect as evidenced by the reduction in IL-6 level ranging from 47 to 80% in lipopolysaccharide-stimulated human monocytes. The potential of SEPD to prevent inflammation and reduce cellular harm in several organs is suggested by its anti-inflammatory activity at the systemic and cellular levels. Due to its inhibitory effect on bradykinin, serotonin, and histamine, it can therefore be hypothesized that SEPD may lessen acute respiratory distress and restrict problems in COVID-19 (Sharma et al., 2021). Collagenases are enzymes that attack peptide bonds in collagen. Sometimes collagen is produced in higher quantity and may not disintegrate after a certain period of time. Collagen degradation in these circumstances may benefit from the use of an injectable collagenase or its ointment. Collagenases are useful in treating a variety of ailments, such as cellulite, lipoma, intervertebral disc herniation, burns, nipple pain, and others (Alipour et al., 2016). It is also used to promote debridement of necrotic tissue in burns and skin ulcers as well as to treat Dupuytren's contracture and Peronei's disease. Table 5.8 summarizes some enzymes exploited as an anti-inflammatory agent.

**TABLE 5.8** Microbial Enzymes Used as Anti-Inflammatory Agent

| S. No. | Name of Microorganism | Anti-inflammatory molecule | Inhibitory effect | References |
|---|---|---|---|---|
| 1. | *Bacillus pumilus* SG2 | Serine protease | Induce hemolysis and protein denaturation | Sangeetha and Arulpandi (2019) |
| 2. | *Serratia marcescens* | Serratiopeptidase | Reduction in inflammatory markers C-reactive proteins, myeloperoxidase, serotonin, histamine | Jadhav et al. (2020); Sharma et al. (2021) |
| 3. | *Clostridium histolyticum* | Collagenase | Breaks peptide bond in collagen | Vachher et al. (2021) |

## 5.8 ENZYMES IN COSMETICS

Due to the increasing demand from consumers for biological ingredients and cosmetic products, the cosmetics industry has been compelled to look into microbiological sources. Microbes are a rich source of enzymes, fatty acids, peptides, lipopolysaccharides, vitamins, and pigments with beneficial properties for aesthetic applications (Gupta et al., 2019). Additionally, enzymes have a significant impact on the cosmetics sector (Table 5.9). Proteins and peptides have been used by humans to improve the appearance of their skin, hair, and nails since the beginning of time. One area where the topical application of enzymes has been shown to have a significant role is skin protection. Some enzymes have the capability to capture free radicals, preventing damage to the skin caused by bacteria, environmental pollution, smoke, sunlight, and other harmful factors. They may also gradually decrease the signs of aging (Satyanarayana et al., 2012). Superoxide dismutase (SOD) is among the most widely used defensive enzymes. Nearly all living organisms contain SOD, which helps to defend the cell from oxygen-free radical damage in the aqueous environment. It works by a process of dismutation, by which a dangerous, highly reactive oxygen-free radical is converted to a less reactive form. It is known that proteases, including keratinases, are used in the repairing of stretch marks and scar tissues. In addition, they help in the regeneration of epithelial cells (Lin et al., 1992). Hyaluronidase, an enzyme that degrades HA, has been used to boost the absorption of drugs into tissue and to lessen tissue damage in situations when the drug is extravasated (Jung et al., 2020). Several issues related to the injection of cosmetic HA fillers can be handled with hyaluronidase (Cohen et al., 2015). A promising method for whitening cosmetics applications involved the decolorization of melanin by lignin peroxidase with *in situ* produced $H_2O_2$ (Sung et al., 2019). Due to its high redox potential to oxidize melanin, lignin peroxidase has a significant role in cosmetics for skin lightening. Tyrosine forms melanin by the enzyme tyrosinase using its oxidizing property. Melanocytes, pigment-producing cells, are the main source of this enzyme. It helps in maintaining the amount of melanin produced. When skin is exposed to UV light, tyrosinase produces melanin in order to prevent UV-induced damage (Agarwal et al., 2019). On the other hand, water-soluble retinol derivatives are made using immobilized lipases. These lipases are used in hair weaving preparation and have also been used as an ingredient of topical anti-obese creams or as oral administration.

**TABLE 5.9** Microbial Enzymes Used in Cosmetics

| S. No. | Enzyme | Source | Cosmetic use | Reference |
|---|---|---|---|---|
| 1. | Keratinase | *Bacillus licheniformis* | Repairing of stretch marks, in hair removing and hair growth | Gupta et al. (2012) |
| 2. | Lignin peroxidase | *Phanerochaete chryosporium* | Decolorization of melanin | Sung et al. (2019) |
| 3. | Tyrosinase | *Agaricus bisporus* | Tanning agent | Sunar et al. (2016) |
| 4. | Superoxide dismutase | Yeast | Antifree radicals | Gupta et al. (2012) |
| 5. | Hyaluronidase | Bacteria | Moisturizing agent | Lods et al. (2000) |
| 6. | Alkaline phosphatase | Yeast | Antiwrinkle agent | Sunar et al. (2016) |

## 5.9 MICROBIAL ENZYMES IN TREATING GASTROINTESTINAL DISTURBANCE

Microbial enzymes require lower effective dosages, have increased specific activity, are resistant to acid inactivation and proteolytic digestion, and are active across a wider pH range.

### *5.9.1 AMYLASE*

The key enzyme for breaking down carbohydrates is called amylase. It can be isolated exogenously from *Bacillus subtilis*, *Aspergillus oryzae*, and barley malt. It is a kind of endoamylase found in human saliva and pancreatic secretion. Amylase, also known as fungal diastase, is derived from a fungus, *Aspergillus oryzae*, and contains the high activity of enzyme α-amylase. Its ability to digest starch is convincingly strong over a wide pH range, with maximum activity at pH 5. For the treatment of dyspepsia, typical components of mixed digestive enzymes are exploited (Swami et al., 2017).

### 5.9.2 LIPASE

Lipase (triacylglycerol acylhydrolases) catalyzes the partial or complete hydrolysis of triacylglycerols. All biological systems, including those of animals, plants, and microbes, are capable of producing lipases. However, microbial lipases are gaining more attention due to their wide range of catalytic activities, higher yields, ease of genetic manipulation, constant supply, multiplication of microorganisms on inexpensive media, and being more stable than the corresponding plant and animal enzymes, and because their production is more practical and secure. Lipase produced by *C. cylindracea* has been used in hydrolytic reactions (Salihu et al., 2012). Lipases play a major role in hydrolysis of fats and form fatty acid and glycerol. Therefore, they can be used as therapeutic agents for many digestive disorders such as, in cases of pancreatic insufficiency, chronic pancreatitis, and following gastric resection.

### 5.9.3 SARCOIDOSIS

Sarcoidosis is an efficient and well-tolerated therapeutic option and a digestive aid for people with CSID (Puntis and Zamvar, 2015). A hereditary disease called congenital sucrase-isomaltose deficiency (CSID) impairs a person's capacity to digest some carbohydrates. Due to their inability to digest simple sugars (carbohydrates) like sucrose and maltose, people with this illness may have symptoms like diarrhea and abdominal pain.

### 5.9.4 PROLYL ENDOPEPTIDASE

The digestive by-products of wheat gluten trigger an immunological reaction that leads to celiac disease. Due to human digestive enzymes' inability to break proteins at proline residues, gluten cannot be fully digested.

Some gluten peptides in susceptible people cause a T-cell reaction, which leads to inflammation of the small intestine. It has been proposed that nonhuman prolyl oligopeptides, which can cleave proteins at proline residues, be added to diets as a form of treatment for celiac disease (Shan et al., 2004; Stepniak et al., 2006). A newly discovered prolyl endopro tease from *Aspergillus niger* (AN-PEP) is active throughout the pH range encountered in the human digestive tract. It has many properties like pepsin resistance, high catalytic rate, activity against intact gluten, and effectiveness against immunostimulatory peptides. In the gastrointestinal tract, proline-containing peptides can be hydrolyzed by prolyl oligopeptides that have been identified from *Flavobacterium mengiosepticum*, *Sphingomonas capsulate*, and *Myxococcus xanthus*. These enzymes are not digested by protease (Amador et al., 2019).

## 5.10 CONCLUSION AND FUTURE PROSPECTIVE

The incidence of viral and bacterial diseases is increasing day by day, and the pathogenic bacteria isolated from patients are showing resistance to the commonly used antibiotics. The problem of antibiotic resistance is not a problem of a single country; it is a problem of many developing countries. The emergence of MDR or XDR is a major health concern in developing countries because they are not controlled by common antibiotics and need broad-spectrum or third-generation antibiotics, which are costly. The microbial enzymes produced by the microorganism have shown promising results in controlling infections caused by pathogens. They have also shown promising anti-cancer properties and anti-inflammatory activity, as well as industrially important products such as additives for detergent, in animal feed, and as a digestive enzyme for proper digestion. The most affordable source of a valuable industrial product that may be used for a variety of tasks is microbial enzymes. Although the isolation and purification of the microbial enzymes is a laborious procedure, once optimization is completed, it is quite simple to generate these enzymes commercially. Through "Make in India" initiatives and financial support for start-up businesses, the Indian government is now supporting entrepreneurship. Genetic engineering, recombinant DNA technology, mutation, and other contemporary techniques can be used to enhance the production from the microbe that has been isolated and has the potential to become industrially significant strains.

## KEYWORDS


- **detergent industry**
- **food industry**
- **industrial applications**
- **lifestyle diseases**
- **microbial enzymes**
- **natural resources**


## REFERENCES


Adeola, O., & Cowieson, A. J. (2011). Board-invited review: opportunities and challenges in using exogenous enzymes to improve non-ruminant animal production. *Journal of Animal Science, 89*, 3189–3218.

Agarwal, P., Singh, M., & Singh, R. P. (2019). In: *Microbial tyrosinases: A novel enzyme, structural features, and applications*. *Applied Microbiology and Bioengineering*, 3–19.

Akesson, M., Dufour, M., Sloan, G. L., Robin, S., & Simmonds, R. S. (2007). Targeting of streptococci by zoocin A. *FEMS Microbiology Letters, 270*(1), 155–161.

Al Farraj, D. A., Kumar, T. S. J., Vijayaraghavan, P., Elshikh, M. S., Alkufeidy, R. M., & Alkubaisi, N. A. (2020). Enhanced production, purification and biochemical characterization of therapeutic fibrinolytic enzyme from a new *Bacillus flexus* from marine environment. *Journal of King Saud University–Science, 232*(7), 3174–3180.

Alipour, H., Raz, A., Zakeri, S., & Djadid, N. D. (2016). Therapeutic applications of collagenase (metalloproteases): a review. *Asian Pacific Journal of Tropical Biomedicine, 6*(11), 975–981.

Alkawash, M. A., Soothill, J. S., & Schiller, N. L. (2006). Alginate lyase enhances antibiotic killing of mucoid *Pseudomonas aeruginosa* in biofilms. *APMIS, 114*, 131–138.

Alrumman, S. A., Mostafa, Y. S., & Al-Izran, K. A. (2019). Production and anticancer activity of an L-asparaginase from *Bacillus licheniformis* isolated from the Red Sea, Saudi Arabia. *Scientific Reports, 9*, 3756.

Alt, E., Leipold, F., Milatovic, D., & Lehmann, G. (1999). Hydrogen peroxide for prevention of bacterial growth on polymer biomaterials. *Annals of Thoracic Surgery, 68*, 2123–2128.

Alves, E. D. P., Morioka, L. R. I., & Suguimoto, H. H. (2019). Comparison of bioethanol and beta-galactosidase production by *Kluyveromyces* and *Saccharomyces* strains grown in cheese whey. *International Journal of Dairy Technology, 72*(3), 409–415.

Anusree, M., Swapna, K., Aguilar, C. N., & Sabu, A. (2020). Optimization of process parameters for the enhanced production of fibrinolytic enzyme by a newly isolated marine bacterium. *Bioresource Technology Reports, 11*.

Ao, X. L., Yu, X., Wu, D. T., Li, C., Zhang, T., Liu, S. L., & Zou, L. K. (2018). Purification and characterization of neutral protease from *Aspergillus oryzae* Y1 isolated from naturally fermented broad beans. *AMB Express, 8*(1), 1–10.

Bhardwaj, N., & Chandra, H. (2021). Impacts of lockdown interventions on the spread of COVID-19 in India. *Journal of Global Infectious Diseases, 13*(1), 61–62.

Boos, C. J., & Lip, G. (2006). Blood clotting, inflammation, and thrombosis in cardiovascular events: perspectives. *Frontiers in Bioscience, 11*, 328–336.

Borysowski, J., Weber-Dabrowska, B., & Górski, A. (2006). Bacteriophage endolysins as a novel class of antibacterial agents. *Journal of Experimental Biology and Medicine, 231*, 366–377.

Brunetti, J., Carnicelli, V., Ponzi, A., Di Giulio, A., Lizzi, A. R., Cristiano, L., Crsti, L., Cappello, G., Pollini, S., Mosconi, L., Rossolini, G. M., Bracci, L., Falciani, C., & Pini, A. (2020). Antibacterial and anti-inflammatory activity of an antimicrobial peptide synthesized with D amino acids. *Antibiotics, 9*, 840–857.

Carniel, A., Valoni, E., Junior, J. N., Da Conceição Gomes, A., & De Castro, A. M. (2017). Lipase from *Candida antarctica* (CALB) and cutinize from *Humicola insolens* act synergistically for PET hydrolysis to terephthalic acid. *Process Biochemistry, 59*, 84–90.

Carswell, E. A., Old, L. J., Kassel, R. L., Green, S., Fiore, N., & Williamson, B. (1975). An endotoxin-induced serum factor that causes necrosis of tumors. *Proceedings of the National Academy of Sciences of the United States of America, 72*(9), 3666–3670.

Chaignon, P., Sadovskaya, I., Ragunah, C., & Ramasubbu, N. (2007). Susceptibility of staphylococcal biofilms to enzymatic treatments depends on their chemical composition. *Applied Microbiology and Biotechnology, 75*, 125–132.

Chandra, H., Bishnoi, P., Yadav, A., Patni, B., Mishra, A. P., & Nautiyal, A. R. (2017). Antimicrobial resistance and the alternative resources with special emphasis on plant-based antimicrobials—A review. *Plants, 6*(2), 16.

Cohen, B. E., Bashey, S., & Wysong, A. (2015). The use of hyaluronidase in cosmetic dermatology: a review of the literature. *Journal of Clinical Investigative Dermatology, 3*(2), 7.

Coley, W. B. (1910). The treatment of inoperable sarcoma by bacterial toxins (the mixed toxins of the *Streptococcus erysipelas* and the *Bacillus prodigiosus*). *Proceedings of the Royal Society of Medicine, 3*(Surg Sect), 1–48.

Duan, X., Hu, S., Qi, X., Gu, Z., & Wu, J. (2017). Optimal extracellular production of recombinant *Bacillus circulans* β-galactosidase in *Escherichia coli* BL21 (DE3). *Process Biochemistry, 53*, 17–24.

Egmond, M., & Vlieg, J. (2000). *Fusarium solani pisi* cutinase. *Biochimie, 82*(11), 1015–1021.

Enzymes market size, share & trends analysis report by application (industrial enzymes, specialty enzymes), by product (carbohydrase, proteases, lipases), by source, by region, and segment forecasts, 2020–2027.

Fang, C., & Chen, X. (2018). Potential biocontrol efficacy of *Trichoderma atroviride* with cellulase expression regulator ace1 gene knock-out. *3 Biotech, 8*(7), 1–10.

Francetic, O., & Pugsley, A. P. (2005). Towards the identification of type II secretion signals in a nonacylated variant of pullulan's from *Klebsiella oxytoca*. *Journal of Bacteriology, 187*(20), 7045–7055.

Gangola, S., Sharma, A., Bhatt, P., Khati, P., & Chaudhary, P. (2018). Presence of esterase and laccase in *Bacillus subtilis* facilitates biodegradation and detoxification of cypermethrin. *Scientific Reports, 8*(1), 1–11.

Gao, X., Yin, Y., Yan, J., Zhang, J., Ma, H., & Zhou, C. (2019). Separation, biochemical characterization and salt-tolerant mechanisms of alkaline protease from *Aspergillus oryzae*. *Journal of the Science of Food and Agriculture, 99*(7), 3359–3366.

Gauterio, G. V., da Silva, L. G. G., Hubner, T., Da Rosa Ribeiro, T., & Kalil, S. J. (2021). Xylooligosaccharides production by crude and partially purified xylanase from *Aureobasidium pullulans*: biochemical and thermodynamic properties of the enzymes and their application in xylan hydrolysis. *Process Biochemistry, 104*, 161–170.

Gitto, L., Bonaccorso, L., & Serinelli, S. (2019). Death due to severe blood loss following an accidental lesion to the femoral vessels. *Medico-Legal Journal, 87*(4), 196–201.

Gupta, P. L., Rajput, M., Oza, T., Trivedi, U. K., & Sanghvi, G. (2019). Eminence of microbial products in cosmetic industry. *Natural Products and Bioprospecting, 9*, 267–278.

Gurung, N., Ray, S., Bose, S., & Rai, V. (2013). A broader view: microbial enzymes and their relevance in industries, medicine, and beyond. *BioMed Research International*.

Hawkey, P. M. (2008). The growing burden of antimicrobial resistance. *Journal of Antimicrobial Chemotherapy, 62*, 1–9.

Heidary Vinche, M., Khanahmadi, M., Ataei, S. A., & Danafar, F. (2021). Optimization of process variables for production of beta-glucanase by *Aspergillus niger* CCUG33991 in solid-state fermentation using wheat bran. *Waste and Biomass Valorization, 12*(6), 3233–3243.

Helal, S. E., Abdelhady, H. M., Abou-Taleb, K. A., Hassan, M. G., & Amer, M. M. (2021). Lipase from *Rhizopus oryzae* R1: in-depth characterization, immobilization, and evaluation in biodiesel production. *Journal of Genetic Engineering and Biotechnology, 19*(1), 1–13.

Hmidet, N., Bayoudh, A., Berrin, J. G., Kanoun, S., Juge, N., & Nasri, M. (2008). Purification and biochemical characterization of a novel α-amylase from *Bacillus licheniformis* NH1: cloning, nucleotide sequence and expression of amyN gene in *Escherichia coli*. *Process Biochemistry, 43*(5), 499–510.

Irfan, M., Asghar, U., Nadeem, M., Nelofer, R., & Syed, Q. (2016). Optimization of process parameters for xylanase production by *Bacillus* sp. in submerged fermentation. *Journal of Radiation Research and Applied Sciences, 9*(2), 139–147.

Jadhav, S. B., Shah, N., Rathi, A., Rathi, V., & Rathi, A. (2020). Serrati peptidase: insights into the therapeutic applications. *Biotechnology Reports (Amsterdam), 28*.

Jain, M. (n.d.). "Amity Institute of Biotechnology. Enzymology Assignment-I, Enzymes used in detergents," Faculty of Enzymology. http://www.scribd.com/doc/11523933/Enzymes-in-Detergents (accessed on 5th November 2025).

Jaiswal, S., & Mishra, P. (2018). Co-delivery of curcumin and serrati peptidase in HeLa and MCF-7 cells through nanoparticles show improved anti-cancer activity. *Materials Science and Engineering: C, Materials for Biological Applications, 92*, 673–684.

Jampala, P., Tadikamalla, S., Preethi, M., Ramanujam, S., & Uppuluri, K. B. (2017). Concurrent production of cellulase and xylanase from *Trichoderma reesei* NCIM 1186: enhancement of production by desirability-based multi-objective method. *3 Biotech, 7*(1), 1–13.

Jung, H. (2020). Hyaluronidase: an overview of its properties, applications, and side effects. *Archives of Plastic Surgery, 47*(4), 297–300.

Kareem, S. O., Adebayo, O. S., Balogun, S. A., Adeogun, A. I., & Akinde, S. B. (2017). Purification and characterization of lipase from *Aspergillus flavus* PW2961 using magnetic nanoparticles. *Nigerian Journal of Biotechnology, 32*, 77–82.

Karlund, A., Moor, U., & Sandell, M. (2014). The impact of harvesting, storage and processing factors on health-promoting phytochemicals in berries and fruits. *Processes, 2*(3), 596–624.

Kim, Y. K., Lee, S. C., Cho, Y. Y., Oh, H. J., & Ko, Y. H. (2012). Isolation of cellulolytic *Bacillus subtilis* strains from agricultural environments. *International Scholarly Research Notices*.

Konishi, T., Aoshima, T., Mizuhashi, F., Choi, S. S., & Roberts, A. (2013). Safety evaluation of glucose oxidase from *Penicillium chrysogenum*. *Regulatory Toxicology and Pharmacology, 66*(1), 13–23.

Kubrak, O. I., Storey, J. M., Storey, K. B., & Lushchak, V. I. (2010). Production and properties of α-amylase from *Bacillus* sp. BKL20. *Canadian Journal of Microbiology, 56*(4), 279–288.

Kunamneni, A., & Singh, S. (2006). Improved high thermal stability of pullulan's from a newly isolated thermophilic *Bacillus* sp. AN-7. *Enzyme and Microbial Technology, 39*(7), 1399–1404.

Kuraishi, C., Yamazaki, K., & Susa, Y. (2001). Transglutaminase: its utilization in the food industry. *Food Reviews International, 17*, 221–246.

Leskovac, V., Trivić, S., Wohlfahrt, G., Kandrac, J., & Peričin, D. (2005). Glucose oxidase from *Aspergillus niger*: the mechanism of action with molecular oxygen, quinones, and one-electron acceptors. *The International Journal of Biochemistry & Cell Biology, 37*(4), 731–750.

Li, D. X., Ni, K. K., Zhang, Y. C., Lin, Y. L., & Yang, F. Y. (2018). Influence of lactic acid bacteria, cellulase, cellulase-producing *Bacillus pumilus* and their combinations on alfalfa silage quality. *Journal of Integrative Agriculture, 17*(12), 2768–2782.

Li, Q., Zhang, M., Li, X., Zhang, Y., Wang, Z., & Zheng, J. (2021). A novel lipase from *Aspergillus oryzae* WZ007 catalyzed synthesis of brivaracetam intermediate and its enzymatic characterization. *Chirality, 33*(2), 62–71.

Liang, Z. (2022). Purification and characterization of a fibrinolytic enzyme from marine *Bacillus velezensis* Z01 and assessment of its therapeutic efficacy *in vivo*. *Microorganisms, 10*(5), 843.

Lin, X., Lee, C. G., Casale, E. S., & Shih, J. C. (1992). Purification and characterization of a keratinase from a feather-degrading *Bacillus licheniformis* strain. *Applied and Environmental Microbiology, 58*(10), 3271–3275.

Liu, W., Ma, C., Liu, W., Zheng, Y., Chen, C. C., Liang, A., Xuegang, L., Zhongyuan, L., Ma, W., Song, Y., Guo, R. T., & Zhang, T. (2021). Functional and structural investigation of a novel β-manganese BaMan113A from *Bacillus* sp. N16-5. *International Journal of Biological Macromolecules, 182*, 899–909.

Lods, L. M., Dres, C., Johnson, C., Scholz, D. B., & Brooks, G. J. (2000). The future of enzymes in cosmetics. *International Journal of Cosmetic Science, 22*(2), 85–94.

Mackman, N. (2018). Triggers, targets and treatments for thrombosis. *Nature, 451*(7181), 914–918.

Mahmoud, A., Kotb, E., Alqosaibi, A. I., Al-Karmalawy, A. A., Al-Dhuayan, I. S., & Alabkari, H. (2021). *In vitro* and *in silico* characterization of alkaline serine protease from *Bacillus subtilis* D9 recovered from Saudi Arabia. *Helion, 7*(10), e08148.

Mehta, P. K., & Sehgal, S. (2019). Microbial enzymes in food processing. In Q. Husain & M. Ullah (Eds.), *Biocatalysis*. Springer, Cham. https://doi.org/10.1007/978-3-030-25023-2_13 (accessed on 5th November 2025).

Molobela, P., Cloete, T., & Beukes, E. M. (2010). Protease and amylase enzymes for biofilm removal and degradation of extracellular polymeric substances (EPS) produced by *Pseudomonas fluorescens* bacteria. *African Journal of Microbiology Research, 4*, 1515–1524.

Monteiro, P. S., Guimarães, V. M., Melo, R. R. D., & Rezende, S. T. D. (2015). Isolation of a thermostable acid phytase from *Aspergillus niger* UFV-1 with strong proteolysis resistance. *Brazilian Journal of Microbiology, 46*, 251–260.

Moreno-Amador, M. L., Arévalo-Rodríguez, M., Durán, E. M., Martínez-Reyes, J. C., & Sousa-Martín, C. (2019). A new microbial gluten-degrading prolyl endopeptidase: potential application in celiac disease to reduce gluten immunogenic peptides. *PLoS One, 14*(6), e0217758.

Mostafa, Y. S., Alamri, S. A., Alfaifi, M. Y., Alrumman, S. A., Elbehairi, S., Taha, T. H., & Hashem, M. (2021). L-glutaminase synthesis by marine *Halomonas meridiana* isolated from the Red Sea and its efficiency against colorectal cancer cell lines. *Molecules, 26*(7), 1963.

Navarre, W. W., Ton-That, H., Faull, K. F., & Schneewind, O. (1999). Multiple enzymatic activities of the murein hydrolase from staphylococcal Phage f11. *Journal of Biological Chemistry, 274*, 15847–15856.

Ncube, T., Howard, R. L., Abotsi, E. K., Van Rensburg, E. L. J., & Ncube, I. (2012). *Jatropha curcas* seed cake as substrate for production of xylanase and cellulase by *Aspergillus niger* FGSCA733 in solid-state fermentation. *Industrial Crops and Products, 37*(1), 118–123.

Nema, A., Patnala, S. H., Mandari, V., Kota, S., & Devarai, S. K. (2019). Production and optimization of lipase using *Aspergillus niger* MTCC 872 by solid-state fermentation. *Bulletin of the National Research Centre, 43*(1), 1–8.

Noori, H., & Aziz, G. (2020). Purification, characterization, and evaluation of fibrinolytic activity of staphylokinase from locally isolated *Staphylococcus aureus* GH38. *Iraqi Journal of Agricultural Sciences, 51*(4), 1195–1203.

Padmapriya, M., & Williams, B. C. (2012). Purification and characterization of neutral protease enzyme from *Bacillus subtilis*. *Journal of Microbiology and Biotechnology Research, 2*(4), 612–618.

Pan, S., Chen, G., Wu, R., Cao, X., & Liang, Z. (2019a). Non-sterile submerged fermentation of fibrinolytic enzyme by marine *Bacillus subtilis* harboring antibacterial activity with starvation strategy. *Frontiers in Microbiology, 10*, 1025.

Pandey, A., & Singhania, R. R. (2008). Production and application of industrial enzymes. *Chemical Industry Digest, 21*, 82–91.

Pandey, P., Summpunn, P., Wiyakrutta, S., Isarangkul, D., & Meevootisom, V. (2011). A thermostable phytase from *Neosartorya spinosa* BCC 41923 and its expression in *Pichia pastoris*. *Journal of Microbiology, 49*, 257–264.

Pant, G., Prakash, A., Pavani, J. V. P., Bera, S., Deviram, G. V. N. S., Kumar, A., & Prasuna, R. G. (2015). Production, optimization and partial purification of protease from *Bacillus subtilis*. *Journal of Taibah University for Science, 9*(1), 50–55.

Pritsa, A. A., Papazisis, K. T., Kortsaris, A. H., Geromichalos, G. D., & Kyriakidis, D. A. (2001). Antitumor activity of L-asparaginase from *Thermus thermophilus*. *Anti-Cancer Drugs, 12*(2), 137–142.

Puntis, J. W., & Zamvar, V. (2015). Congenital sucrase-isomaltose deficiency: diagnostic challenges and response to enzyme replacement therapy. *Archives of Disease in Childhood*, 869–871.

Purushothaman, K., Bhat, S. K., Singh, S. A., Marathe, G. K., & Rao, A. R. G. A. (2019). Aspartic protease from *Aspergillus niger*: molecular characterization and interaction with pepstatin A. *International Journal of Biological Macromolecules, 139*, 199–212.

Raveendran, S., Parameswaran, B., Ummalyma, S. B., Abraham, A., Mathew, A. K., Madhavan, A., Rebello, S., & Pandey, A. (2018). Applications of microbial enzymes in food industry. *Food Technology and Biotechnology, 56*(1), 16–30.

Recsei, P. A., Gruss, A. D., & Novick, R. P. (1987). Cloning, sequence, and expression of the lysostaphin gene from *Staphylococcus simulans*. *Proceedings of the National Academy of Sciences of the United States of America, 84*, 1127–1131.

Reda, F. M. (2015). Kinetic properties of *Streptomyces canarius* L-glutaminase and its anticancer efficiency. *Brazilian Journal of Microbiology, 46*, 957–968.

Sabu, A. (2003). Sources, properties and applications of microbial therapeutic enzymes. *Indian Journal of Biotechnology, 2*, 334–341.

Salihu, A., Alam, M. Z., Abdul Kalim, M. I., & Salleh, H. M. (2012). Characterization of *Candida cylindracea* lipase produced from palm oil mill effluent based medium. *IJCBS, 2*, 24–31.

Sangeetha, R., & Arulpandi, I. (2019). Anti-inflammatory activity of a serine protease produced from *Bacillus pumilus* SG2. *Biocatalysis and Agricultural Biotechnology, 19*, 101162.

Satyanarayana, T., Johri, B. N., & Prakash, A. (2012). *Microorganisms in Environmental Management: Microbes and Environment*. Springer, Dordrecht.

Selle, P. H., Ravindran, V., & Partridge, G. G. (2009). Beneficial effects of xylanase and/or phytase inclusions on ileal amino acid digestibility, energy utilization, mineral retention and growth performance in wheat-based broiler diets. *Animal Feed Science and Technology, 153*, 303–313.

Selvakumar, P., Ashakumary, L., & Pandey, A. (1996). Microbial synthesis of starch saccharifying enzyme in solid-state fermentation. *Journal of Scientific and Industrial Research, 55*(5–6), 443–449.

Shan, L., Marti, T., Sollid, L. M., Gray, G. M., & Khosla, C. (2004). Comparative biochemical analysis of three bacterial prolyl endopeptidases: implications for coeliac sprue. *Biochemical Journal, 383*, 311–318.

Sharma, C., Jha, N. K., Meeran, M. F. N., Patil, C. R., Goyal, S. N., & Ojha, S. (2021). Serrati peptidase, a serine protease anti-inflammatory, fibrinolytic, and mucolytic drug, can be a useful adjuvant for management in COVID-19. *Frontiers in Pharmacology, 12*, 603997.

Shivakumar, S. (2012). Production and characterization of an acid protease from a local *Aspergillus* sp. by solid substrate fermentation. *Archives of Applied Science Research, 4*(1), 188–199.

Shrivastava, S., Shukla, P., & Mukhopadhyay, K. (2011). Purification and preliminary characterization of a xylanase from *Thermomyces lanuginosus* strain SS-8. *3 Biotech, 1*(4), 255–259.

Singh, R. S., Singh, T., & Pandey, A. (2019). Microbial enzymes—An overview. In *Advances in Enzyme Technology*, 1–40.

Stepniak, D. (2006). Highly efficient gluten degradation with a newly identified prolyl Endo protease: implications for celiac disease. *American Journal of Physiology–Gastrointestinal and Liver Physiology, 291*, 621–629.

Straksys, A., Kochane, T., & Budriene, S. (2016). Catalytic properties of maltogenic α-amylase from *Bacillus stearothermophilus* immobilized onto poly (urethane urea) microparticles. *Food Chemistry, 211*, 294–299.

Stressler, T., Ewert, J., Merz, M., Funk, J., Claaßen, W., Lutz-Wahl, S., Schmidt, H., Kuhn, A., & Fischer, L. (2016). A novel glutamyl (aspartyl)-specific aminopeptidase A from *Lactobacillus delbrueckii* with promising properties for application. *PLoS One, 11*(3), e0152139.

Suganthi, R., Benazir, J. F., Santhi, R., Ramesh Kumar, V., Hari, A., Meenakshi, N., Nidhiya, K. A., Kavitha, G., & Lakshmi, R. (2011). Amylase production by *Aspergillus niger* under solid state fermentation using agro-industrial wastes. *International Journal of Engineering Science and Technology, 3*(2), 1756–1763.

Sulyman, A., Igunnu, A., & Malomo, S. (2020). Isolation, purification and characterization of cellulase produced by *Aspergillus niger* cultured on *Arachis hypogaea* shells. *Helion, 6*(12), e05668.

Sunar, K., Kumar, U., & Deshmuk, S. (2016). Recent applications of enzymes in personal care products. In *Agro-Industrial Wastes as Feed Stock for Enzyme Production* (pp. 1–20).

Sung, J. H., Khan, M. F., & Kim, Y. H. (2019). Recombinant lignin peroxidase-catalyzed decolorization of melanin using *in-situ* generated $H_2O_2$ for application in whitening cosmetics. *International Journal of Biological Macromolecules, 136*, 20–26.

Swami, O. C., & Shah, N. J. (2017). Functional dyspepsia and the role of digestive enzymes supplement in its therapy. *International Journal of Basic and Clinical Pharmacology, 6*, 1035–1041.

Thomas, L., Arumugam, M., & Pandey, A. (2013a). Production, purification characterization and overexpression of xylanases from actinomycetes. *Indian Journal of Experimental Biology, 51*(6), 875–884.

Thomas, L., Parameswaran, B., & Pandey, A. (2016). Hydrolysis of pretreated rice straw by an enzyme cocktail comprising acidic xylanase from *Aspergillus* sp. for bioethanol production. *Renewable Energy, 98*, 9–15.

Tiwari, M. (2017). The role of serrati peptidase in the resolution of inflammation. *Asian Journal of Pharmaceutical Sciences, 12*, 209–215.

Uday, U. S. P., Majumdar, R., Tiwari, O. N., Mishra, U., Mondal, A., Bandyopadhyay, T. K., & Bhunia, B. (2017). Isolation, screening and characterization of a novel extracellular xylanase from *Aspergillus niger* (KP874102.1) and its application in orange peel hydrolysis. *International Journal of Biological Macromolecules, 105*, 401–409.

Unissa, R., Varma, D. B., Kesana, N. S., Srinivas, C., & Raj, B. S. (2018). *In vitro* cytotoxicity of L-glutaminase against Hep-G2 cell lines. *Research Journal of Pharmacy and Technology, 11*(6), 2213–2216.

Vachher, M., Sen, A., Kapila, R., & Nigam, A. (2021). Microbial therapeutic enzymes: A promising area of biopharmaceuticals. *Current Research in Biotechnology, 3*, 195–208.

Wang, J., Jiang, M., Chen, X., & Montaner, L. J. (2020). Cytokine storm and leukocyte changes in mild versus severe SARS-CoV-2 infection: Review of 3939 COVID-19 patients in China and emerging pathogenesis and therapy concepts. *Journal of Leukocyte Biology, 108*(1), 17–41.

Yassin, S., Jiru, T., & Indracanti, M. (2021). Screening and characterization of thermostable amylase-producing bacteria isolated from soil samples of Adera, afar region, and molecular detection of amylase-coding gene. *International Journal of Microbiology*, 5592885.

Zhou, Y., Chen, H., Yu, B., Chen, G., & Liang, Z. (2022). Purification and characterization of a fibrinolytic enzyme from marine *Bacillus velezensis* Z01 and assessment of its therapeutic efficacy *in vivo*. *Microorganisms, 10*(5), 843.

CHAPTER 6

# Microbial Technology Interventions to Increase Productivity of Maize Crop

ALOK KUMAR SINGH,[1,2] ALOK KUMAR SRIVASTAVA,[1,*] and MALA TRIVEDI[2,*]

[1]*ICAR–National Bureau of Agriculturally Important Microorganisms (NBAIM), Mau, Uttar Pradesh, India*

[2]*Amity Institute of Biotechnology, Amity University Uttar Pradesh, Lucknow Campus, Lucknow, Uttar Pradesh, India*

*Corresponding author

## ABSTRACT

With the growing challenges of climate change, there is an urgent need to develop crop cultivars with higher genetic yield potential and improved stress tolerance to support global food security. India, the world's third-largest producer of cereals, relies heavily on crops such as *Zea mays* L. (maize), an important source of nutrition. As the global population continues to rise, traditional farming practices can no longer meet increasing food demands. Modern agriculture has also become dependent on chemical fertilizers, which negatively impact soil health, natural microflora, and the environment. Microbial technology offers a sustainable solution for enhancing agricultural productivity without compromising soil fertility. Native microbial consortia, rather than single strains, are particularly effective in improving crop growth through enhanced metabolism and beneficial gene transfer. These microorganisms can promote plant growth, protect crops from stress, and enhance nutrient uptake, making them a valuable alternative to chemical fertilizers.

Industrial Biotechnology: Current Progress and Novel Technologies.
Prakash Kumar Sarangi, Akhilesh Kumar Singh, Rajesh Kumar Srivastava, and Brijesh Pandey (Eds.)


DOI: 10.1201/9781779642233-6

This chapter explores microbial technologies used for maize crop protection and improvement, with a focus on identifying plant growth–promoting (PGP) genes. Understanding maize's nutritional and health benefits may further encourage its consumption and support future research. Overall, the chapter emphasizes the role of microbial systems in boosting maize yield and ensuring sustainable crop enhancement.

## 6.1 INTRODUCTION

The world population and global food demands are increasing day by day. Therefore, to fulfill these demands, improved production and protection of crops is important and can be mainly accomplished through microbial technology. While in India, farmers are using chemicals and/or pesticides on a large scale due to a lack of scientific knowledge. In the current decade, synthetic pesticides are used for controlling crop pathogens, viz., weeds and pests, to increase food production. The large-scale use of synthetic xenobiotics is no longer sustainable for the environment (Oerke, 2006). Scientists emphasize alternative solutions in the form of bio-pesticides and plant growth-promoting microorganisms (PGPMs) for the improvement and protection of crops (Berg, 2009; Lehr, 2010). Legumes have been inoculated with nitrogen-fixing bacteria for a very long period, and they play a significant role in the worldwide food supply. Therefore, adding beneficial microorganisms to seeds and cereal crops is not a novel concept; rather, it is an active method for introducing microbial inoculum into the soil, and these organisms have a significant role in seedling root colonization and correspondence with soil-dwelling invertebrate pests that consume plant roots (Graham and Vance, 2003).

The beneficial microorganisms are applied during planting as liquids (in culture media) or dry formulations placed in the furrow; however, there are still relatively few commercially available microbial crop and seed inoculants. With the aid of these helpful microorganisms, crops, products, and their functionality in the target environment are all optimized. According to the literature, a variety of microorganisms were used to inoculate crops, but only a small number of strains—including those of *Bacillus, Pseudomonas, Xanthomonas,* and *Achromobacter* spp.—were chosen for commercial applications and to increase crop production. Today, however, farmers need a specific strain or consortium of microorganisms to boost crop growth and yield. The PGPR (plant growth-promoting rhizobacteria) activity is caused by the rhizospheric microflora, which is significant for the crop in terms of biogeochemical cycles, such as nitrogen fixation, carbon, and phosphorous cycles. Rhizospheric microflora can also be crucial for the survival of endangered plant species (Pankaj, 2012; Pankaj et al., 2016). To increase crop yield and decrease the usage of synthetic chemical fertilizers, it is currently necessary to identify microbial cultures and create ways for mass-producing microbial consortium from natural microflora. Crop improvement may benefit from genetic modification and the microbial consortium. Microbiological technology refers to the large-scale use of living things and their byproducts in industrial processes. Microbial technology is a branch of technology that includes the application of microorganisms for various economic applications. Sometimes, microbial technology is also known as industrial microbiology, particularly when microbes are used for large-scale production of enzymes and other pharmaceutical products. Researchers can now use microbes to manufacture novel chemicals that they were unable to produce naturally thanks to genetic engineering. Microbial technology can be classified into two divisions: (1) Products are normally produced by microorganisms at a large scale by traditional microbial technology. (2) New genes are inserted or deleted in the organism by microbial technology with genetically engineered microorganisms (Luciana et al., 2017).

Cereals are the essence of human subsistence, and their consolidation into a broad range of commodities is of prominent economic significance. From ancient times, maize has become the most fruitful cereal crop, directly or indirectly, in the feeding of human beings and massively plays a significant role in human life. It is one of the most widely grown crops in the world, used for food, fuel, and the production of industrial goods. It is essential for supplying the world's increasing food requirements. Overall, 967 million metric tons (MMT) of maize production were obtained in the world; it is ranked third among major cereal crops and in India was 23 MMT in 2013–14. *Zea mays* is known globally as the queen of cereals due to the highest yield potential among the cereals. It is ranked third among major cereal crops. The United States of America (USA) contributes about 35% of the total world maize production; it is the largest producer of maize (Sandhu et al., 2007). Maize is the driver of the US economy and known as the mother grain of Americans. Uttar Pradesh, Bihar, Rajasthan, Madhya Pradesh, Punjab, Haryana, Maharashtra, Andhra Pradesh, Himachal

Pradesh, West Bengal, Karnataka, and Jammu and Kashmir are the major maize-growing states in India and jointly account for over 95% of the national maize production (Mehta and Dias, 1999; Milind et al., 2013). A major focus of various studies in the phytochemical compounds and health properties is the development of nutraceuticals in cereal crops viz. maize. The various nutrients and other food components like phytochemicals are present in cereals and play an important contribution to the diet, but lysine amino acid remains absent in most of the cereals. Increasing levels of specific vitamins in the fortified cereals would have a significant impact on nutritional benefits (Wally et al., 2017). Maize is a significant staple cereal crop with a wider range of uses than other cereals (Oliver, 2014). In agricultural sciences, the identification and development of new microbial technologies will be helpful for the improvement and protection of crops, and these techniques will greatly contribute to food security. In this chapter, we are going to discuss an array of microbial technologies for enhanced crop protection of the maize crop, thus better realization of yields.

## 6.2 TRANSGENIC APPROACHES FOR CROP IMPROVEMENT

The microorganisms have a variety of naturally advantageous genes that can be introduced to crop plants via genetic engineering methods. The gene transfer from microorganisms to plants is a very common practice by *Agrobacterium tumefaciens*-mediated gene transfer. In general, genetically engineered cultivars have increased nutrition, yield, and resistance to biotic and abiotic stressors. The most significant abiotic environmental stressor among these is drought, which lowers the output of cultivated crops (Arafa et al., 2009; Kamthan et al., 2016). Developing nitrogen-fixing cereals by direct *nif*-gene is another important factor for cereal crop improvement. Transferring genes of interest by using recombinant DNA technology has many ethical issues. However, genome-editing techniques pave the way to use nucleases that allow change or mutation of important genes without introducing foreign DNA for the development of plants, and this technology might be acknowledged as non-transgenic genetically reconstructed plants (Table 6.1). Genome editing can be helpful where GM crops are poorly accepted and pave the way for the establishment and marketing of transgenic plants with excellent phenotypes, even in countries (India). GM crops can easily fulfill the need for hunger in India (Kamthan et al., 2016).

**TABLE 6.1** Transgenic (GM) Maize Varieties for Commercial Cultivation

| Gene | Causal Organism | Varieties | Year of release | Releasing Country |
|---|---|---|---|---|
| **Resistance of Insecticides and Pesticides of *Zea mays* (Maize)** | | | | |
| *Bacillus thuringiensis* (Bt gene Cry3Bb1), a soil bacterium | *Ostrinia nubilalis* (European Corn borer) | Bt-176 "Maximizer" | 1995 | Northrup King |
| Bt gene (Cry3Bb1) | *Ostrinia nubilalis* | MON 810 (YieldGard® Corn Borer | 1996 | Monsanto |
| Bt gene (Cry3Bb1) | *Diabrotica virgifera virgifera* (corn root worm) | MON 863 (YieldGard® Rootworm) | 2003 | United States |
| **Resistance of Herbicides of *Zea mays*** | | | | |
| Glufosinate | Attack on Combat missed weeds | Libertylink (non-selective herbicide) | 1996 | AgeEvo |
| Sethoxydim | Attack on post-emergent herbicide | SR | 1994 | BASF |
| Glufosinate | Attack on Combat missed weeds | Non-selective foliar herbicide | 1996 | Dekaib Genetics |
| Glyphosate or Roundup Ready | Attack on pre- and post-emergence herbicide | Non-selective foliar herbicide | 1970 | Monsanto |
| Glyfosinate | Attack on Combat missed weeds | Non-selective weed control | 1970 | Plant Genetic Systems |
| **Resistance of Glyphosate Herbicides of GM lines of *Zea mays*** | | | | |
| Modified 5-enolpyruvylshikimate-3-phosphate synthase (*EPSPS*) enzyme | *Ostrinia nubilalis* | Roundup Ready™ Maize, Agrisure™GT (GA21) | 1996/1997 | France, Spain, Germany, U.K., and Canada |

## 6.3 TECHNIQUES FOR CROP TRANSFORMATION

Genetic transformation is the process of integrating external DNA into the germ line of entire organisms; as a result, it will be passed on to succeeding generations. In order to create transgenic plants, genetic transformation techniques are currently often used in a wide variety of plant species. *Agrobacterium*-mediated transformation, biolistic technique, silicon whisker, liposomes, and microinjection are a few examples. The most practical method for introducing the genes in plants is through biolistic-mediated transformation and *Agrobacterium tumefaciens* (Hwang et al., 2017).

### 6.3.1 DEVELOPMENT OF MAIZE TRANSFORMATION

Since the mid-1990s, the first transgenic of (*Bacillus thuringiensis* (*'Bt'*) genes (*Cry1Ab, Cry1F*) maize products were launched in the market. A critical step in the development of transgenic plants is the introduction of novel biotech traits or products, producing maize plants with highly desirable traits and their commercial applications. Rhodes et al. (1988) reported the use of protoplasts for developing transgenic maize plants. The advanced technologies for the development or improvement of *Agrobacterium*-mediated and biolistic (also known as microparticle bombardment) methods of transformation were effectively exhibited to generate extremely fertile maize transgenics using embryogenic suspension cell cultures as an explant, and *ALS* (*acetolactate synthase*), *HPT* (*hygromycin phosphotransferase*), or *BAR* (*bialaphos resistance*) genes as selectable markers have made the production of transgenic maize more manageable and more stable (Gordon-Kamm et al., 1990; Ishida et al., 2003). A selectable marker *BAR* was used for establishing hybrid Hi-II (Frame et al., 2006). The inbred line A188 (Ishida et al., 1996), Hi-II (Zhao et al., 2002), and A188/Hi-II hybrids were used in the efficient *Agrobacterium*-mediated transformation systems. The most important step is to first examine the following available factors as described previously ( Lowe et al., 2018; Mookkan et al., 2017) such as:

1. Tissue culture techniques.
2. Identify regeneration methods.
3. Identify prospective explants.
4. Determine the location of the cells involved.
5. Improve tissue culture conditions to increase cell numbers or accessibility.
6. Create conditions for the nonlethal transfer of DNA into a large number of target cells per bombardment.

One of the most important components is an effective selection system with an efficient transformation. In the presence of the selection agents, it permits the preferred proliferation of transformed cells while suppressing or eliminating untransformed cells. In addition, the ideal selection agent shouldn't have a detrimental impact on subsequent regeneration, rooting, or plant development. The evolution optimization of selectable markers and gene delivery methods has been an essential element of developing efficient maize transformation systems, as selection agents such as antibiotics and herbicides have been widely used in maize transformation system development.

### 6.3.2 TRANSFORMATION OF TARGET VARIETY AND EXPLANT

Development of maize transformants inbred lines with outstanding agronomic features would be ideal for commercial use. The creation of maize lines that are highly transformable, affordable, and readily accessible in significant amounts all year round should be used as the mother plant (Jones et al., 2019). Agrobacterium-mediated transformation technologies have effectively generated transgenic plants from many inbred genotypes of maize immature embryos (Frame et al., 2006; Gordon-Kamm et al., 2002; Huang et al., 2005). Callus formation is also considered a noteworthy transformation factor, and the callus of maize immature embryos are classified into two types of embryogenic (Jones et al., 2019). Immature embryos from several maize inbred genotypes respond to stimulation by producing type I calluses, which are more difficult to convert. The transformation of *Agrobacterium*-mediated inbred genotypes that produce type I callus has been substantially improved by the optimization of the media component (Gordon-Kamm et al., 2002; Ishida et al., 2003). The majority of investigations used type II callus; however, some transformation experiments used type I callus, which is produced from the immature embryonic scutellum and is fragile, quickly developing, and highly regenerable (Armstrong, 1991). These characteristics facilitate the collection and improvement of transformants, and as a result, the friable and target tissues in maize have changed into type II callus and its liquid suspension (Frame et al., 2006; Fromm et al., 1990; Gordon-Kamm et al., 1990). Type II callus development is strongly reliant on genotype. Only a few genotypes, including A188, Hi-II, A188Hi-II, B73, and Cz643, are known to produce type II callus development (Armstrong, 1991; Frame et al., 2000; Green et al., 2009). Hi-II, a hybrid line, is the most commonly used for genotypes producing type II callus, as of its dependability and great efficiency of transformation in laboratories. Identification for the genetic loci responsible for embryogenic callus formation is a considerable effort, and it makes non-responsive inbred lines transformable are shown in Jones et al. (2019).

### *6.3.3 TRANSFORMATION OF BINARY VECTOR SYSTEM HAS ALSO BEEN ACHIEVED*

According to Frame et al. (2002), normal maize transformation uses the model binary (non-super binary) vector system of *Agrobacterium tumefaciens* (Zea mays). According to the existing convention, the average stable transformation performance (the number of bialaphos-safe functions increased per 100 embryos undeveloped organisms tainted) was 5.5%. Integration, expression by the southern blot, and progeny analysis of fertile, stable transgenic maize employing an *A. tumefaciens* standard binary vector system have all been used to demonstrate the *bar* and *gus* transgenes inheritance in the R0, R1, and R2 generations of transgenic events (Raruang et al., 2020).

## 6.4 CROP PROTECTION THROUGH MICROBIAL TECHNOLOGY

For the production of crops and yields, soil is one of the most crucial elements. Because elements can be disintegrated from the soil due to the transformations that predispose nutrients to loss, soil microbes play a critical role in recycling nutrients as well as making them available to plants. They also convert elements into gaseous form (Jacoby et al., 2017). Nowadays, researchers are focusing on pesticidal activity, mainly herbicidal, insecticidal, and nematocidal, of microorganisms having numerous types of compounds. European corn borer (*Ostrinia nubilalis*) and Mediterranean corn borer (*Sesamia nonagrioides*) are found in winter seasons in India. It is commonly known as pink borer and is nocturnal. On the lower leaf sheath, *Sesamia* lays eggs, and *Sesamia* larva enters into the plant near the base and causes damage to the stem. In India, *Chilo partellus* is one of the major insects, which are found in stems of maize. It is commonly known as stalk borer. During the monsoon seasons, this insect is obtained throughout the country. After the germination of the lower side of the leaves, it is suitable for the *Chilo* to lay eggs for 10–25 days. The *Chilo* larva enters the whole plant and damages the whole plant, especially the leaves. In South India, *Atherigona* sp., sometimes known as the shoot fly, is a major pest that affects North Indian maize crops in the spring and summer. Attacks of shoot fly, especially on the seedling stage, mainly affect the core branch or primary growth point and cause dead heart formation. The larvae of American bollworm (*Helicoverpa armigera*, novel *cry2AX1* gene to impart insect resistance), chaffer beetle (*Chiloloba acuta*), and termites (*Odontotermes obesus*) are unconventional pests that are also causing damage to maize crop (Table 6.2). In the Southern part of India, American bollworm and termites mainly damage the cob of maize. In the Northern part of India, the chaffer beetle pest is feeding only on pollen of maize and mainly affects pollination. These diseases are cured by genetic engineering and produced transgenic maize traits including *Bacillus thuringiensis* ('*Bt*') genes (*Cry1Ab and Cry1F*) that code for *lepidopteran*-specific protein toxins for protection against *lepidopteran* pests like European corn borer (*Ostrinia nubilalis*) and Mediterranean corn borer (*Sesamia nonagrioides*) (Sarwar, 2015). Around 75% of maize advance production is reflected in the United States containing biotech traits, which are contributed by technology.

In different parts of India, the *Macrophomina phaseolina* (charcoal rots), *Fusarium moniliforme* (foot rots and wilting), and *Fusarium graminearum* (root rots, stalk rots, and wilting), and so forth, pests cause substantial damage to the maize. The development of bio-control agents is the best alternative source to minimize the incidence of these diseases because the soil-borne fungal pathogen can easily infest the crop. By the combined applications of the two *Bacillus* as well as *Pseudomonas* sp., two *Bacillus* obtained from maize rhizosphere significantly reduced (56.04%) charcoal rots of maize. The collar rots, root, and foot rots, and wilting of maize caused by *F. moniliforme* and *F. graminearum* are significantly reduced when treated with the *Bacillus* and *Pseudomonas* species (Chang et al., 1968; Pal et al., 2001).

## 6.5 IMPACTS OF STRESS IN ZEA MAYS YIELD

Yield of any crop depends on many factors, and stress is one of them. Stresses are majorly two types: biotic and abiotic. Abiotic stresses such as salinity, drought, nutrient deficiency, and high and low temperatures are the significant environmental factors that negatively affect maize yields.

**TABLE 6.2** Relationship Between Maize Microbial Diseases and Pathogen

| S. No. | Name of Crop | Microbial Inoculants | Environmental Conditions | Significance |
|---|---|---|---|---|
| 1. | Maize | *Bacillus subtilis, Pseudomonas corrugate* | Cool regions (22°C) | Grain yields are increased in size and resistance to pathogen |
| **Fungal Disease** | | | | |
| **S. No.** | **Crop** | **Plant Disease and Pathogen** | **Bio-Control Agents** | **Management Approaches** |
| 1. | Maize | Fusarium wilt<br>*Fusarium* Spp. | *Bacillus subtilis*<br>*Trichoderma* spp., *Penicillium, Rhizobium* and *Pseudomonas* spp., and so forth. These bio-control agents are promoting PGPF and PGPR these are boosting defense mechanism | Chemical fertilizers and cultural including soil disinfection (fumigants, hot water treatment, and solarisation) and resistant cultivars |
| 2. | Maize | Pythium stalk rot<br>*Pythium aphanidermatum* | Can use *Trichoderma* spp. and *PGPF* | Remove low areas in the field and improvement in drainage |
| 3. | Maize | Head smut<br>*Sphacelotheca reiliana* | Can use *Trichoderma* spp. and *PGPF* | Seed treatment with triadimenol (Baytan), tebuconazole (Raxil-50), and Sumi-8 (diniconazole) and take resistance variety including Commander, Rapidpak, Style-pak, and Reliance |
| 4. | Maize | Anthracnose stalk rot<br>*Colletotrichum graminicola* | Not reported | Hybrids resistance variety, residue management, stress mitigation, and crop rotation |
| 5. | Maize | Ear rot<br>*Fusarium verticillioides* and *Fusarium graminearum* | Biocontrol (PGPR and PGPF) | Chemical fertilizers and cultural including soil disinfection (fumigants, hot water treatment, and solarisation) and resistant cultivars |
| 6. | Maize | Ergot<br>*Claviceps gigantea* | Not reported | Field control methods for ergot disease are not developed. Sclerotia can be removed before planting. |

**TABLE 6.2** *(Continued)*

| S. No. | Crop | Plant disease and Pathogen | Bio-Control Agents | Management Approaches |
|---|---|---|---|---|
| **Bacterial Disease** | | | | |
| 1. | Maize | Bacterial stalk rot *Erwinia carotovora* | VAM fungi (*Glomus fasciculatum*) and Antagonistic bacteria (*Bacillus subtilis, Pseudomonas fluorescens*) | Cultural practices (avoid flooding and excessive irrigation), chemical (tried streptomycin and ter-ramycin), and biological control |
| 2. | Maize | Stewart's wilt *Pantoea stewartii* | *P. stewartii* sub spp. *stewartii* might be effectively reduced within its vector (beetle) by virulent bacteriophages. | Through chemical control |
| 3. | Maize | Bacteria leaf stripe *Xanthomonas vasicola* | No bio-agents | Cultural and physical control and sanitary measures |
| **Viruses and Mollicutes Disease** | | | | |
| 1. | Maize | Corn stunt Spiroplasma kunkelii | Not reported | Control the vector and no significant approaches are developed |
| 2. | Maize | Maize bushy stunt Phytoplasma | For control leafhoppers (vector) through parasitic fungi including *Beauveria bassiana, Metarhizium anisopliae, Verticillium lecanii,* and *Paecilomyces fumosoroseus* | Chemical control |

Abiotic stresses are an important limiting factor in agricultural production. To cope with these edaphic and environmental factors, plants modify their metabolic system, in that microbes present in the vicinity play an important role. The interaction between plants and microorganisms, which modifies local and systemic systems in plants to provide nourishment in challenging environmental situations, is a crucial component of the living ecosystem (Meena et al., 2017). Under the constant strain of growing environmental changes, the interactions between plants and microbes in terms of defense against abiotic stressors are rising. The major bacterial species such as *Rhizobium* spp., *Bacillus* sp., *Acetobacter* spp., *Azotobacter* spp., fungal species *Fusarium* spp., *Aspergillus* spp., *Trichoderma* spp., and cyanobacterial species *Nostoc* spp., *Oscillatoria* sp., *Anabaena* spp., *Cylindrospermum* spp., *Lyngbya* spp., *Scytonema* spp., *Calothrix* spp., and *Fischerella* spp., and so forth, are found in *Zea mays* root (Meena et al., 2017).

### 6.5.1 ROLE OF ENDOPHYTES AND PGPR IN CROP PRODUCTION UNDER STRESS

Endophytes are organisms that include fungi and bacteria, which spend their whole lifecycle in living plant cells. They establish varied types of relationships with the plant, from symbiotic to bordering on pathogenic. Such a heterogeneous group is called Plant Growth Promoting Rhizobacteria (PGPR); these are root-associated bacteria that enhance plant health and/or growth by several mechanisms (Santos et al., 2018) (Figure 6.1). Some of the rhizospheric bacteria enhance productivity due to their phosphate solubilization abilities, by acetylene reduction activities, or by indole acetic acid production potential. These isolates significantly enhanced shoot and root fresh and dry biomass of maize plants, compared to the non-inoculated control under greenhouse requirements (Majeed et al., 2015). *Bacillus* species like *B. polymyxa, B. pantothenticus, B. anthracis, B. thuringiensis,* and *B. circulans,* three *Pseudomonas* species (*P. cichorii, P. putida,* and *P. syringae),* and *Serratia marcescens* were identified from maize root of five agro-ecological zones as PGPR (Agbodjato et al., 2015; Akinrinlola et al., 2018). In another study, Kuan et al. (2016) identified PGPR strains of bacteria viz. *Klebsiella* sp. (*Br1*), *Klebsiella pneumoniae* (*Fr1*), *Bacillus pumilus* (*S1r1*), and *Acinetobacter* sp. (*S3r2*), and a reference strain used was *Bacillus subtilis* (*UPMB10*) to enhance yield in maize.

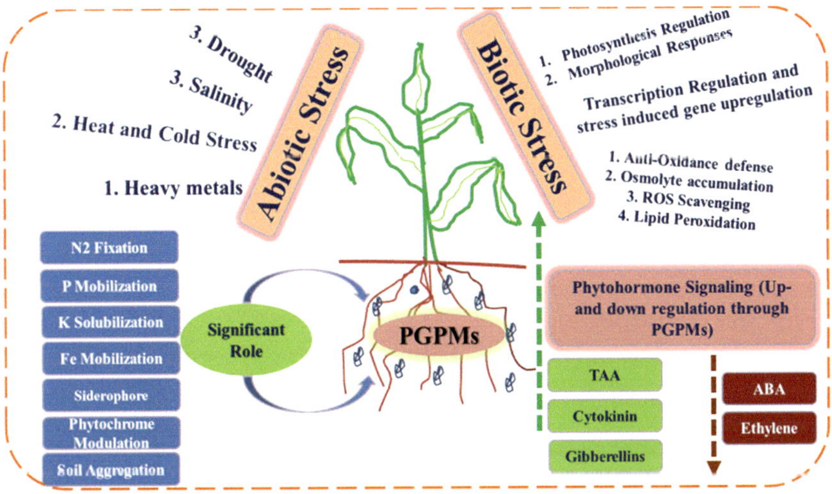


**FIGURE 6.1** A schematic approach of microbial community-based under biotic and abiotic stress conditions.

## 6.6 CONCLUSIONS

In ancient times, agricultural crops were grown under the natural system (without the use of pesticides), but the crop yield was not sufficient for the increasing world population, so agriculture shifted toward a load of chemical fertilizers. Crop yield was obtained sufficiently, but the natural microflora and other living systems were affected. Pollution is now one of the leading causes of human mortality. Excessive chemical fertilizers were used to feed the growing population of the world. The world population depends directly or indirectly on agriculture to fulfill all types of requirements. Therefore, to solve such problems, scientists are focusing on bio-fertilizers for crop improvement on a large scale. Many scientific reports have shown and confirmed that bio-fertilizers are more advantageous than chemical fertilizers and obtain higher crop yields. A consortium of natural bacterial cultures is more propitious than the free strain. Microbial technology is another pathway for improvement and protection of crop predictability. Till now, a total of 251 beneficial genes has been transferred through these techniques to crops using microorganisms, which are beneficial in providing biotic and abiotic resistance. Through the development of microbial technology, a new microbial consortium will significantly increase agricultural yield. Correct communication clarification in consortium inoculants will improve rhizosphere acclimation. Industrial and municipal wastewater-irrigated maize plants' rhizosphere and endorhiza are home to heavy metals-resistant bacteria that have a variety of positive impacts and the capacity to produce PGP characteristics.

## KEYWORDS

- **bio-fertilizers**
- **consortium microbial technologies**
- **microbial services**
- **improvement**
- **protection**
- **plant-microbe interactions**

## REFERENCES


Agbodjato, N. A., Noumavo, P. A., Baba-Moussa, F., Salami, H. A., Sina, H., Sèzan, A., & Baba-Moussa, L. (2015). Characterization of potential plant growth promoting rhizobacteria isolated from maize (*Zea mays* L.) in central and northern Benin (West Africa). *Applied and Environmental Soil Science, 2015.*

Akinrinlola, R. J., Yuen, G. Y., Drijber, R. A., & Adesemoye, A. O. (2018). Evaluation of *Bacillus* strains for plant growth promotion and predictability of efficacy by *in vitro* physiological traits. *International Journal of Microbiology*. https://doi.org/10.1155/2018/5686874 (accessed on 5th November 2025).

Arafa, A. A., Khafagy, M. A., & El-Banna, M. F. (2009). The effect of glycine betaine or ascorbic acid on grain germination and leaf structure of sorghum plants grown under salinity stress. *Australian Journal of Crop Science, 3*(5), 294–304.

Armstrong, C. (1991). Development and availability of germplasm with high type II culture response. *Maize Genetics Cooperation Newsletter, 65*, 92–93.

Basu, S. K., Dutta, M., Goyal, A., Bhowmik, P. K., Kumar, J., Nandy, S., Kumar, R., & Prasad, R. (2010). Is genetically modified crop the answer for the next green revolution? *GM Crops, 1*(2), 68–79. https://doi.org/10.4161/gmcr.1.2.11877 (accessed on 5th November 2025).

Berg, G. (2009). Plant–microbe interactions promoting plant growth and health: perspectives for controlled use of microorganisms in agriculture. *Applied Microbiology and Biotechnology, 84*(1), 11–18.

Chang, I., & Kommedahl, T. (1968). Biological control of seedling blight of corn by coating kernels with antagonistic microorganisms. *Phytopathology, 58*, 1395–1401.

Frame, B. R., McMurray, J. M., Fonger, T. M., Main, M. L., Taylor, K. W., Torney, F. J., & Wang, K. (2006). Improved *Agrobacterium*-mediated transformation of three maize inbred lines using MS salts. *Plant Cell Reports, 25*(10), 1024–1034.

Frame, B. R., Paque, T., & Wang, K. (2006). Maize (*Zea mays* L.). In *Agrobacterium Protocols* (pp. 185–200).

Frame, B. R., Shou, H., Chikwamba, R. K., Zhang, Z., Xiang, C., Fonger, T. M., & Wang, K. (2002). *Agrobacterium tumefaciens*-mediated transformation of maize embryos using a standard binary vector system. *Plant Physiology, 129*(1), 13–22. https://doi.org/10.1104/pp.000653 (accessed on 5th November 2025).

Frame, B. R., Zhang, H., Cocciolone, S. M., Sidorenko, L. V., Dietrich, C. R., Pegg, S. E., & Wang, K. (2000). Production of transgenic maize from bombarded type II callus: effect of gold particle size and callus morphology on transformation efficiency. *In Vitro Cellular & Developmental Biology–Plant, 36*(1), 21–29.

Fromm, M. E., Morrish, F., Armstrong, C., Williams, R., Thomas, J., & Klein, T. M. (1990). Inheritance and expression of chimeric genes in the progeny of transgenic maize plants. *Bio/Technology, 8*(9), 833–839.

Gordon-Kamm, W. J., Spencer, T. M., Mangano, M. L., Adams, T. R., Daines, R. J., Start, W. G., & Lemaux, P. G. (1990). Transformation of maize cells and regeneration of fertile transgenic plants. *The Plant Cell, 2*(7), 603–618.

Gordon-Kamm, W., Dilkes, B. P., Lowe, K., Hoerster, G., Sun, X., Ross, M., & Larkins, B. A. (2002). Stimulation of the cell cycle and maize transformation by disruption of the plant retinoblastoma pathway. *Proceedings of the National Academy of Sciences, 99*(18), 11975–11980.

Graham, P. H., & Vance, C. P. (2003). Legumes: importance and constraints to greater use. *Plant Physiology, 131*(3), 872–877.

Green, J. M., Hale, T., Pagano, M. A., Andreassi, J. L., & Gutteridge, S. A. (2009). Response of 98140 corn with gat4621 and hra transgenes to glyphosate and ALS-inhibiting herbicides. *Weed Science, 57*(2), 142–148.

Huang, X., & Wei, Z. (2005). Successful *Agrobacterium*-mediated genetic transformation of maize elite inbred lines. *Plant Cell, Tissue and Organ Culture, 83*(2), 187–200.

Hwang, H. H., Yu, M., & Lai, E. M. (2017). *Agrobacterium*-mediated plant transformation: biology and applications. *The Arabidopsis Book, 15*. https://doi.org/10.1199/tab.0186 (accessed on 5th November 2025).

Ishida, Y., Saito, H., Hiei, Y., & Komari, T. (2003). Improved protocol for transformation of maize (*Zea mays* L.) mediated by *Agrobacterium tumefaciens*. *Plant Biotechnology, 20*(1), 57–66.

Ishida, Y., Saito, H., Ohta, S., Hiei, Y., Komari, T., & Kumashiro, T. (1996). High efficiency transformation of maize (*Zea mays* L.) mediated by *Agrobacterium tumefaciens*. *Nature Biotechnology, 14*(6), 745–750.

Jacoby, R., Peukert, M., Succurro, A., Koprivova, A., & Kopriva, S. (2017). The role of soil microorganisms in plant mineral nutrition—current knowledge and future directions. *Frontiers in Plant Science, 8*, 1617. https://doi.org/10.3389/fpls.2017.01617 (accessed on 5th November 2025).

Jones, T., Lowe, K., Hoerster, G., Anand, A., Wu, E., Wang, N., & Gordon-Kamm, W. (2019). Maize transformation using the morphogenic genes Baby Boom and Wuschel2. In *Transgenic Plants* (pp. 81–93). Humana Press, New York, NY.

Kamthan, A., Chaudhuri, A., Kamthan, M., & Datta, A. (2016). Genetically modified (GM) crops: milestones and new advances in crop improvement. *Theoretical and Applied Genetics, 129*(9), 1639–1655. https://doi.org/10.1007/s00122-016-2747-6 (accessed on 5th November 2025).

Kuan, K. B., Othman, R., Abdul Rahim, K., & Shamsuddin, Z. H. (2016). Plant growth-promoting rhizobacteria inoculation to enhance vegetative growth, nitrogen fixation and nitrogen remobilisation of maize under greenhouse conditions. *PLOS ONE, 11*(3), e0152478.

Lehr, P. (2010). *Biopesticides: The Global Market*. Report code CHM029B, BCC Research, Wellesley, Massachusetts.

Lowe, K., La Rota, M., Hoerster, G., Hastings, C., Wang, N., Chamberlin, M., & Gordon-Kamm, W. (2018). Rapid genotype "independent" *Zea mays* L. (maize) transformation via direct somatic embryogenesis. *In Vitro Cellular & Developmental Biology–Plant, 54*(3), 240–252. https://doi.org/10.1007/s11627-018-9905-2 (accessed on 5th November 2025).

Majeed, A., Abbasi, M. K., Hameed, S., Imran, A., & Rahim, N. (2015). Isolation and characterization of plant growth-promoting rhizobacteria from wheat rhizosphere and their effect on plant growth promotion. *Frontiers in Microbiology, 6*, 198. https://doi.org/10.3389/fmicb.2015.00198 (accessed on 5th November 2025).

Meena, K. K., Sorty, A. M., Bitla, U. M., Choudhary, K., Gupta, P., Pareek, A., & Minhas, P. S. (2017). Abiotic stress responses and microbe-mediated mitigation in plants: the omics strategies. *Frontiers in Plant Science, 8*, 172. https://doi.org/10.3389/fpls.2017.00172 (accessed on 5th November 2025).

Mehta, D. C., & Dias, F. F. (1999). Maize: perspectives and applications in India. *Starch-Stärke, 51*(2, 3), 52–57. https://doi.org/10.1002/(ISSN)1521-379X (accessed on 5th November 2025).

Milind, P., & Isha, D. (2013). *Zea mays*: A modern craze. *International Research Journal of Pharmacy, 4*(6), 39–43.

Mookkan, M., Nelson-Vasilchik, K., Hague, J., Zhang, Z. J., & Kausch, A. P. (2017). Selectable marker independent transformation of recalcitrant maize inbred B73 and sorghum P898012 mediated by morphogenic regulators BABY BOOM and WUSCHEL2. *Plant Cell Reports, 36*(9), 1477–1491. https://doi.org/10.1007/s00299-017-2169-1 (accessed on 5th November 2025).

Oerke, E. C. (2006). Crop losses to pests. *The Journal of Agricultural Science, 144*(1), 31–43.

Oliver, M. J. (2014). Why we need GMO crops in agriculture. *Missouri Medicine, 111*(6), 492.

Pal, K. K., Tilak, K. V. B. R., Saxena, A. K., Dey, R., & Singh, C. S. (2001). Suppression of maize root diseases caused by *Macrophomina phaseolina*, *Fusarium moniliforme* and *Fusarium graminearum* by plant growth promoting rhizobacteria. *Microbiological Research, 156*(3), 209–223.

Pankaj, B. (2012). Isolation and characterization of rhizobia isolate from the rhizosphere soil of *Meizotropis pellita*. *Asian Journal of Microbiology Biotechnology and Environmental*

*Sciences, 16*(2), 301–306. https://www.researchgate.net/publication/267635876_Isolation_and_characterization_of_rhizobial_isolates_from_the_rhizospheric_soil_of_an_endangered_plant_Meizotropis_pellita (accessed on 5th November 2025).

Pankaj, S. A., Gangola, S., Khati, P., Kumar, G., & Srivastava, A. (2016). Novel pathway of cypermethrin biodegradation in a *Bacillus* sp. strain SG2 isolated from cypermethrin-contaminated agriculture field. *3 Biotech, 6*(1), 1–11. https://doi.org/10.1007/s13205-016-0372-3 (accessed on 5th November 2025).

Raruang, Y., Omolehin, O., Hu, D., Wei, Q., Han, Z. Q., Rajasekaran, K., & Chen, Z. Y. (2020). Host-induced gene silencing targeting *Aspergillus flavus* aflM reduced aflatoxin contamination in transgenic maize under field conditions. *Frontiers in Microbiology, 11*, 754. https://doi.org/10.3389/fmicb.2020.00754 (accessed on 5th November 2025).

Rhodes, C. A., Pierce, D. A., Mettler, I. J., Mascarenhas, D., & Detmer, J. J. (1988). Genetically transformed maize plants from protoplasts. *Science, 240*(4849), 204–207.

Sandhu, K. S., Singh, N., & Malhi, N. S. (2007). Some properties of corn grains and their flours I: Physicochemical, functional and chapati-making properties of flours. *Food Chemistry, 101*(3), 938–946. https://doi.org/10.1016/j.foodchem.2006.02.040 (accessed on 5th November 2025).

Santos, M. L. D., Berlitz, D. L., Wiest, S. L. F., Schünemann, R., Knaak, N., & Fiuza, L. M. (2018). Benefits associated with the interaction of endophytic bacteria and plants. *Brazilian Archives of Biology and Technology, 61*. https://doi.org/10.1590/1678-4324-2018160431 (accessed on 5th November 2025).

Sarwar, M. (2015). Biopesticides: an effective and environmentally friendly insect-pests inhibitor line of action. *International Journal of Engineering and Advanced Research Technology, 1*(2), 10–15.

Vitorino, L. C., & Bessa, L. A. (2017). Technological microbiology: development and applications. *Frontiers in Microbiology, 8*, 827. https://doi.org/10.3389/fmicb.2017.00827 (accessed on 5th November 2025).

Wally, A., & Beillard, M. J. (2017). Egypt's wheat and corn imports hold steady; rice exports remain restricted. *United States Department of Agriculture (USDA), Foreign Agricultural Service.*

Zhao, Z. Y., Gu, W., Cai, T., Tagliani, L., Hondred, D., Bond, D., & Pierce, D. (2002). High throughput genetic transformation mediated by *Agrobacterium tumefaciens* in maize. *Molecular Breeding, 8*(4), 323–333.

CHAPTER 7

# Contemporary Role of Biotechnology in Agriculture and Food Industries

SASHI SONKAR,[1] AKHILESH KUMAR SINGH,[2,*]
PRAKASH KUMAR SARANGI,[3,*] and LAXUMAN SHARMA[4]

[1]*Department of Botany, Bankim Sardar College, Tangrakhali, West Bengal, India*

[2]*Department of Biotechnology, School of Life Sciences, Mahatma Gandhi Central University, Motihari, Bihar, India*

[3]*College of Agriculture, Central Agricultural University, Imphal, Manipur, India*

[4]*Department of Horticulture, Sikkim University, Gangtok, Sikkim, India*

*Corresponding author

## ABSTRACT

Biotechnology refers to any technological application that uses living organisms or their derivatives to produce or modify goods for a specific use. The biotechnologist's unique approaches can help science, agriculture, and other crucial fields. Since the beginning of time, there has been biotechnology. When Edward Jenner developed vaccines and Alexander Fleming discovered antibiotics, the potential of biotechnology was recognized. Unquestionably, the processes of fermentation that generated beer, wine, and cheese are essential to modern society. The importance of food biotechnology is demonstrated by recent advancements in the food sector. Genetically modified (GM) plants are used to enhance the flavor, shelf life, nutrition, and value of food. The enzyme production in the food industry

Industrial Biotechnology: Current Progress and Novel Technologies.
Prakash Kumar Sarangi, Akhilesh Kumar Singh, Rajesh Kumar Srivastava, and Brijesh Pandey (Eds.)


DOI: 10.1201/9781779642233-7

has been carried out by involving transgenic yeast and bacteria. Biotechnological techniques, principally genetic engineering, are used to create these GM foods. Integrating advantageous foreign genes into an organism is the aim of genetic engineering. This foreign gene has been introduced in an effort to increase food production and quality. In this chapter, the applications of biotechnology in food and agriculture are discussed.

## 7.1 INTRODUCTION

Since ancient times, products derived from natural resources have been utilized. Across every scientific period, utilizing natural resources to obtain considerable benefits has always been of the utmost importance (Ranjha et al., 2022). Biotechnology is the use of any technological method to produce products for a specified purpose using biological organisms or their derivatives (GBO Report, 2007). Microorganisms, as well as human and animal contributions to every part of our life, are integrated via biotechnology. Different industries, including medical, environmental sciences, plant sciences, cell biology, animal sciences, agriculture, and food technology, have benefited greatly from biotechnology. For instance, food technology is a promising field of study that uses biotechnology to advance some of the oldest methods of food processing, including plant preservation, enzyme manufacturing, and fermentation (Yu, 2017).

Biotechnology is an essential tool in food industries to manipulate the genetic makeup of the sources of food, such as microorganisms, plants, and animals, to produce new species of plants and animals (Pal, 2017). Food industries utilize biotechnology to transform dietary components into other marketable and appealing value-added goods that are affordable, secure, nourishing, and healthful to promote human health. For instance, it has been demonstrated that the use of genetic engineering with the fermentation process is beneficial to produce "green" products like antioxidants, as well as the safeguarding of agricultural products. Therefore, by recycling food wastes using fermentation and enzymatic technologies, food biotechnology contributes to advances in resource utilization rates and decreases ecological pollution. Biotechnological methods are utilized to improve the quality, shelf life, nutrient content, and flavor of food items by the exploitation of genetically modified (GM) animals as well as plants. Nevertheless, GM bacteria and yeast are utilized to improve the production of food, particularly using genetic engineering methods (Enitan-Folami and Swalaha, 2020). Moreover, the utilization of biotechnology also comprises the cultivation of plants to increase and stabilize productivity by increasing their resistance to various insects, pests, and other potential threats, as well as various environmental factors like drought, cold, and acidic soil. Besides, modern biotechnology is also used to improve the nutritional value of various food crops (Khan and Khan, 2010; Ranjha et al., 2022). Overall, this chapter covers the application of biotechnology in the food and agricultural industries.

## 7.2 APPLICATIONS OF BIOTECHNOLOGY IN AGRICULTURE AND FOOD PRODUCTION

The potential uses of biotechnology in the field of agriculture and food sectors are discussed in subsections.

### *7.2.1 DISEASE-FREE CROP*

Plants are vulnerable to several viral and microbial infections and illnesses, which have a negative impact on plant yield, production, and global food security. Traditional breeding techniques have been used for years to create disease-free crops, but these techniques are often labor-intensive and costly. As a result, several cutting-edge technologies have been created to assist in combating viruses that cause disease. An extremely important utilization of biotechnology is the production of disease-free crops using the micropropagation technique. Disease-free plantlets of banana can be developed through micropropagation from healthy banana plant tissues. It has all the benefits of a cutting-edge technology and is also inexpensive and easy to use (Jain et al., 2021).

### *7.2.2 CULTIVATION ON ACIDIC SOIL*

Plant development is not hampered by soil acidity in and of itself. Instead, acidity can have a detrimental impact on biological activities that are beneficial to the growth of plants. Besides enhancing the accessibility of certain components to hazardous levels, especially manganese as well as aluminum, it diminishes the accessibility of plant nutrients like molybdenum as well as phosphorus. The beneficial habitat for earthworms, bacteria, and other soil organisms can be damaged by acidity. Moreover, the plant nutrients essential for growth can be leached underneath the rooting zone. Additionally, severely acidic soils can stop the survival of advantageous bacterial strains/species, such as the *Rhizobia* sp., which carry out the nitrogen fixation of legumes. To maintain the soil pH, lime can be administered. Although this method turns out to be fantastic, it is both costly and short-lived. An alternative is to develop enhanced varieties that are resistant to aluminum (Ranjha et al., 2022).

### 7.2.3 BIOENERGY

The availability of affordable, environmentally friendly, and fairly distributed energy will be a major determinant of any nation's economic security. The development of bioenergy in the form of biofuel is one of the newest developments to emerge. Biofuel is a feasible and developing substitute for fossil fuels. In order to increase lipid productivity, Sonkar and Mallick (2018) looked at four distinct phosphate application procedures in five green microalgae (*Chlamydomonas* sp., *Chlorella minutissima*, *Chlorella vulgaris*, *Tetradesmus lagerheimii*, and *Tetradesmus obliquus*). The two key factors that affect the final lipid production from algal biomass are cellular lipid content and biomass productivity. So, of the five test microalgae, *Chlorella minutissima* may be used as a source of feedstock for the production of biodiesel.

### 7.2.4 BIOFORTIFICATION OF EDIBLE CROPS

The terms biological fortification or biofortification relate to edible crops that have been designed and cultivated utilizing agronomic practices, traditional plant breeding, and advanced biotechnology techniques which are nutritionally enriched with greater accessibility to the world population (Garg et al., 2018). Growing malnourished children in developing nations with severe food shortages can benefit greatly from nutrient-supplemented foods like biofortified crops. One of these examples of biofortified crops is "potato." This GM potato, which is higher in protein than conventional potatoes, is widely grown and eaten in India. This GM potato contains substantial levels of all the essential amino acids, including methionine and lysine (Ranjha et al., 2022). Table 7.1 presented some of the plant species under biofortification of nutrients created by genetically engineered organisms to improve the nutritional quality.

**TABLE 7.1** The GM Plant Species with Enhanced Nutritional Value

| GM Plant Species | Type of Biofortification | References |
|---|---|---|
| Rice | Beta-carotene (pro-vitamin A) | Paine et al. (2005) |
| Sorghum | Protein digestibility improved | Elkonin et al. (2016) |
| Barley | Polyunsaturated fatty acids | Mihalik et al. (2014) |
| Maize | Pro-vitamin A | Decourcelle et al. (2015) |
| Wheat | Pro-vitamin A | Wang et al. (2014) |

### 7.2.5 AQUACULTURAL REPRODUCTION

Aquaculture has witnessed that biotechnology has a wide range of practical applications, which has increased aquaculture output. To increase output and enhance quality, scientists can find and combine features in fish and shellfish using biotechnology. Researchers are looking at genes that will boost the synthesis of chemicals that help marine species fight against microbial diseases and increase the natural growth hormones (GH) for fish. Research in this area is still ongoing in an effort to produce aquatic creatures safer and more effectively that can be consumed by humans (Jin et al., 2021).

### 7.2.6 SALINITY OR DROUGHT TOLERANCE

In most nations, starvation might come from the demolition or transformation of cropland; thus, farmers are obliged to cultivate their crops in areas that are largely unsuited for agricultural growth. Agricultural plants are created or developed to withstand greater salt content in soil, groundwater, as well as prolonged drought periods in order to assist people in agricultural output, particularly in unfavorable conditions (Maryam et al., 2017). The two basic strategies used in biotechnology techniques are short and targeted-gun methods. These methods are used to create GM crops with the capacity to confer drought tolerance (Khan and Khan, 2010). The GM

AgbO103 is a drought resistance variety of rice. The antinutrients, amino acids, proximate components, vitamins, and lipid profile of this resistant rice are identical to those of the parental rice cultivar (Cho, 2016).

### 7.2.7 FEEDING ANIMAL

Animal feed may be improved through biotechnology in three primary ways, which includes modifying rumen microorganisms to increase feed consumption, creating feed additives, and adding value to forage used as animal feed (Getabalew and Alemneh, 2019). In developed nations, genetically engineered crops are essentially in use. Such plants have a great potential to supply more nourishment than conventional crops (Kumar et al., 2020).

### 7.2.8 PRODUCTION OF INDUSTRIAL ENZYMES

For many years, people have employed enzymes as biological catalysts to speed up the metabolic processes of living things. They are proteins that are employed in several food sectors as raw materials and in the manufacture, processing, and preservation of food. They are employed in the preparation of a variety of foods, including beverages, baked goods, mayonnaise, cheese, and dairy products. Historically, enzymes were extracted from plants, but nowadays they may be found in microbes, plants, and animals. Microorganisms such as bacterial, yeast, and fungal strains/ species are key sources of the numerous commercial enzymes that are available in the market, depending on the substrate used and the ecological circumstances of the fermentation process. Some microorganism strains have undergone genetic modification in order to improve their capability for optimal enzyme synthesis. Using GM organism as a culture starter, a variety of industrial enzymes, including glucoamylase, lipase, amylase, pectinase, antibiotics, amino acids, lactic acid, nucleic acid, and polysaccharides have been generated (Enitan-Folami and Swalaha, 2020).

### 7.2.9 INSECTICIDE OR PESTICIDE RESISTANCE

Farmers suffer a financial loss when insects and other pests destroy their crops. Consumers are worried as toxic doses of synthetic pesticides are applied to agricultural fields every year, which might endanger human health. In light of this, development and research have led to the creation of GM foods like *Bacillus thuringiensis* (Bt) corn. This GM not only lowers the price of crop production and transportation to the market, but also assists in the reduction of the exploitation of chemically originated pesticides. Additionally, it aids in reducing any health concerns (Maryam et al., 2017). As a result, farmers no longer always need to use insecticides or pesticides, or they need to use them less frequently. This safeguards plants from hazardous pests (Enitan-Folami and Swalaha, 2020).

### 7.2.10 FOOD FERMENTATION

Fermentation is primarily responsible for the production/development of breweries. Commercial brewers use a range of yeast strains to manufacture beer. It is possible to produce light wine by genetic engineering. It is now possible to modify yeast using glucoamylase-encoded foreign genes. Glucoamylase is produced by yeast during alcoholic fermentation, which has been proven to convert starch into glucose. Yeast varieties that can initiate the malolactic fermentation process are used to make wine. There are two processes involved in wine synthesis. Firstly, yeast is used in primary fermentation to turn glucose into alcohol. Secondly, lactic acid with the highest amount of acidity is produced by secondary fermentation employing bacteria. To solve this problem, expensive divergent techniques are used. To remedy this issue, a malolactic gene from *Lactobacillus delbrueckii* is introduced. This gene inhibits the production of malate, reducing the acidity of the wine (Haroon and Ghazanfar, 2016; Ranjha et al., 2022).

### 7.2.11 VACCINE RESEARCH AND DEVELOPMENT

Synthetic antibiotics were developed in the 1950s, while DNA polymerase was discovered in 1955. The first polio vaccine, created by Dr. Jonas Salk in the same year, opened the door for the first application of mammalian cells and cell culture approaches towards vaccine manufacturing (Enitan-Folami and Swalaha, 2020). Biotechnology has created a potentially useful platform for scientists to create a variety of vaccines in big quantities and with high quality and dependability (de Sa and Keshavarz-Moore, 2021).

### 7.2.12 IMPROVE SHELF LIFE OF FOOD

By producing secondary metabolites, bacteria increase the shelf life of fermented foods and drinks. As an illustration, lactic acid bacteria, which includes the species *Streptococcus, Pediococcus, Lactococcus,* and *Lactobacillus* generate metabolites including lactic acid, hydrogen peroxide, and bacteriocins (pediocin PA-1 and nisin), that are used as natural preservatives in food (Enitan-Folami and Swalaha, 2020). The utilization of lactic acid bacteria as a starter or their byproducts is safe for food preparation (Enitan-Folami and Swalaha, 2020). The fermenting of milk can also benefit from the use of a lactic acid bacteria that produces nisin. Additionally, biotechnological methods to lengthen the duration that tomatoes may be stored have been created and patented (Zhao, 2007). This is accomplished by decreasing the enzymes that cause ripe tomato fruit to soften, which leads to the tomato's early degradation during the postharvest period or during storage (Deltsidis et al., 2018). Nevertheless, a lengthy shelf life for ripe tomatoes has been created, and margarine and canned goods have gained acceptance on a global scale (Monteiro, 2019).

### 7.2.13 SWEETENERS AND FLAVORS FOR FOOD

The manufacture of food components such as sweeteners, flavors, and amino acids is one of biotechnology's additional advantages. More than 100 commercial aroma compounds derived from biotechnological applications are currently vying with traditional agriculturally produced sources of taste to manufacture flavor generated by microorganisms. Utilizing transgenic technology, microorganisms are more effective at producing flavor-enhanced glutamate, thaumatin, aspartame, and other non-nutritive sweeteners. High-performance strains of *Corynebacterium glutamicum* and *E. coli* are used to do this while fermenting sugar sources such as molasses, sucrose, and glucose (Enitan-Folami and Swalaha, 2020).

### 7.2.14 IMPROVING PRODUCTIVITY OF CROPS

Healthy eating is known to be important for human growth and development. Adverse ecological factors, such as drought, floods, severe heat, and other similar conditions, have a greater impact on crop production than diseases and pests do. Hence, two primary objectives of plant scientists are to generate crops with enhanced nutritional content as well as strategies to maintain high productivity during stress. To meet the need for high-quality food around the world, GM crops might prove to be valuable alternatives to those grown employing conventional methods. The GM crops can be used to improve yields, nutritive value, and susceptibility to a range of biotic and abiotic challenges. Although there have been several biosecurity and health issues expressed in respect to GM crops, there is no reason to be wary of feeding items that have undergone careful research and testing. It is possible to achieve the goal of ensuring food security for both the present and future generations by sustainably combining contemporary biotechnology with conventional agronomic practices (Datta, 2013). Scientists introduced *Escherichia coli* with the bovine somatotropin genome. Nowadays, milk production is increased by 10–12 percent because of this hormone. Further, nine billion people are projected to inhabit the planet by the year 2050. Therefore, the same amount of land will therefore require a higher yield of milk. In this context, biotechnology may be the most effective way to address several difficulties with food productivity (Haroon and Ghazanfar, 2016; Ranjha et al., 2022). The four main GM crops include canola, cotton, maize, and soybeans. They were the most widely adopted GM crop among 26 nations. Soybeans, for example, accounted for 50% of the usage of genetically engineered crops worldwide with 95.9 million hectares, a 2% increase from 2017. They were followed by maize (58.9 million hectares), cotton (24.9 million hectares), and canola (10.1 million hectares) (Enitan-Folami and Swalaha, 2020).

## 7.3 FUTURE PROSPECTS

As biotechnology development and research progress, experts may find a quicker method to identify potentially harmful viruses and bacteria in food, which may help to keep food safe to consume and reduce the risk of food-borne diseases. Biotechnology is also being used to create crops that can thrive in challenging environmental circumstances like drought and high heat. This might result in the growing of crops on ground that was previously unsuited for cultivation. Nutritive food may be produced by employing food biotechnology for animals as well as humans. The store shelves will soon be stocked with foods that have improved nutritional qualities. By supplying more beneficial chemicals, such as higher levels of vitamins and antioxidants and lower levels of harmful fats, food biotechnology may help to fight against chronic diseases, which cause illnesses.

## 7.4 CONCLUSIONS

It might be argued that the use of biotechnological methods in the global food sectors has unquestionably advanced humanity up until this point. It is important to note that advantages outweigh any known limits, even though there is evidence of flaws in some sectors in which the technology from the biotechnology field has indeed been implemented. For instance, current concerns of hunger, malnutrition, poverty, and illnesses are being effectively handled with the use of modern biotechnology in food processing, such as enzyme synthesis, fermentation, and high nutritious foods and drinks. The development of GM crops using food biotechnology to improve the shelf life, yields, and nutritional qualities has greatly aided in addressing the demand for food self-sufficiency among several populations, particularly in Third World nations. All GM foods made by manufacturers, or the food industry, must have the appropriate labels. So that individuals may make an informed decision, awareness of the possible benefits and drawbacks of GM foods should be increased. To spread the advantages of GM foods, seminars and discussions should be held. While biotechnological application aids in raising food production, specialists in the area should step up their research output for more worthwhile discoveries and to eliminate any potential risks associated with foods created using biotechnology. To develop or manufacture more nutritious meals through the use of biotechnological skills, it is evident that collaboration between the food industry and scientists in universities and research centers be strengthened.

## KEYWORDS

- **biofortification**
- **biotechnology**
- **disease-resistant crops**
- **food and agriculture**
- **genetic engineering**
- **genetically modified organisms**

## REFERENCES

Cho, K., Lee, H. J., Jo, Y. M., Lim, S. H., Rakwal, R., Lee, J. Y., & Kim, Y. M. (2016). RNA interference-mediated simultaneous suppression of seed storage proteins in rice grains. *Frontiers in Plant Science, 7*, 1624.

Datta, A. (2013). Genetic engineering for improving quality and productivity of crops. *Agriculture & Food Security, 2*, 15. https://doi.org/10.1186/2048-7010-2-15 (accessed on 5th November 2025).

de Sa, M. S., & Keshavarz-Moore, E. (2021). *Pichia pastoris* (*Komagataella phaffii*) as a cost-effective tool for vaccine production for low- and middle-income countries (LMICs). *Bioengineering, 8*, 119.

Decourcelle, M., Perez-Fons, L., Baulande, S., Steiger, S., Couvelard, L., Hem, S., Zhu, C., Capell, T., Christou, P. F., & Sandmann, G. (2015). Combined transcript, proteome, and metabolite analysis of transgenic maize seeds engineered for enhanced carotenoid synthesis reveals pleotropic effects in core metabolism. *Journal of Experimental Botany, 66*, 3141–3150. https://doi.org/10.1093/jxb/erv120 (accessed on 5th November 2025).

Deltsidis, A. I., Sims, C. A., & Brecht, J. K. (2018). Ripening recovery and sensory quality of pink tomatoes stored in controlled atmosphere at chilling or nonchilling temperatures to extend shelf life. *Hort Science, 53*, 1186–1190.

Elkonin, L. A., Italianskaya, J. V., Domanina, V. N., Selivanov, N. Y., Rakitin, A. L., & Ravi, N. V. (2016). Transgenic sorghum with improved digestibility of storage proteins obtained by *Agrobacterium*-mediated transformation. *Russian Journal of Plant Physiology, 63*, 678–689. https://doi.org/10.1134/S1021443716050046 (accessed on 5th November 2025).

Enitan-Folami, A. M., & Swalaha, F. M. (2020). 10 Application of biotechnology in the food industry. *Food Science and Technology*, 235–278. https://doi.org/10.1515/9783110667462-010 (accessed on 5th November 2025).

Garg, M., Sharma, N., Sharma, S., Kapoor, P., Kumar, A., Chunduri, V., & Arora, P. (2018). Biofortified crops generated by breeding, agronomy, and transgenic approaches are improving lives of millions of people around the world. *Frontiers in Nutrition, 5*, 12. https://doi.org/10.3389/fnut.2018.00012 (accessed on 5th November 2025).

Getabalew, M., & Alemneh, T. (2019). The application of biotechnology on livestock. *Archives in Biomedical Engineering & Biotechnology, 1*. https://doi.org/10.33552/ABEB.2019.01.000522 (accessed on 5th November 2025).

Global Biodiversity Outlook (GBO) report. (2007). Convention on Biological Diversity, Chapter 2. https://www.cbd.int/gbo1/summary.shtmL (accessed on 5th November 2025).

Haroon, F., & Ghazanfar, M. (2016). Applications of food biotechnology. *Journal of Ecosystem & Ecography, 6*, 1000215. https://doi.org/10.4172/2157-7625.1000215 (accessed on 5th November 2025).

Jain, A., Singh, N., Kumari, S., & Khan, S. (2021). Bio entrepreneurship in agricultural biotechnology. In Agarwal, S., Kumari, S., & Khan, S. (Eds.), *Bio Entrepreneurship and Transferring Technology into Product Development* (pp. 183–200). IGI Global, Hershey, PA, USA.

Jin, Y. H., Robledo, D., Hickey, J. M., McGrew, M. J., & Houston, R. D. (2021). Surrogate broodstock to enhance biotechnology research and applications in aquaculture.

*Biotechnology Advances, 49*, 107756. https://doi.org/10.1016/j.biotechadv.2021.107756 (accessed on 5th November 2025).

Khan, S., & Khan, J. (2010). Drought tolerant wheat cultivar (raj) for rainfed areas of Kpk, Pakistan. *Pakistan Journal of Agricultural Sciences, 47*, 355–359.

Kumar, K., Gambhir, G., Dass, A., Tripathi, A. K., Singh, A., Jha, A. K., Yadava, P., Choudhary, M., & Rakshit, S. (2020). Genetically modified crops: current status and future prospects. *Planta, 251*, 91. https://doi.org/10.1007/s00425-020-03372-8 (accessed on 5th November 2025).

Maryam, B. M., Datsugwai, M. S. S., & Shehu, I. (2017). The role of biotechnology in food production and processing. *Industrial Engineering, 1*, 24–35.

Mihalik, D., Gubisova, M., Klempova, T., Certik, M., Ondreickova, K., Hudcovicova, M., Klcova, L., Gubis, J., Dokupilova, I., Ohnoutkova, L., & Kraic, J. (2014). Transgenic barley producing essential polyunsaturated fatty acids. *Biological Plantarum, 58*, 348–354. https://doi.org/10.1007/s10535-014-0406-9 (accessed on 5th November 2025).

Monteiro, C. A., Cannon, G., Levy, R. B., Moubarac, J. C., Louzada, M. L., Rauber, F., Khandpur, N., Cediel, G., Neri, D., Martinez-Steele, E., Baraldi, L. G., & Jaime, P. C. (2019). Ultra-processed foods: what they are and how to identify them. *Public Health Nutrition, 22*, 936–941. https://doi.org/10.1017/S1368980018003762 (accessed on 5th November 2025).

Paine, J. A., Shipton, C. A., Chaggar, S., Howells, R. M., Kennedy, M. J., Vernon, G., Wright, S. Y., Hinchliffe, E., Adams, J. L., Silverstone, A. L., & Drake, R. (2005). Improving the nutritional value of golden rice through increased pro-vitamin A content. *Nature Biotechnology, 23*, 482–487. https://doi.org/10.1038/nbt1082 (accessed on 5th November 2025).

Pal, M., Patel, A. S., Bariya, A. R., Godishala, V., & Kandi, V. (2017). A review of biotechnological applications in food processing of animal origin. *American Journal of Food Technology, 5*, 143–148.

Ranjha, M. M. A. N., Shafique, B., Khalid, W., Nadeem, H. R., Mueen-ud-Din, G., & Khalid, M. Z. (2022). Applications of biotechnology in food and agriculture: a mini-review. *Proceedings of the National Academy of Sciences, India Section B: Biological Sciences, 92*, 11–15. https://doi.org/10.1007/s40011-021-01320-4 (accessed on 5th November 2025).

Sonkar, S., & Mallick, N. (2018). An alternative strategy for enhancing lipid accumulation in chlorophycean microalgae for biodiesel production. *Journal of Applied Phycology, 30*, 2179–2192.

Wang, C., Zeng, J., Li, Y., Hu, W., Chen, L., Miao, Y., Deng, P., Yuan, C., Ma, C., Chen, X., Zang, M., Wang, Q., Li, K., Liu, K., Chang, J., Wang, Y., Yang, G., & He, G. (2014). Enrichment of provitamin A content in wheat (*Triticum aestivum* L.) by introduction of the bacterial carotenoid biosynthetic genes *CrtB* and *CrtI*. *Journal of Experimental Botany, 65*, 2545–2556. https://doi.org/10.1093/jxb/eru138 (accessed on 5th November 2025).

Yu, P. (2017). Food biotechnology–an important and promising research field. *Journal of Food Biotechnology Research, 1*, 1.

Zhao, J. (2007). Nutraceuticals, nutritional therapy, phytonutrients, and phytotherapy for improvement of human health: a perspective on plant biotechnology application. *Recent Patents on Biotechnology, 1*, 75–97.

# CHAPTER 8

# Fungal Cell Factories: Producers of Industrially Important Proteins

SOMALI SANYAL,* ARJUN SINGH KOHLI, and PRITI PAL

*Amity Institute of Biotechnology, Amity University Uttar Pradesh, Lucknow Campus, Lucknow, India*

*Corresponding author

## ABSTRACT

A huge and diversified taxonomic category of microorganisms, known as filamentous fungi, is present in all types of ecosystems around the world. They develop as a hyphal network, which is a network of cells. Since filamentous fungi inhabit a variety of settings, they create numerous enzymes to break down materials for their food, such as hydrolytic enzymes to break down various types of bio-masses. Many of them are simple to cultivate in a variety of established environments (such as submerged fermentation and solid-state fermentation), and they often secrete proteins and enzymes that are much greater than those produced by yeast and bacteria. Consequently, these fungal species have been proved to be effective fabricators of proteins with substantial industrial, commercial, therapeutic, and/or medicinal significance. Also, there has been a significant shift in the recent past in the way that fungal species are harvested and exploited. The properties and characteristics of fungal species that make them important sources of proteins have sparked better and advanced research, as well as analytical studies into the various ways that these advantages might be utilized to meet the needs of the general public. This chapter highlighted the filamentous fungal strains/species as efficient protein producers along with potential commercial applications.

Industrial Biotechnology: Current Progress and Novel Technologies.
Prakash Kumar Sarangi, Akhilesh Kumar Singh, Rajesh Kumar Srivastava, and Brijesh Pandey (Eds.)


DOI: 10.1201/9781779642233-8

## 8.1 INTRODUCTION

For the manufacturing of a broad range of products, filamentous fungi make excellent cell factories. They are efficient at breaking down and converting biological material and naturally fabricate effective enzymes (Lübeck and Lübeck, 2022). Additionally, they generate various chemicals, several of which have intriguing industrial uses. As their heterogenic lifestyle needs accessibility to organic carbon, filamentous fungi are found practically everywhere in a variety of environments (Papagianni, 2004). The inorganic material that fungi consume allows them to produce the necessary biomolecules, including all of the amino acids. Further, submerged fermentation (SMF) and solid-state fermentation (SSF) are two different fermentation approaches that can be used for fungus cultivation and production (Lee, 2022). Unlike SSF, which uses solid substrates for its fungal cultivation, SF uses free-flowing liquid substrates. Both methods are frequently employed for the cultivation and production of fungal species/strains (Barzee et al., 2021). Due to their quick growth, effective use of resources, and ability to transform complicated substrates into fermentable sugars, fungi have demonstrated their efficiency as industrial cell factories to generate a variety of different chemicals. Complex secondary metabolites including antibiotics (like penicillin), organic acids (like citric acid), and numerous extracellular enzymes, like amylases and cellulases, are among the most well-known ones as detailed previously (Madhavan et al., 2022; Meyer, 2021, Wei et al., 2021). Overall, fungi have been recognized and acknowledged as huge and prolific providers of numerous significant enzymes and proteins (Ahmed et al., 2017).

Researchers have focused their attention on filamentous fungi in particular because they are thought to possess two qualities that make them particularly well-suited for use as efficient protein manufacturers shown in Figure 8.1. High protein secretion efficiency is one benefit, and the ability to perform post-translational changes is another (Bergquist et al., 2002). Interestingly, filamentous fungi produced more than half of the proteins that are currently sold commercially. These facts show that fungi are potent, effective, and incredibly helpful factories for the secretion, manufacture, and release of proteins, which have now come to be recognized and valued on an industrial scale. Several filamentous fungi have been classified as Generally Regarded as Safe (GRAS) because specific species of these fungi show improved protein secretory capabilities. For instance, a number of commercial filamentous fungi like *Aspergillus niger*, *A. oryzae*, and *Trichoderma reesei*, have been approved as GRAS strains (Frisvad et al., 2018). The *T. reesei* and *A. niger* were both capable of producing 25 to 30 g/L of glucoamylase and 100 g/L of cellulose in their respective fermentation media (Ward, 2012). In addition to possessing developed post-translation processing (like glycosylation, protease cleavage, and disulfide bond formation) as well as modification systems, filamentous fungi exhibit a variety of skills by effectively producing protein using a variety of monosaccharides (Cavka and Jönsson, 2014; Karnaukhova et al., 2007). Their glycoproteins undergo less extensive hyper-mannosylation, which can be transformed into mammalian-type glycoproteins for medicinal use (Deshpande et al., 2008; Punt et al., 2002a). Recombinant proteins are now used at exceptionally high levels across a variety of industries, and this trend is expected to continue. Such instances can be observed in a number of industries. The chemical

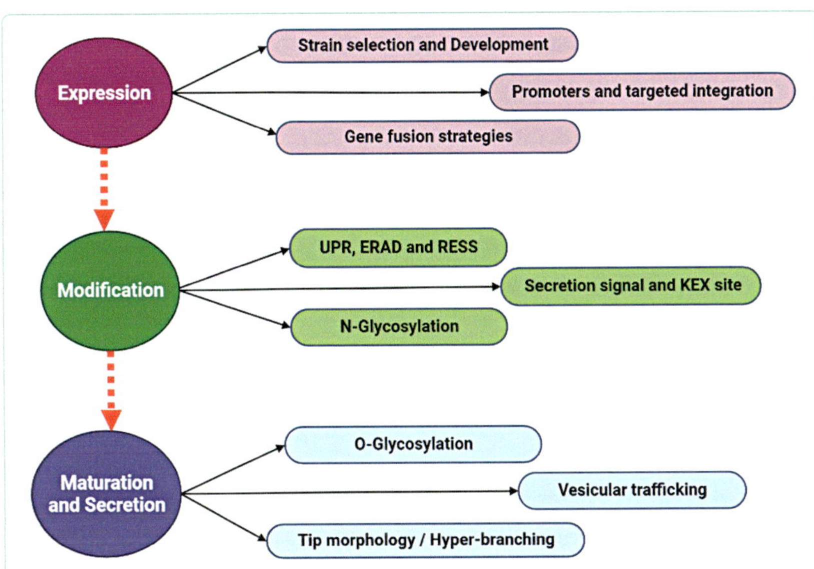


**FIGURE 8.1** Flow chart for the expression and secretion of fungal proteins. In filamentous fungi, the metabolic pathway for protein secretion has three main stages, starting with the gene of interest and ending with the secretion of the mature protein. Also shown are various events and optimization techniques.

industry seeks out creative ways to maintain sustainability while also improving process performance and safety. Similar to this, protein-based treatments are used in the medical field to guarantee accurate diagnosis as well as precision medicine. Overall, the present chapter highlights the advantages of employing filamentous fungi as effective protein fabricators and discusses possible commercial uses.

## 8.2 FUNGAL SPECIES/ STRAINS MEDIATED PRODUCTION OF PROTEIN

Over many decades, several filamentous fungi have been exploited for their efficiency in the secretion of native proteins. Glucoamylase from *A. niger* and cellulases from *T. reesei* are some of the most common examples. It has been projected that with an improving wealth of experience obtained from large-scale culture and downstream processing of these microbes; heterologous proteins of commercial importance can be produced. The problems associated with the expression of such proteins, it has been realized, that since intracellular compartmentalization in recombinant proteins presents less of a problem in filamentous fungi, the problems lie with either the secretion pathway or the extracellular environment (Wang et al., 2020; Ward, 2012). Numerous benefits have been found in this concern if the protein of interest is released into the growth media rather than intracellular synthesis. If the protein is secreted, both the potentially harmful effects of intracellular product build-up and the time and money required to recover an internal product are minimized. The filamentous fungi produce different types of industrially important proteins, which are discussed below.

### *8.2.1 SACCHAROMYCES CEREVISIAE AND PICHIA PASTORIS MEDIATED HETEROLOGOUS PROTEIN PRODUCTION*

In order to express a gene product in an organism or system where it is not typically produced or naturally formed, heterologous or recombinant proteins are created or developed utilizing recombinant DNA technology. However, producing recombinant proteins is more complex than producing recombinant DNA molecules because the heterologous DNA must be translated into a suitably folded protein with the right biological activity after being transcribed (Punt et al., 2011b; Sakekar et al., 2021). The capacity of filamentous fungi to accurately carry out diverse post-translational modifications of eukaryotic proteins, such as glycosylation as well as disulfide bond formation, like mammalian cells, is one of the biggest justifications for employing them as expression hosts for the recombinant production of particular target protein molecules (Van Den Hombergh et al., 1997; Zhang et al., 2020). Even while genetic alterations are simpler and faster in the model organisms, *E. coli* as well as yeasts, it has become obvious over time that they provide certain distinct benefits over other microbial protein expression systems. One benefit is that released protein levels may be attained that are 10–1000 times higher than those possible with bacterial, yeast, or mammalian cell secretion. Protein secretion levels in these cells are frequently lesser than a few g/L (Meyer, 2021). The construction of filamentous fungal expression platforms is far more difficult, time-consuming, and requires considerable development compared to expression platforms employing bacteria (particularly *E. coli*) or yeast like *Saccharomyces cerevisiae*, and so forth (Funk et al., 2002; Juturu et al., 2018; Ki and Pack, 2020). Numerous reviews have analyzed various facets of recombinant protein synthesis utilizing filamentous fungus because of the tremendous potential as well as industrial interests (Lübeck and Lübeck, 2022). As a result, systems of heterologous gene expression have been used with a variety of fungi, including *S. cerevisiae*, *Pichia pastoris*, and so on (Table 8.1) (Wang et al., 2020).

**TABLE 8.1** Therapeutic Use of the Heterologous Proteins Generated By Some Fungal Strains/Species

| Host | Product | Origin | Therapeutic Use |
|---|---|---|---|
| *S. cerevisiae* | Human Papillomavirus Vaccine | Human Papillomavirus | A vaccine to protect against papillomavirus infection |
| *S. cerevisiae* | Glucagon | Human cDNA | Hormone involved in blood glucose level regulation |
| *S. cerevisiae* | Hepatitis B Vaccine | Hepatitis Virus | A vaccine to protect against Hepatitis B infection |
| *P. pastoris* | Hepatitis B Vaccine | Hepatitis Virus | A vaccine to protect against Hepatitis B infection |
| *P. pastoris* | Ecallantide | Human cDNA | A 60-Amino acid protein inhibitor of plasma kallikrein |

The process of making heterologous proteins involves several steps, that is (i) insertion of the desired heterologous DNA coding sequence into the proper regulatory sequences in specialized expression vectors; (ii) transformation to introduce the construct into the desired host species;

and (iii) transcription and translation of this sequence into biologically active protein molecules (Wei et al., 2021). Further, *S. cerevisiae* was acknowledged as the first eukaryotic cell to be engineered to express heterologous proteins since it shared many characteristics with *Escherichia coli* that made it a desirable host for recombinant DNA technology. *S. cerevisiae* has various interesting features like it can be transformed while still intact, it can grow quickly by cell division, it can form distinct colonies on clearly defined media, it can carry out post-translational modifications on expressed proteins, and it can secrete a small number of proteins that can be used to accelerate the production of heterologous proteins. These characteristics enabled *S. cerevisiae* as an excellent choice for producing heterologous proteins. In general, *S. cerevisiae* has been utilized in industrial fermentation techniques for a very long time. It is a good option for the secure production of heterologous proteins due to all these factors (Anssi et al., 2019). On the other hand, *Pichia pastoris*, a member of the methylotrophs group, has gained recognition as a preferred option for producing heterologous proteins with significant therapeutic potential (Punt et al., 2011b). Over 100 distinct heterologous proteins have been expressed in *P. pastoris* over the years for both research and industrial uses. Compared to *S. cerevisiae*, it is regarded as a more reliable and effective glycosylator of secreted proteins (Sakekar et al., 2021). *Pichia* has produced a number of therapeutically significant goods, including insulin, interferons, *ecallantide* (a protein inhibitor of plasma kallikrein), and the hepatitis B vaccine. This yield is expected to rise as *Pichia* has undergone numerous in-depth genetic manipulation experiments to create yeast strains that can produce human glycoproteins that are in every way comparable to those found in human bodies (Figure 8.2). Interestingly, *P. pastoris* has been able to replicate the necessary pattern of sugar moieties on heterologous proteins, unlike yeast cells (Punt et al., 2011b; Sakekar et al., 2021).

### 8.2.2 TRICHODERMA HARZIANUM MEDIATED PROTEIN PRODUCTION

The fact that microorganisms are prevalent in nature makes it obvious that they are the source of enzymes, which are known to be incredibly important and essential for the conversion of biomass. Fungi have been used for more than 50 years to build proteins and enzymes with industrial importance. In fungal biomass, there exist high concentrations of crude protein,

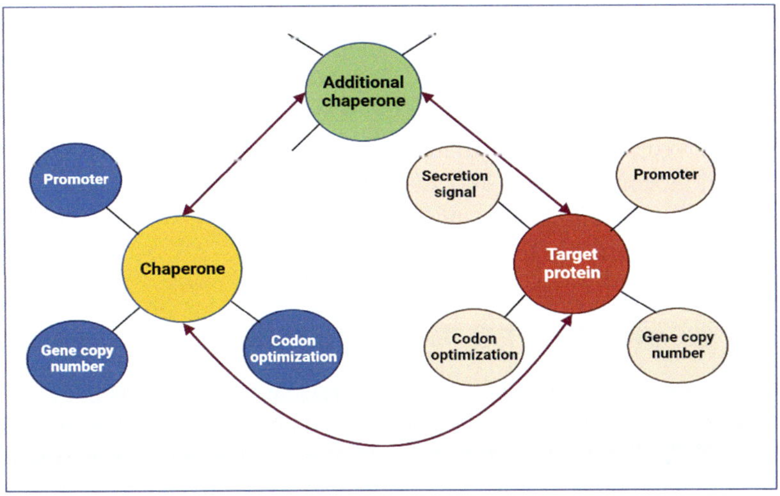


**FIGURE 8.2** Combinatorial map of a co-expression strategy in *P. pastoris* for genes encoding the target protein and chaperones. Along with the selection of the proper promoter and secretion signal sequences, codon optimization, and optimized copy number of the gene, co-expression of a chaperone gene is one approach that might be used to improve the production or secretion of a target recombinant protein. It is important to think about and test various chaperone genes with diverse promoter strengths that have codon-optimized sequences and optimized gene copy numbers (strong, moderate, weak). It is possible that the promoter used to regulate the target gene's expression is different from the promoter used with chaperones. The chaperon that functions inside the cell is not required for the recombinant protein, which also requires a secretion signal.

up to 45%, along with a balanced ratio of essential amino acids. From a biotechnological perspective, *Trichoderma harzianum* has been used for this specific purpose and has produced a number of promising outcomes in the direction of Fungal Biomass Protein (FBP) production (Punt et al., 2002a). The ability of *T. harzianum* to create FBP from rice polishings was investigated in a study by Ahmed et al. (2017). After 72 hours of incubation at 28°C and pH 4, the highest biomass output was attained using 5% (w/v) rice polishings. A 20:1 carbon: nitrogen ratio resulted in noticeably greater fungal biomass protein (FBP) synthesis. The 75 L fermenter's FBP had a content of 49.5% crude protein, 32% true protein, 19.45% crude fiber, 9.62% ash, 11.5% cellulose, and 0.325% RNA. The final FBP's amino acid profile showed that all of the necessary amino acids were present in significant amounts. It has been demonstrated that the FBP generated by this fungus is a good source of additional nutrients for chickens. This study's findings are applicable in that rice polishing might be utilized to successfully create FBP utilizing the fungus *T. harzianum*. Such an investigation concludes that the creation of FBP from rice polishings not only elaborates the effectiveness of filamentous fungi in protein production but also underlines the viability of this process as a means of bioconversion of agricultural wastes (Ward, 2012). *Aspergillus, Chaetomium, Paecilomyces,* and *Penicillium* species of filamentous fungi have also been utilized for biomass generation.

### 8.2.3 TRICHODERMA REESEI MEDIATED PROTEIN PRODUCTION

Due to its great and innate potential to secrete and manufacture cellulolytic enzymes, the *Trichoderma reesei* has been widely identified and used as a source of industrial enzymes. As a result, *T. reesei* is now a desirable host for usage in numerous industrial applications (Ahmed et al., 2017). Today, *T. reesei* is used as a host to manufacture a variety of enzymes, including cellulases, xylanases, amylases, and proteases. In a recent development, it has been suggested that *T. reesei* can generate vital biopharmaceuticals like interferons since it can do so at a low cost with the capacity to provide a platform for their synthesis (Punt et al., 2002a). It has been revealed through the several strategic analyses carried out to assess the productivity potential of this organism that it can produce total secreted protein titers above 100g/L (Archer et al., 1994). *T. reesei* uses strategies based on using native cellulolytic gene promoters, which are considered to be the most widely used expression system for proteins. These promoters are said to be activated by the presence of inducing chemicals, which are often lactose and cellulose or any of its derivatives (Punt et al., 2002a). Because of this, it is noteworthy that a variety of cellulolytic and hemicellulolytic enzymes are expressed and secreted at the same time when the promoters are exposed to the inducing substances (Jeenes et al., 1991).

### 8.2.4 ASPERGILLUS AND RHIZOPUS MEDIATED PROTEIN PRODUCTION

Ascomycetes have been identified and demonstrated to grow on a range of diverse substrates, demonstrating their enormous adaptability. For its industrial uses, *Aspergillus oryzae* has been the subject of the greatest research in this area. In addition, the focus has switched to zygomycetes due to their broad capacity to thrive on substrates with low or no cost. *R. oryzae* has been seen to grow on such substrates, including residues and agro-waste. It is noteworthy that wastewater has worked well as a platform for the cultivation of these microbes. Large amounts of wastewater generated by starch plants must first be treated and disposed of before being dumped. Due to environmental concerns and regulations, wastewater cannot be released without appropriate treatment; therefore, this treatment and disposal process imposes additional costs on the sector. The hunt for options to handle this wastewater without rising prices or harming the environment has been prompted by stricter restrictions and guidelines. In line with this advancement, *A. oryzae* and *R. oryzae* were grown and cultivated using wastewater from a wheat-starch plant as a substrate. Due to the fact that these microbes not only minimized the negative environmental effects of the residues emitted by the industry but also produced value-added bio-products, it was determined that the agro-industrial residue provided the nutrients necessary for the growth of microorganisms (Kavanagh, 2011). In order to determine and predict the protein content, which is a key factor in determining whether the experiments produced biomass suitable for use in animal feed formulations, the biomass that was generated as a result of the experiment was analyzed as well as weighed. The growth of *A. oryzae* at pH value of 3.85 produced the most biomass, while *R. oryzae* produced the biomass with the highest protein content (Kavanagh, 2011). The various types of heterologous proteins produced in *Aspergillus* species are revealed in Table 8.2.

## 8.3 BIOTECHNOLOGICAL APPLICATIONS OF EXPRESSION TECHNOLOGY

The filamentous fungal protein expression system, like *Saccharomyces cerevisiae*, can be modified to prepare as well as supply *in vivo* technologies, in addition to fabricating proteins with medicinal and commercial value. Biotechnologists can use these expression systems' ability to re-engineer promoter elements, transcription factors, and signal cascade proteins to translate heterologous molecular interactions into quickly measurable phenotypes to screen for molecules that hinder or improve these interactions and serve as key lead molecules in drug development technology (Wei et al., 2021). In order to investigate the molecular

**TABLE 8.2** Examples of Filamentous Fungi that Have Been Genetically Modified to Produce More Protein

| Host | Origin | Protein | Strategy | Fold-Change of Protein Secretion | References |
|---|---|---|---|---|---|
| A. *niger* | *Trametes versicolor* | Laccase | Constructing a protease-deficient strain by deletion of pepAa, pepAb, or pepAd | 1.21–1.42-fold increase | Wang et al. (2008) |
| A. *niger* | A. *niger* | β-Glucuronidase | Regulating the UPR and ERAD by overexpression of sttC and deletion of dorA | Not quantified | Jacobs et al. (2009) |
| A. *oryzae* | *bovine* | Chymosin | Fusing target protein with a naturally secreted protein α-amylase | 2-fold increase | Ohno et al. (2011) |
| A. *niger* | *bovine* | Prochymosin | Optimizing the intracellular transport process by deletion of Aovip36 or Aoemp47, and fusing the target protein with α-amylase | Approximately 2-fold increase | Hoang et al. (2015) |
| T. *reesei* | A. *niger* | Glucose oxidase | Regulating the UPR and ERAD by overexpression of bip1 or hac1 | 1.5–1.8-fold increase | Wu et al. (2017) |
| T. *reesei* | T. *reesei* | Glucose oxidase | Optimizing the intracellular transport process by overexpression of snc1 | 2.2-fold increase | Wu et al. (2017) |
| T. *reesei* | T. *reesei* | Cellulase | Constructing a protease-deficient strain by deletion of res-1, cre-1, gh1-1, and alp-1 | 5-fold increase | Liu et al. (2017) |
| A. *niger* | A. *niger* | Glucoamylase | Regulating mycelium morphology by deletion of racA | 4-fold increase | Fiedler et al. (2018) |
| A. *niger* | A. *niger* | α-Galactosidase | Replacing the original signal peptide with a glucoamylase (GlaA) signal peptide in A. *niger* | Approximately 9-fold increase | Xu et al. (2018) |

biology of expressed heterologous steroids as well as peptide receptor protcins, reporter genes, as well as a selective growth medium, have been employed.

## 8.4 CONCLUSION AND FUTURE PERSPECTIVES

Filamentous fungi are desirable cell factories for protein expression and secretion because of their potent protein secretion mechanism. There are many aspects to the successful synthesis of heterologous proteins from filamentous fungus. It is important to keep in mind that target proteins made with a fungal host must be seen favorably by the general public and economically feasible to create (Mackenzie et al., 1993; Souza Filho et al., 2012; Wösten, 2019). These systems aim to take advantage of the fungal species' inherent capacity to manufacture high to extremely high levels of proteins with the appropriate degrees of purity. To improve the choices for the industrial synthesis of heterologous proteins from filamentous fungi, more knowledge on transcriptional regulation, introns, mRNA stability and processing, translational efficiency, protein secretion, glycosylation, and proteolysis is needed (Souza Filho et al., 2012; Sun et al., 2019). The product's genuineness will become more significant over time, and therapeutic proteins in particular will be subject to deeper investigation. Based on the level and pattern of glycosylation, the product's legitimacy must also be determined. It is already possible to manufacture novel modified proteins on a therapeutic and commercial scale. The most notable instance is the effective reengineering of the yeast *Pichia pastoris* to create human proteins with more consistent glycosylation patterns than those made by mammalian host cells. More of these strategies are anticipated to take the central stage in transcriptome research-based activity, and the production of proteins from fungi hosts is predicted to remove all present and previous obstacles in heterologous protein secretion routes. Further, the development of the CRISPR/Cas9 technology and its steadfast performance across a wide range of species have opened up new opportunities for precise genome modification. Such new approaches potentially expand the use of fungi in bioprocesses for the synthesis of compounds and proteins. In addition to these, there is a growing need to find novel fungal species/ strains to employ as effective future cell factories for the production of proteins and chemicals with added value.

## KEYWORDS


- **enzymes**
- **fermentation**
- **filamentous fungi**
- **heterologous/recombinant proteins**
- **industrial applications**
- **protein production**


## REFERENCES


Ahmed, S., Mustafa, G., Arshad, M., & Rajoka, M. I. (2017). Fungal biomass protein production from *Trichoderma harzianum* using rice polishing. *BioMed Research International, 2017*, 6232793.

Archer, D. B., Jeenes, D. J., & Mackenzie, D. A. (1994). Strategies for improving heterologous protein production from filamentous fungi. *Antonie van Leeuwenhoek, 65*(3), 245–250.

Barzee, T. J., Cao, L., Pan, Z., & Zhang, R. (2021). Fungi for future foods. *Journal of Future Foods, 1*, 25–37.

Bergquist, P. L., Te'O, V. S. J., Gibbs, M. D., Cziferszky, A. C. E., De Faria, F. P., Azevedo, M. O., & Nevalainen, K. M. H. (2002). Production of recombinant bleaching enzymes from thermophilic microorganisms in fungal hosts. *Applied Biochemistry and Biotechnology, 98–100*, 327–340.

Cavka, A., & Jönsson, L. J. (2014). Comparison of the growth of filamentous fungi and yeasts in lignocellulose-derived media. *Biocatalysis and Agricultural Biotechnology, 3*, 197–204.

Deshpande, N., Wilkins, M. R., Packer, N., & Nevalainen, H. (2008). Protein glycosylation pathways in filamentous fungi. *Glycobiology, 18*, 626–637.

Fiedler, M. R. M., Barthel, L., Kubisch, C., Nai, C., & Meyer, V. (2018). Construction of an improved *Aspergillus niger* platform for enhanced glucoamylase secretion. *Microbial Cell Factories, 17*, 95.

Frisvad, J. C., Møller, L. L. H., Larsen, T. O., Kumar, R., & Arnau, J. (2018). Safety of the fungal workhorses of industrial biotechnology: Update on the mycotoxin and secondary metabolite potential of *Aspergillus niger*, *Aspergillus oryzae*, and *Trichoderma reesei*. *Applied Microbiology and Biotechnology, 102*, 9481–9515.

Funk, M., Niedenthal, R., Mumberg, D., Brinkmann, K., Rönicke, V., & Henkel, T. (2002). Vector systems for heterologous expression of proteins in *Saccharomyces cerevisiae*. *Methods in Enzymology, 350*, 248–257.

Hoang, H. D., Maruyama, J. I., & Kitamoto, K. (2015). Modulating endoplasmic reticulum-Golgi cargo receptors for improving secretion of carrier-fused heterologous proteins in the filamentous fungus *Aspergillus oryzae*. *Applied and Environmental Microbiology, 81*, 533–543.

Jacobs, D. I., Olsthoorn, M. M. A., Maillet, I., Akeroyd, M., Breestraat, S., Donkers, S., et al. (2009). Effective lead selection for improved protein production in *Aspergillus niger* based on integrated genomics. *Fungal Genetics and Biology, 46*(1, Suppl.), S141–S152.

Jeenes, D. J., Mackenzie, D. A., Roberts, I. N., & Archer, D. B. (1991). Heterologous protein production by filamentous fungi. *Biotechnology and Genetic Engineering Reviews, 9*, 327–367.

Juturu, V., & Wu, J. C. (2018). Heterologous protein expression in *Pichia pastoris*: Latest research progress and applications. *ChemBioChem, 19*, 7–21.

Karnaukhova, E., Ophir, Y., Trinh, L., Dalal, N., Punt, P. J., Golding, B., et al. (2007). Expression of human α1-proteinase inhibitor in *Aspergillus niger*. *Microbial Cell Factories, 6*, 34.

Kavanagh, K. (2011). *Fungi: Biology and Applications*. Hoboken, NJ: Wiley. https://doi.org/10.1002/9781119976950 (accessed on 5th November 2025).

Ki, M. R., & Pack, S. P. (2020). Fusion tags to enhance heterologous protein expression. *Applied Microbiology and Biotechnology, 104*, 2411–2425.

Lee, B. H. (2022). *Advanced Fermentation and Cell Technology*. Wiley-Blackwell: Hoboken, NJ, USA.

Liu, Q., Gao, R., Li, J., Lin, L., Zhao, J., Sun, W., et al. (2017). Development of a genome-editing CRISPR/Cas9 system in thermophilic fungal *Myceliophthora* species and its application to hyper-cellulase production strain engineering. *Biotechnology for Biofuels, 10*, 1.

Lübeck, M., & Lübeck, P. S. (2022). Fungal cell factories for efficient and sustainable production of proteins and peptides. *Microorganisms, 10*, 753.

MacKenzie, D. A., Jeenes, D. J., Belshaw, N. J., & Archer, D. B. (1993). Regulation of secreted protein production by filamentous fungi: Recent developments and perspectives. *Journal of General Microbiology, 139*(10), 2295–2307.

Madhavan, A., Arun, K., Sindhu, R., Jose, A. A., Pugazhendhi, A., Binod, P., Sirohi, R., Reshmy, R., & Awasthi, M. K. (2022). Engineering interventions in industrial filamentous fungal cell factories for biomass valorization. *Bioresource Technology, 344*, 126209.

Meyer, V. (2021). Metabolic engineering of filamentous fungi. In *Metabolic Engineering: Concepts and Applications* (1st ed.). WILEY-VCH GmbH: Hoboken, NJ, USA.

Ohno, A., Maruyama, J. I., Nemoto, T., Arioka, M., & Kitamoto, K. (2011). A carrier fusion significantly induces unfolded protein response in heterologous protein production by *Aspergillus oryzae*. *Applied Microbiology and Biotechnology, 92*, 1197–1206.

Papagianni, M. (2004). Fungal morphology and metabolite production in submerged mycelial processes. *Biotechnology Advances, 22*, 189–259.

Punt, P. J., Levasseur, A., Visser, H., Wery, J., & Record, E. (2011). Fungal protein production: Design and production of chimeric proteins. *Annual Review of Microbiology, 65*, 57–69.

Punt, P. J., van Biezen, N., Conesa, A., Albers, A., Mangnus, J., & van den Hondel, C. (2002). Filamentous fungi as cell factories for heterologous protein production. *Trends in Biotechnology, 20*, 200–206.

Rantasalo, A., Vitikainen, M., Paasikallio, T., Jäntti, J., Landowski, C. P., & Mojzita, D. (2019). Novel genetic tools that enable highly pure protein production in *Trichoderma reesei*. *Scientific Reports*, *9*(1), 5032.

Sakekar, A. A., Gaikwad, S. R., & Punekar, N. S. (2021). Protein expression and secretion by filamentous fungi. *Journal of Biosciences*, *46*(5).

Souza Filho, P. F., Zamani, A., & Taherzadeh, M. J. (2019). Edible protein production by filamentous fungi using starch plant wastewater. *Waste and Biomass Valorization*, *10*, 2487–2496.

Sun, X., & Su, X. (2019). Harnessing the knowledge of protein secretion for enhanced protein production in filamentous fungi. *World Journal of Microbiology and Biotechnology*, *35*(4), 54.

Van Den Hombergh, J. P. T. W., Gelpke, M. D. S., Van De Vondervoort, P. J. I., Buxton, F. P., & Visser, J. (1997). Disruption of three acid proteases in *Aspergillus niger*: Effects on protease spectrum, intracellular proteolysis, and degradation of target proteins. *European Journal of Biochemistry*, *247*, 605–613.

Wang, Q., Zhong, C., & Xiao, H. (2020). Genetic engineering of filamentous fungi for efficient protein expression and secretion. *Frontiers in Bioengineering and Biotechnology*, *8*. https://doi.org/10.3389/fbioe.2020.00293 (accessed on 5th November 2025).

Wang, Y., Xue, W., Sims, A. H., Zhao, C., Wang, A., Tang, G., et al. (2008). Isolation of four pepsin-like protease genes from *Aspergillus niger* and analysis of the effect of disruptions on heterologous laccase expression. *Fungal Genetics and Biology*, *45*, 17–27.

Ward, O. P. (2012). Production of recombinant proteins by filamentous fungi. *Biotechnology Advances*, *30*(5), 1119–1139.

Wei, H., Wu, M., Fan, A., & Su, H. (2021). Recombinant protein production in the filamentous fungus *Trichoderma*. *Chinese Journal of Chemical Engineering*, *29*(2), 74–81.

Wösten, H. A. B. (2019). Filamentous fungi for the production of enzymes, chemicals and materials. *Current Opinion in Biotechnology*, *59*, 65–70.

Wu, Y., Sun, X., Xue, X., Luo, H., Yao, B., Xie, X., et al. (2017). Overexpressing key component genes of the secretion pathway for enhanced secretion of an *Aspergillus niger* glucose oxidase in *Trichoderma reesei*. *Enzyme and Microbial Technology*, *106*, 83–87.

Xu, Y., Wang, Y., Liu, T., Zhang, H., Zhang, H., & Li, J. (2018). The GlaA signal peptide substantially increases the expression and secretion of α-galactosidase in *Aspergillus niger*. *Biotechnology Letters*, *40*, 949–955.

Zhang, T., Liu, H., Lv, B., & Li, C. (2020). Regulating strategies for producing carbohydrate active enzymes by filamentous fungal cell factories. *Frontiers in Bioengineering and Biotechnology*, *8*, 691.

## CHAPTER 9

# Microbial Lipases and Their Industrial Applications

PRITI PAL,[1] AKHILESH KUMAR SINGH,[2,*] LAXUMAN SHARMA,[3] BRIJESH PANDEY,[2] PRAKASH KUMAR SARANGI,[4] and SASHI SONKAR[5]

[1]*Amity Institute of Biotechnology, Amity University Uttar Pradesh, Lucknow Campus, Lucknow, India*

[2]*Department of Biotechnology, School of Life Sciences, Mahatma Gandhi Central University, Motihari, Bihar, India*

[3]*Department of Horticulture, Sikkim University, Gangtok, Sikkim, India*

[4]*College of Agriculture, Central Agricultural University, Imphal, Manipur, India*

[5]*Department of Botany, Bankim Sardar College, Tangrakhali, West Bengal, India*

*Corresponding author

## ABSTRACT

Microbial lipases have gained significant attention due to their high substrate specificity, rapid processing time, low energy requirements, and stable performance under diverse conditions. Their production is cost-effective, supported by the use of inexpensive and readily available raw materials. Owing to their exceptional stability, microbial lipases are widely applied in industries producing oleochemicals, surfactants, pharmaceuticals, and various bioactive compounds. These enzymes primarily catalyze the hydrolysis of triacylglycerols into free fatty acids and glycerol, but their versatility allows them to participate in numerous other reactions,

Industrial Biotechnology: Current Progress and Novel Technologies.
Prakash Kumar Sarangi, Akhilesh Kumar Singh, Rajesh Kumar Srivastava, and Brijesh Pandey (Eds.)


DOI: 10.1201/9781779642233-9

even under extreme pH, temperature, and solvent conditions. Their broad applicability makes microbial lipases essential in food processing, pharmaceutical manufacturing, detergent formulations, pulp and paper industries, biodiesel production, and environmental applications. This chapter highlights recent advancements in microbial lipase research, focusing on industrial and commercial uses, emerging technologies, and future prospects. It also explores how metagenomics, nanotechnology, OMICs tools, and machine learning approaches contribute to discovering novel lipases. Additionally, topics such as microbial sources, enzyme immobilization strategies, and applications in agrochemicals, biosensors, cosmetics, perfumery, and bioremediation are discussed, emphasizing the expanding significance of microbial lipases in modern biotechnology.

## 9.1 INTRODUCTION

Lipases (EC 3.1.1.3) are a class of vital bio-catalysts that have a variety of industrial uses and resemble esterases. In 1935, *Aspergillus flavus* and *Penicillium oxalicum* produced the first microbial lipase (Kirsh, 1935). According to Verger's definition from 1997, true lipases are carboxyl esterases that can hydrolyze long-chain acylglycerols. The majority of lipases used in industry are derived from bacteria, fungi, and yeast and are of microbial origin. Lipase's importance stems from its adaptability, particularly concerning the catalytic reactions of esterification, transesterification, interesterification, alcoholysis, acidolysis, and amylolysis other than hydrolysis (Sarmah et al., 2017). Applications for lipases include the production of bio-diesel through lipase-catalyzed transesterification, ester synthesis (flavor compounds) in food, cosmetics, perfumery, and medicine, bioremediation through lipid hydrolysis, and more in the production of vital medications like Diltiazem hydrochloride, Epothilone A, and Nikkomycin, as degreasing agents in tanneries, for pitch treatment in the paper industry, as dewaxing, desiring, and scouring agents in textiles, and in detergent formulation for hydrolyzing greasy and oily stains (Chandra et al., 2020). Utilizing esterification, interesterification, and 1, 3 regio-specific activity properties, lipase is used to degum vegetable oil, modify oil and fats for higher value products rich in polyunsaturated fatty acids (PUFA), and produce substitutes for coco butter and human milk fat (Chandra et al., 2020). Other significant uses include the production of bio-lubricants, an excellent substitute for traditional petroleum lubricants, through esterification and transesterification, the degradation of plastics, the production of agrochemicals, waxes, and biopolymers, the processing of tea, and the development of biosensors (Bolina et al., 2021). Only a small portion of the numerous microbial lipases that have been isolated and characterized have been used commercially. The primary cause of this is the aforementioned inability of the majority of common enzymes to withstand demanding reaction conditions. There has been a search for new enzymes with specific properties regarding thermostability, enatio-selectivity, and stability in the presence of organic solvents, as well as increased activity, higher productivity, and re-usability to meet the demands of the ever-increasing industrial sector and overcome these drawbacks. Since lipase production has the benefits of being active at the interfaces of organic compounds, producing a high yield at a low production cost, being simple to genetically modify, and having a wide substrate range, interest in it has recently increased significantly. The microbial lipase enzymes are highlighted in this chapter along with their industrial uses and current position in the enzyme market. The global lipase market is projected to reach USD 797.7 million by 2025, growing at a 6.2% compound annual growth rate between 2017 and 2025. The creation of new and improved lipases using molecular techniques is a recent development in the field of lipase research. For instance, combining directed enzyme evolution with rational enzyme design to give lipases the desired properties. Usually, a multi-step process is required to achieve significant lipase purification. This multi-step method of lipase purification includes both traditional and cutting-edge methods. The current review aims to present an overview of various aspects of lipase production, including fermentation techniques, factors affecting lipase production, and purification strategies, to assist researchers in selecting an appropriate method for the production and purification of lipase.

## 9.2 MICROBIAL LIPASES

Microorganisms can produce lipases, and industries are particularly interested in this source of the enzyme because it is used so frequently in biotechnology (Bharathi et al., 2019). The yeast, bacterial, and fungal lipases are examples of microbial lipases. Because they are stable at high temperatures, have a wide range of substrate selectivity, are amenable to genetic manipulation, are stable in organic solvents, do not require co-factors, are abundant and simple to grow in microorganisms, and have the potential for high yield, microbial lipases are crucial in biotechnology. Microbial lipases are preferred over plant and animal lipases due to several traits that make them more desirable. Microorganisms can be easily genetically altered, and this source provides high enzyme yields that make it possible to make incredibly stable lipases (Thapa et al., 2019). Their tolerance to organic solvents is one factor that makes them necessary to perform biotechnological processes (Salihu and Alam et al., 2015). Microbial lipases can exhibit regioselectivity, chemo selectivity, and enantioselectivity in addition to being active over a wide pH and temperature range. Lipases are versatile enzymes that can catalyze both hydrolysis and synthesis reactions, as shown by the fact that they accounted for about 20% of the bio-transformations carried out in 2019 (Chandra et al., 2020). Fungi, bacteria, and yeasts are some of the microorganisms that produce lipase. Bacterial lipases are resistant to the conditions used in the industry and can be found intracellularly, extracellularly, or attached to the membrane (Javed et al., 2018). Fungi are the most desirable group of lipase-producing microorganisms for industrial use because these sources are frequently extracellular and make extraction easier (Ferraz et al., 2018). The biotechnology industry has specific requirements for fungi lipases, including stability, specificity, and ease of production (Sarmah et al., 2018). Numerous microorganisms are capable of producing lipase. Among them, *Rhizopus, Aspergillus, Penicillium, Geotrichum, Mucor,* and *Rhizomucor* fungi, *Candida, Yarrowia, Pichia, Rhodotorula,* and *Saccharomycopsis* yeasts, and *Bacillus, Pseudomonas, Burkholderia*, and *Staphylococcus* bacteria stand out (Liu and Kokare, 2017). Around 57.14% of the fungi and 71.43% of the bacteria both produced extracellular lipase. Numerous microbes have been found to produce lipases, but only a small number of these have been thoroughly studied, purified, and used in industry (Sarmah et al., 2018). *Bacillus*, *Staphylococcus*, *Arthrobacter*, *Achromobacter*, and *Pseudomonas* are some of the most important lipase-producing bacterial genera.

## 9.3 SCREENING PROCEDURES FOR MANUFACTURERS OF LIPASE

Numerous approaches have been proposed and used for screening lipase enzymes, including the identification of microorganisms that produce lipases, which necessitates the culture of microbial strains on solid agar medium or in liquid media containing various substrates. Direct and indirect screening methods are the two main types of lipase production capability screening.

### 9.3.1 DIRECT METHOD (QUALITATIVE-ON AGAR MEDIUM)

A solid agar medium with additional substrates or indicator dyes can be used to screen lipolytic microorganisms. It is a helpful, fast screening technique to assess each microorganism's capacity to produce lipase enzyme (Mateos-Díaz et al., 2012). Based on how substrates and indicator dyes are used, the direct plate assay is further divided into two types, which are as follows:

#### 9.3.1.1 ASSESSMENTS FOR GEL DIFFUSION USING DIFFERENT LIPID SUBSTRATES

These techniques are used to identify lipolytic microbial strains based on their capacity to degrade lipids incorporated into solid media and create a distinct lipolysis zone (Lee et al., 2015). Different agar plate assays have been developed based on the substrates used, and it has been found that many researchers strongly prefer substrates like olive oil, tributyrin, Tween 20, and Tween 80 (Bharathi et al., 2018). Tributyrin agar plate assay has been used frequently for detecting the production of lipase among those substrate assays because it is quick and simple to prepare (Bharathi et al., 2018). de Souza et al. (2019) studied a variety of marine fungi cultures (181) for their ability to secrete hydrolytic enzymes and found that a sizable portion of isolated fungi had lipolytic activity. They did this using nutrient agar supplemented with tributyrin as a substrate.

#### 9.3.1.2 APPLICATION OF DIFFERENT INDICATOR DYES IN GEL DIFFUSION ASSAYS

These techniques involve screening the lipase-producing microbial strains using a variety of indicator dyes and substrates. As an indicator dye for screening, colors like phenol red, Rhodamine B, Victoria blue, and night blue can be used. An extremely popular, sensitive, and reliable assay for determining active lipases is an olive oil agar plate with Rhodamine B added. This method's fundamental idea and mechanism involve the interaction of hydrolyzed substrates with the fluorescent dye Rhodamine B, which produces orange fluorescent halo-like structures around microbial colonies that are visible when exposed to UV light (Dhiman and Chapadgaonkar, 2013). According to Abrunhosa et al. (2013), *Aspergillus ibericus* produced lipase when Rhodamine B and olive oil were combined. It is also common practice to screen for lipolytic microbes using an indicator dye like phenol red.

### *9.3.2 INDIRECT METHOD*

Numerous quantitative techniques, including the titrimetric method, the spectrophotometric method, the chromatographic method, and molecular screening techniques, can be used to assess a microorganism's capacity to produce lipase. For more than 50 years, titrimetric methods have been regularly used to estimate lipase activity. Alkali titration was used by Dayanandan et al. (2013) to identify potential lipases that produced *Penicillium crustosum* and *Aspergillus carneus*, respectively. Due to its straightforward procedures, the spectroscopic method recently popularized uses p-NPP (p-nitrophenyl palmitate) and olive oil as a substrate for quantitative lipase procedure screening (Romero et al., 2012). Alkaline lipase from *Aspergillus fumigates* MTCC 9657 produced liberated FFAs, which Rajan et al. (2011) measured using HPTLC.

## 9.4 PRODUCTION OF MICROBIAL INDUSTRIAL LIPASES BY MICROORGANISMS

Most of the microbial lipase is extracellular and secreted into the medium used to make lipase. The production of lipase enzyme from microorganisms is frequently accomplished using SmF and SSF systems shown in Figure 9.1.

### *9.4.1 SUBMERGED FERMENTATION SYSTEM*

A liquid fermentation system is another name for a SMF system. A method of growing microorganisms in a liquid broth medium, known as

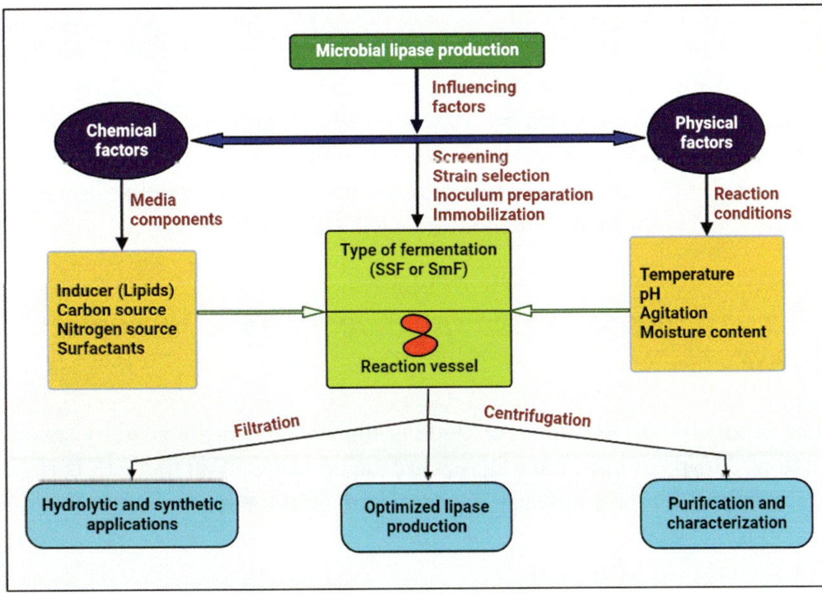


**FIGURE 9.1** Schematic representation of the fermentation process for the production of lipase from the microorganism.

SMF, converts the nutrients provided to compounds (Costa et al., 2017). Furthermore, SmF-produced lipases can be recovered and purified in a fairly straightforward manner. The SmF system is primarily employed to produce lipase from bacterial strains. Due to their sticky nature, oil carbon sources like vegetable oil, olive oil, and coconut oil are frequently influencing factors in SmF systems. Despite this, many oils have been used as carbon sources to produce lipase enzymes from microbial strains, with olive oil, palm oil, sunflower oil, and almond oil having the highest yields (Colla et al., 2016).

### *9.4.2 SOLID-STATE FERMENTATION SYSTEM*

To produce compounds from microorganisms on solid substrate media, several industries, including the food and pharmaceutical sectors, use solid-state fermentation (SSF) systems (also known as solid substrate fermentation systems (Barrios-González et al., 2012)). Most commonly, SSF uses a variety of solid substrates to produce mycelial, yeast, and fungal lipases. For instance, in both SSF and liquid fermentation, *Aspergillus* sp. produced lipase using mustard oil as the substrate, with SSF producing the best results. Along with the lower production costs, the benefits of producing lipase enzymes by SSF have been highlighted. An affordable alternative to using fungi to produce enzymes on a large scale is SSF. As a result, SSF is a good and preferred method for producing lipases as opposed to submerged fermentation (FMF) (Colla et al., 2015).

### 9.4.3 FACTORS AFFECTING THE PRODUCTION OF MICROBIAL LIPASE

The production of the lipase enzyme is significantly influenced by several factors. The most important factors are the presence of an inducer, particularly carbon sources, nitrogen sources, and temperature.

#### 9.4.3.1 CARBON SOURCE

The induction of genes that produce lipase typically results in the production of microbial lipase. All types of microbial lipases are induced to produce lipase enzymes by carbon sources, particularly olive oil. However, the recovery has been impacted by the use of oil carbon sources (olive oil, palm oil, and other vegetable oils) for the induction of lipases. When mustard seed oil was used as a carbon source, *Aspergillus terreus* produced a good yield of lipase (Sethi et al., 2013). The production of the lipase enzyme in fungal strains is increased when sugar cane bagasse and olive oil cake are combined. When using olive oil as opposed to other types, bacterial strains have been shown to produce more lipase (Zarevúcka et al., 2012). On the other hand, using Tween 80 has also helped to improve the recovery of *Acinetobacter* sp. lipase (Li et al., 2001). Due to their low cost and availability, vegetable oils are also widely used to improve the yield of higher lipases (Messias et al., 2009).

#### 9.4.3.2 NITROGEN SOURCE

The improvement of microbial lipase production and microbial growth depends on nitrogen sources. Peptone, tryptone, yeast extract, sodium nitrate, urea, and other organic and inorganic nitrogen sources have all been used to produce higher lipases from various types of microorganisms (Priyanka et al., 2019). *Rhizopus* sp. was cultured with increased lipolytic activity after urea was added to the medium to produce lipase (Rodriguez et al., 2006). Similarly, *Aspergillus* sp. has produced lipase by combining peptone with other nitrogen extracts (Colonia et al., 2019).

#### *9.4.3.3 EFFECT OF TEMPERATURE ON LIPASE PRODUCTION*

Microbial lipases are produced in large part as a function of temperature. In the shake flask method, the ideal temperature is essential for the secretion of the enzyme. At 37°C, a higher biomass concentration of lipase was seen (Bharathi et al., 2018). Researchers found that the production of lipase was enhanced by a slight temperature increase up to 38°C (de Souza et al., 2019). The production of the lipase enzyme is decreased at lower temperatures, and the activity of the enzyme is influenced by higher temperatures.

#### *9.4.3.4 EFFECT OF PH ON LIPASE PRODUCTION*

Bacterial lipases typically have neutral pH or alkaline pH optimums. According to research, bacterial and yeast cells produce more lipase when the pH is alkaline or neutral (Bharathi et al., 2018). When the pH of the production medium was kept at a nearly neutral pH, *Rhodotorula glutinis* HL25 produced a good yield of lipase (Taskin et al., 2016). On the other hand, an acidic pH promotes the production of fungal lipases. In 2019, Turati et al. observed increased lipase activity and production while keeping the pH of the reaction medium at 4. Both the production of the lipase enzyme and the activity of the enzyme are influenced by temperature, as shown in Table 9.1.

## 9.5 PURIFICATION OF MICROBIAL LIPASE ENZYME

Purification of microbial lipases involves various steps depending on the intracellular or extracellular nature of the enzyme. In either scenario, produced proteins are further salted out through precipitation methods

**TABLE 9.1** Lipase-Producing Microorganisms and Some Biochemical Characteristics

| Lipase Source | Optimal Temperature | Optimal pH | Substrate Specificity | References |
|---|---|---|---|---|
| *Pseudomonas protegens* Pf-5 | 55°C | 9.5 | Medium and short chain long pNP-esters | Zha et al. (2014) |
| *Pseudomonas moraviensis* M9 | 65°C | 8.0 | Medium long chain pNPesters (C8-C16) | Yang et al. (2015a) |
| *Geobacillus stearothermophilus* AH22 | 50°C | 8.0–9.0 | Short-chain methyl ester Substrate (C4) | Ekinci et al. (2016) |
| *Janibacter* sp. R02 | 80°C | 8.0–9.0 | MUF-butyrate | Castilla et al. (2016) |
| *Rhizomucor miehei* NRRL5282 | 40°C | 7.0 | Medium long chain pNP-esters | Takó et al. (2017) |
| *Thermomyces Lanuginosus* | 60°C | 8.5 | Short-stranded pNP-esters | Xin et al. (2017) |
| *Candida viswanathii* | 45°C | 4.0 | Long-chain methyl ester substrate (C16) | Almeida et al. (2018) |
| *Paenibacillus pasadenensis* CS0611 | 50°C | 7.0 | pNP-esters (C8) | Gao et al. (2018) |
| *Aeribacillus pallidus* | 65°C | 10.0 | short chain triacylglycerols | Ktata et al. (2019) |
| *Thermomyces lanuginosus* | 60°C | 8.5 | olive oil | Kumar et al. (2019) |
| *Halocynthiibacter arcticus* | 20°C | 8.0 | p-nitrophenyl butyrate (p-NB, C4) | Le et al. (2020) |
| *Aspergillus niger* GZUF36 | 35°C | 4.0 | – | Xing et al. (2020) |
| *Bacillus licheniformis* NCU CS-5 | 40°C | 8.0 | Medium- and long-chain fatty acids (C6-C18) | Zhao et al. (2021) |
| *Streptomyces bacillaris* | 45°C | 9.0 | p-nitrophenyl phosphate (p-NPP) | Gao et al. (2021) |
| *Geobacillus kaustophilus* DSM 7263*T* | 50°C | 8.0 | short-chain fatty acid (C4) | Özdemir et al. (2021) |

utilizing ammonium sulphate (Yang et al., 2016). Additionally, chromatography and dialysis processes are applied to the precipitated protein. The method of chromatography chosen varies depending on the origin of the microorganisms and the size of the proteins, with chromatography being primarily used to purify lipases. Finally, using additional separation techniques like ion exchange, DEAE-Sepharose, and gel filtration chromatography, the crude fractions thus obtained are tested for the presence of enzyme using a variety of assay protocols (Unni et al., 2016). Through precipitation with ammonium sulphate, DEAE-Sepharose FF (ion exchange), and Sephadex G-75, a lipase from *Aspergillus niger* F044 was purified (gel filtration). The yield was 33%, and the purification factor was 73 (Zheng-Yu et al., 2007). Every microorganism has a different size for its microbial lipases. *Pseudomonas aeruginosa*-produced bacterial lipase expressed an average molecular weight of 29 kDa in this case (Unni et al., 2016), while the average weight of fungal lipase was discovered to be 27 kDa (Zhou et al., 2012). Kumar et al. (2014) reported that yeast lipase also exists as a monomer with an average weight of 46 kDa.

## 9.6 ENZYME IMMOBILIZATION

Some negative aspects of these biomolecules have made it more difficult to use enzymes in the industrial sector. Their application in the free form is difficult due to the possibility of denaturation caused by their low stability and the complexity of recovering the enzyme for subsequent uses (Sirisha et al., 2016). Since one issue with using enzymes in the free form is their low stability in factors like temperature and pH, enzyme immobilization techniques aim to make the steps of enzyme separation and recovery easier. Cross-Linked Enzyme Aggregates (CLEAs) are a method of immobilization that has gained attention. It is a beneficial method because its execution is quick and requires little technical expertise (Cui et al., 2017). Sheldon and Roger (2011) proposed CLEAs, which have intriguing properties that are desired in industrial biotransformation's. The technique is simple to use, does not require the use of transporters, allows for the co-immobilization of two or more enzymes, is inexpensive, allows for the retention of high enzymatic activities, has good thermal stability, and is highly resistant to organic solvents. There are two stages to CLEAs. Precipitating substances, including inorganic salts, polymers, and organic solvents, among others, first cause the enzyme to precipitate. After that, cross-linking agents, of which glutaraldehyde is most frequently used as a bi-functional reagent or multifunctional agent, act by reacting with the amino groups on the enzyme's surface (Bilal et al., 2018). Additionally, this approach combines purification and immobilization in a single step, speeding up and simplifying the process (Samoylova et al., 2018). Using ammonium sulphate and glutaraldehyde, the CLEAs method immobilized lipase B from *Candida antarctica*. They discovered that the enzyme could be used repeatedly with 100% of its initial activity, allowing for up to 10 catalytic cycles of bio-diesel conversion. In a different investigation, sodium tripolyphosphate was used to cross-link an *A. niger* lipase that had been precipitated using ammonium sulphate (TPP). When compared to free enzymes, TPP provided highly stable enzymes over a wider temperature and pH range, which led to favorable results (Qian et al., 2020). This method's capacity to increase the pH stability of the enzyme is a benefit. JiaoJiao et al. (2022) demonstrated that *Candida rugosa* lipase (CRL) could be immobilized by the CLEAs technique and that the behavior of the enzyme improved as it became more stable at a given pH than the free enzyme. The use of CLEAs and combi-CLEAs is a promising immobilization technique, particularly because it eliminates the need for previously purified enzymes. However, it is essential to optimize the cross-linking and precipitation parameters as well as their interactions. They can benefit bioprocesses in industrial applications by increasing enzyme stability. The protein forms a bond with the surface of an insoluble matrix in this immobilization process (solid support) (Eş et al., 2015). Adsorption, covalent bonding, entrapment/encapsulation, and cross-linking are the techniques for immobilizing enzymes, as shown in Figure 9.2. There is not a single immobilization technique that can be used for all enzymes, so when choosing a method, certain factors must be considered, including the ease of the process, the cost, and choosing a procedure that offers a satisfactory level of catalytic activity in addition to a technique that allows for good operational stability.

## 9.7 INDUSTRIAL APPLICATIONS OF MICROBIAL LIPASES

This multifaceted enzyme, for which there are numerous application strategies, is one of the essential enzymes in the hydrolase's enzyme class. The food, pharmaceutical, oil and fats, oleo-chemicals, leather, bio-diesel, paper and pulp, dairy, fine chemicals, cosmetics, and perfume industries are just a few of the numerous applications (Sarmah et al., 2018). In some industries, lipases are used, and the most recent research on them is covered in detail.

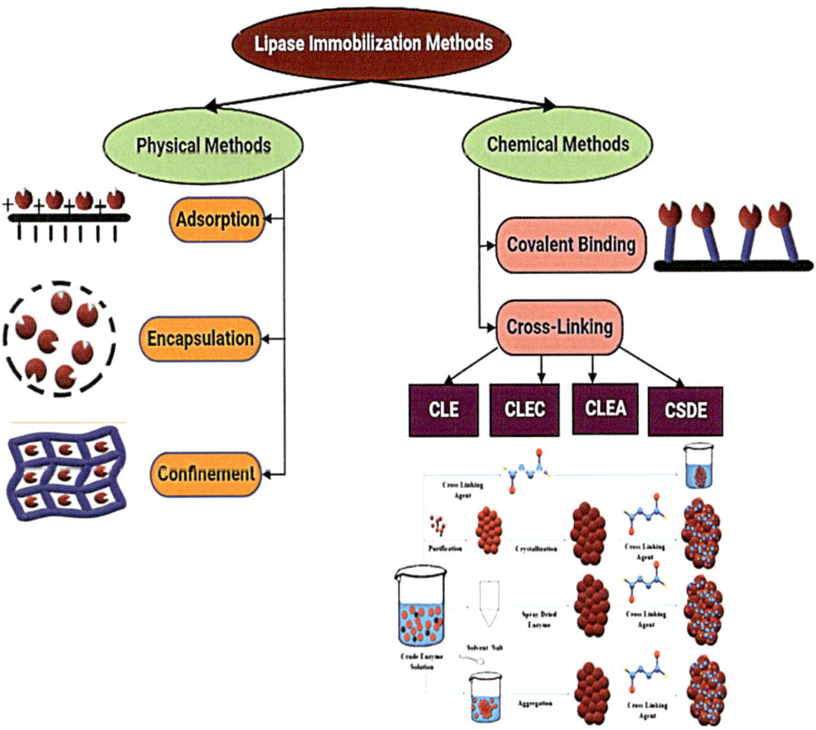


**FIGURE 9.2** Methods of enzyme immobilization: adsorption, entrapment, covalent bonding, and cross-linking. CLE: Cross-Linked Enzyme CLEAs: Cross-Linked Enzyme Aggregates.

### *9.7.1 LIPASES IN THE FOOD INDUSTRY*

Lipase is used in the food industry for several processes, including raising food quality and yield, giving some products aromas, and removing oils and fats. It is employed, among other things, in the production of dairy goods, baking, brewing, and meat processing (Salihu et al., 2016). Lipase hydrolyzes the milk fat in the dairy industry. Additionally, cheese's flavor is improved, and the ripening process is sped up by lipase (Memarpoor-Yazd et al., 2018). Fish meat frequently undergoes the biolipolysis process, in which lipases are added to remove fat from the meat during processing to produce lean meat. Additionally, microbial lipases are used to enhance the flavor of rice, and lipase can be used to create omega-3 fatty acids (Kumar et al., 2018). Esters are flavoring agents that can be used in food, cosmetics, and pharmaceutical products. These esters are found in natural sources, such as fruits. However, they produce little fruit, and the composition of the fruit changes as the fruit ripens. Therefore, using these enzymes to create these aromatic esters is a viable alternative (Su et al., 2016). The production of PUFAs and the synthesis of esters and alcohols are both aided by the potent biocatalysts known as lipases. These substances produced by lipase action are used to create nutritious foods and even in the creation of nutritional supplements (de Jesus et al., 2016). A lipase from *Yarrowia lipolytica*, which was produced by SMF with soybean meal, was used by de Souza et al. (2019) to synthesize a variety of flavoring esters with commercial value in the food industry. The enzymatic synthesis of isoamyl acetate and isopentyl acetate esters was catalyzed by free and immobilized lipases. According to a study by Bayramoglu et al. (2022), the ester conversions for isoamyl acetate and isopentyl acetate were 98.4% and 73.7%, respectively. These findings show that lipases can function as potential biocatalysts for the use of aromatic esters. The use of lipase to extend the shelf life of some shelf goods, such as bakery goods, and to enhance the flavor of juices, soups, sauces, cheeses, and baked goods is another very significant function. The addition of lipase improved some aspects of noodles (Ray, 2012). In their study, Cao et al. (2014) discovered an improvement in blue cheese through the application of lipase, which affected the cheese's distinctive aroma in addition to adding to its distinctive flavor by synthesizing methyl ketones. In a study published in 2014, Schaffarczyk et al. assessed the impact of using lipase in baking. Depending on the type and concentration of the lipase added, the addition of this enzyme increased the volume of bread from 56% to 58%. Some lipases have multiple uses, such as CRL, which can improve the flavor and aroma of food as well as be used in the fats and oils industry in addition to other uses (Melis et al., 2017).

### 9.7.2 LIPASES IN BIO-DIESEL PRODUCTION

In particular, renewable energy sources are being researched to replace the use of non-renewable energy sources, which are quickly running out of resources. The use of degradable oils and fats with a high FFA content for the production of bio-diesel using enzymes has received attention for being a highly feasible and environmentally friendly process.

The final product is bio-diesel because these compounds are transformed through esterification and transesterification reactions mediated by biocatalysts like lipases (Sandoval et al., 2017). Fan et al. (2017) described the lipases from *Burkholderia cepacia, Rhizomucor miehei*, and *Candida rugosa* as promising catalysts for the production of bio-diesel. The produc tion of bio-diesel by these three lipases was compared using soybean oil and leftover vegetable oil. The outcomes demonstrated that the lipase of *Rhizomucor miehei* can efficiently convert the leftover vegetable oil into bio-diesel through the transesterification process. By converting grains used in breweries into bio-diesel in the presence of methanol, Luliano et al. (2020) produced bio-diesel using the lipase of *Candida rugosa*. High yield (98%) and good results were obtained, and the process was also inexpensive because the catalyst could be used again even after four cycles. Amini et al. (2017) claim that a new source of bio-diesel, the oil from the seeds of *Ocimum basilicum*, can be produced effectively. Methanol and immobilized lipase (Novozym 435) were used in the production process. Up to seven cycles of reuse were allowed for the immobilized lipase. Lipases are effective biocatalysts that can be used to make bio-diesel. There are, however, some drawbacks to this practice. For instance, the bio-diesel produced using this method has a low yield, and using it in machines could harm that machinery. Additionally, it is challenging to remove the untreated methanol while producing bio-diesel in one of the final production steps. As a result, additional methods must be employed to eliminate impurities and produce high-quality fuel (Pérez et al., 2019). However, many studies have indicated that using lipases as catalysts in the production of bio-diesel has produced promising results. For instance, in a study by Costa et al. (2020), the researchers looked into the reactions of hydrolysis and esterification as they relate to the production of bio-diesel. Soybean oil was hydrolyzed using *Geotrichum candidum* lipases, and *Pseudomonas fluorescens* immobilized lipase was used to mediate the subsequent step in FFA esterification (PEL). High-quality bio-diesel was produced by the hydro esterification mechanism used in the study, and the reactions showed favorable viscosity and purity. The hydrolysis reactions allowed for the swift conversion of the soybean oil to FFAs without the need for purification, which was advantageous because it cut down on costs. Shalini et al. (2021) studied the transesterification-based synthesis of bio-diesel, which is catalyzed by an *Aspergillus niger* lipase. The immobilized enzyme had a total bio-diesel yield of 90% and could be used five times to make bio-diesel without losing any of its effectiveness. As a result, it works well as a catalyst in the production of bio-diesel. Catalyst research has advanced thanks to the success of laboratory studies, pilot projects, and process optimization. These investigations aid in increasing enzyme productivity and activity (Pasha et al., 2021). The use of lipases as biocatalysts has many benefits, but it is necessary to examine the current approaches and look for new ones to increase the use of lipases in the production of this biofuel (Sankaran et al., 2016).

### 9.7.3 LIPASES IN THE PHARMACEUTICAL INDUSTRY

Since a significant portion of the drugs currently under development is chiral, one of the most important methodologies in the pharmaceutical industry is the production of pure enantiomers. Therefore, the action of biocatalysts, particularly lipases, is what allows for the production of pure enantiomers (Sawant et al., 2016). Chemical processes can also be used to carry out this process, but because of their effectiveness and selectivity, enzymatic catalysts are preferred. These enzymes can also produce a large number of enantiomers (Bhardwaj et al., 2017). Enantiomers can be created by lipases. Ibuprofen, atenolol, and milnacipran, a drug used in the treatment of fibromyalgia, can all be produced using lipases. For instance, ibuprofen can be produced from specific compounds using a lipase of *Rhodothermus marinus* (Memarpoor-Yazdi et al., 2017); atenolol can be produced using a lipase of *Candida rugosa* (Sikora et al., 2017). Other medications made with various types of lipases include nobiletin, naproxen, ascorbic acid, quinolone derivatives, ketoprofen, and chloramphenicol (Carvalho et al., 2015). These enzymes are widely used in the pharmaceutical industry because they possess desirable properties for biocatalysts used to synthesize pharmaceutical products, such as regioselectivity and stereospecificity (Stauch et al., 2015). Future research on biocatalysis may place a greater emphasis on the creation of pharmaceutical intermediates and finished drugs (Sun et al., 2018).

### 9.7.4 LIPASES IN THE DETERGENT INDUSTRY

Among the many uses for lipases, the production of detergents is highlighted (Rahman et al., 2013). Triglycerides can be removed more easily and with less emulsion when they are broken down into fatty acids by lipases (Rahman et al., 2013). Since the aqueous medium is alkaline in the detergent industry, the lipases used in the detergent formulation must be alkalophilic (Bhosale et al., 2016). Some benefits of using enzymes in the formulation of detergents include a decrease in the amount of time needed for washing and an increase in the fabric's lifespan (Agobo et al., 2017).

Microbial lipases can effectively remove fat, according to studies. An olive oil triacylglycerol was successfully removed from cotton fabric by García-Silvera et al. (2018) using lipase from *Serratia marcescens*. Positive results were found when a detergent made with shrimp hepatopancreas lipases was compared to commercial laundry detergents in terms of effectiveness (Kuepethkaew et al., 2017). *Bacillus subtilis* lipase demonstrated favorable characteristics for use in the manufacture of detergents. It was extremely resistant to oxidizing agents, commercial detergents, and surfac tants, making it a promising application in the cleaning sector (Saraswat et al., 2017). Alkaline lipase can help reduce the need for surfactants and other unfavorable substances from an ecological standpoint when used in the manufacture of detergents (Niyonzima and More, 2015). Commercial detergents contain hazardous chemical compounds that are bad for both human and environmental health, so lipases are a better alternative because they can be applied at room temperature and maintain fabric quality (Javed et al., 2018).

### 9.7.5 LIPASES IN THE TREATMENT OF EFFLUENTS

Because many industrial residues contain oily compounds that hinder oxygen diffusion in the water, when they are released into aquatic environments, they kill aquatic organisms. Enzymes help reduce the number of oils and fats present in these residues to address this environmental issue (Hu et al., 2018). The biological treatment of wastewater was carried out by Ktata et al. (2020) using the lipase produced by *Aeribacillus pallidus*. When lipase was used to hydrolyze wastewater at 50°C for 1 h, the treatment of the effluents produced by the canned tuna industry was very effective (96.11%). The ability of the *Bacillus* sp. lipase to hydrolyze fats in various industrial effluents were assessed (dairy, bakery, and poultry). The enzyme was thought to be a good alternative for pretreating these effluents because it could hydrolyze more than 50% of the initial fat present in all of them

(Balaji et al., 2020). When a lipase from *Fusarium verticillioides* was used in the pretreatment of the effluent from a slaughterhouse, a reduction of fat by three times was observed. The enzyme was stable over a wide pH range and had an optimal temperature and pH of 45°C and 5.5, respectively, for enzymatic activity (4.0 to 8.0). For industrial applications, these qualities are advantageous (Facchini et al., 2016). Since enzymatic hydrolysis makes the subsequent step of the treatment by microbes easier, this pretreatment step using lipases is highly feasible (Soares et al., 2019). In addition to being environmentally friendly, studies and new technologies have demonstrated that the use of enzymes in the pretreatment of industrial effluents lowers the costs associated with this process (Garrido and Silva, 2016). Although lipases are frequently used in the industry, their use in treating effluents is constrained by their high cost. Further research is therefore required into the use of these biocatalysts to remove the lipids from effluents, given the potential economic impact and attraction of obtaining high-value by-products from lipid-rich waters (Nimkande and Bafana, 2022).

### 9.7.6 LIPASES IN COSMETICS

Lipases have been utilized in the cosmetics industry to catalyze the creation of chemical products like esters, aromas, and active agents as well as active compounds (Ansorge-Schumacher and Thum, 2013). Lipases are particularly effective in the formulation of cleaning products and creams for cellulite treatment in the field of enzymocosmetics (Beli et al., 2019). Because they can dissolve fat deposits, lipases are also used to prepare slimming products. In addition, lipases also produce hair and makeup products. The catalytic action of lipases has been used to synthesize numerous products, many of which have been put on the market (Ansorge-Schumacher and Thum, 2013). The creation of aromas, which are used in fragrances and other products, is a concern of the cosmetic industry. This is a crucial factor, particularly for the consumers. As a result, the industry looks for biotechnological alternatives to create natural aromas (Baránková et al., 2016). The cosmetics industry has studied biotechnological procedures, and the application of biotechnology has resulted in the development of new products as well as the improvement of current methodologies. Enzymes have enabled this industry to offer consumers better products (Dias et al., 2017).

### 9.7.7 LIPASES IN THE PRODUCTION OF BIOSENSORS

Since lipases have properties that make them desirable for the production of these materials, they can be used to make biosensors. These devices are developed using a variety of microbial lipases (Priyanka et al., 2019). High specificity and selectivity, the potential for regeneration, high yields, and real-time diagnosis are all benefits of using enzymes in the production of biosensors. Numerous enzymatic biosensors are employed in the field of medicine, including portable clinical analyzers and home blood glucose monitors (glucometers) (Nguyen et al., 2019). *Aspergillus oryzae* and *Candida antarctica* lipases were utilized by Hasanah et al. (2019) to create an optical biosensor to identify triglycerides (TGs). Triglycerides can be hydrolyzed by the immobilized lipases, releasing glycerol and FFA. An optical pH sensor detects the medium's decreased acidity and pH after the released acid has been released. In some studies, other lipase-based biosensors have been described. Using a lipase from *Candida rugosa*, Zehani et al. (2015) created a conductometric enzymatic biosensor (CRL). Diazinon, methyl parathion, and methyl paraoxon were three organophosphate pesticides that this apparatus was capable of finding in an aqueous medium. In this apparatus, diazinon hydrolysis was catalyzed by lipase. Since the biosensor could measure concentrations as low as 60 μg, the results were encouraging. Additionally, lipases from *Ceratobasidium* sp. were used to create a biosensor for the detection of pesticides. Lipase hydrolyzed the substrate p-nitrophenyl acetate in this sensor, which was developed by Barboza et al., 2019 for the determination of carbendazim (pNPA). In these devices, enzymatic biosensors must be stable, and their specificity is a crucial factor in preventing false signals. The collaboration between the biological sciences and engineering can be seen in the creation of these biosensors. Health monitoring with biosensors is possible both at home and in medical facilities (Sonawane et al., 2017).

### 9.7.8 LIPASE IN THE TEXTILE INDUSTRY

The treatment of fabric is one of the applications for lipases in the textile industry. Some conventional treatments employ substances that have a higher likelihood of making the patient itchy and may cause a loss of fabric weight. By replacing these substances with lipases, both the likelihood of a reaction and the weight loss of the fabric are decreased. This enzymatic treatment effectively modifies the fabric's properties and softens some fabrics, like polyester (Kumar and Kumar, 2020). Lipases can digest natural fats and oils.

Additionally, this enzyme performs a lot of dyeing and cleaning, which gives cellulosic textiles a lot of hydrophilicity (Kalantzi et al., 2010).

Lipases were used by El-Shemy et al. (2016) to treat polyester fabrics. Better dyeing capacity, higher wettability, and better moisture recovery were all provided by the enzymatic treatment, and the lipase's action did not worsen the fabric's condition during the reaction. Using *Bacillus aryabhattai*, Taleb et al. (2022) successfully produced a lipase with a potent ability to dissolve the lipid barrier from the surface of wool fibers. The enzyme demonstrated up to five times greater bio-cleaning efficiency for wool. The application of the lipase was successful because it did not cause the fiber's properties to degrade. Lipases have been used in several studies to restore, clean, and preserve vintage textiles (Darwish et al., 2020). The benefit of using enzymes to treat fabric over traditional methods is that the polyethylene terephthalate's properties are preserved because enzymes are large proteins and do not penetrate the fabric. Lipases also prevent the fabric from corroding, which happens when other substances are used, like in alkaline treatments (Choudhury, 2020).

### 9.7.9 LIPASES IN BIOREMEDIATION

The bioremediation of lipid residues is possible with the aid of lipases (Lan et al., 2016). By transforming these contaminants into nontoxic substances, they can clean and decontaminate soil contaminated with greasy residues (Larik et al., 2019). Sahoo et al. (2020) used *Pseudomonas* sp. lipase for the bioremediation of soil contaminated with hydrocarbons from automobile oils. The enzyme used mediated the degradation of this oil, resulting in the degradation of 92.6% of the automotive oil, proving its effectiveness in this process. However, there are some drawbacks to using enzymes in bioremediation as well, including the high cost of enzyme production, the possibility that the conditions used in the process could inactivate the enzyme, and a lack of understanding of how the enzymes behave when they interact with pollutants. To improve the technique and optimize the parameters, more research on the use of enzymes in bioremediation is required (Kumar et al., 2020). The methodologies used have been researched and improved upon because biocatalysis mediated by lipase is used in many industrial sectors. The combination of biotechnology, genetic engineering, and protein engineering has improved lipases and enabled the production of many high-quality goods. Although there are still some restrictions, as new technologies are created, these inconveniences can be eliminated (Kirana et al., 2016).

## 9.8 CONCLUSION

Along with other microbial enzymes, lipases are highly beneficial biomolecules with significant biotechnological potential. At the industrial level, different microbial sources of lipase are used to produce enzymes at comparatively lower costs. Researchers have taken advantage of the fact that lipases do not require co-factors and can easily be immobilized on support materials, and they have developed methods for fabricating these enzymes on inexpensive carrier materials for efficient product recovery with reuse (of enzyme). When it comes to utilizing different substrates, lipases exhibit versatility and turn them into highly valuable products that cannot be produced using regular chemical processes. Further engineering of these enzymes, both in terms of quality and quantity, is necessary for proper enzymatic operations on an industrial scale. This engineering includes steps for protein engineering, enzyme immobilization, standardization, and media optimization. Metagenomic library screening, directed evolution, and rational design have a big role to play in this field. Due to its properties, including enantio-, stereo-, and regio-selectivity, solvent stability, compatibility with a variety of substrates for immobilization, and wide range of applications in the detergent, food, bio-diesel, cosmetics, pharmaceutical, and other industries, lipases have established themselves as a versatile enzyme over time. Although numerous microbial strains, such as cold-adapted, thermotolerant, alkaline, and acidic lipases, have been identified, more research is required to fully exploit their potential for use in the context of industrial sustainability. Similar to this, there is still much to learn about engineered lipases that have a variety of properties suitable for bio-process and environmental applications. Therefore, it is necessary to investigate every action that could be taken to increase microbial lipase production, not only to meet the current demand but also to achieve the objective of industrial sustainability.

## 9.9 FUTURE PROSPECTS

Greener technologies are becoming increasingly important and necessary to combat the harmful effects of carbon emissions and the greenhouse effect without slowing down the rate of industrialization and global development. The identification and use of microbial lipases for industrial reactions have eliminated the use of strong acids and alkalis, as well as the application of high temperature and pressure during various reactions.

This is the result of efforts to find substitute technologies for existing ones that are equally effective and less harmful. Even though such research has been going on for many years and has led to the creation and commercialization of enzyme formulations, it has only had a small impact thus far. Cost of production, maintenance, the inadequacy of available technology, and poor commercial competitiveness are the main restrictions. With the current rate of advancement in modern science, the ongoing development of cutting-edge technology, the well-established method of enzyme research, and the data already available, these problems can be systematically addressed in the future, leading to industrial reactions for rational creations in a more environmentally friendly way for a bio-based economy.

## KEYWORDS

- **enzyme production**
- **fermentation**
- **industrial applications**
- **microbial lipases**
- **screening methods**
- **substrate specificity**

## REFERENCES

Abou Taleb, M., Gomaa, S. K., Wahba, M. I., Zaki, R. A., El-Fiky, A. F., El-Refai, H. A., et al. (2022). Bio scouring of wool fibers using immobilized thermophilic lipase. *International Journal of Biological Macromolecules*, *194*, 800–810.

Abrunhosa, L., Oliveira, F., Dantas, D., Gonçalves, C., & Belo, I. (2013). Lipase production by *Aspergillus ibericus* using olive mill wastewater. *Bioprocess and Biosystems Engineering*, *36*(3), 285–291.

Agobo, K. U., Arazu, V. A., Uzo, K., & Igwe, C. N. (2017). Microbial lipases: A prospect for biotechnological industrial catalysis for green products: A review. *Fermentation Technology*, *6*, 2.

Almeida, A. F. D., Terrasan, C. R. F., Terrone, C. C., Tauk-Tornisielo, S. M., & Carmona, E. C. (2018). Biochemical properties of free and immobilized *Candida viswanathii* lipase on octyl-agarose support: Hydrolysis of triacylglycerol and soy lecithin. *Process Biochemistry*, *65*, 71–80.

Amini, Z., Ong, H. C., Harrison, M. D., Kusumo, F., Mazaheri, H., & Ilham, Z. (2017). Biodiesel production by lipase catalyzed transesterification of *Ocimum basilicum* L. (sweet basil) seed oil. *Energy Conversion and Management*, *132*, 82–90.

Ansorge-Schumacher, M. B., & Thum, O. (2013). Immobilized lipases in the cosmetics industry. *Chemical Society Reviews*, *42*, 6475–6490.

Balaji, L., Chittoor, J. T., & Jayaraman, G. (2020). Optimization of extracellular lipase production by halotolerant *Bacillus* sp. VITL8 using factorial design and applicability of enzyme in pretreatment of food industry effluents. *Preparative Biochemistry & Biotechnology*, *50*, 708–716.

Baránková, E., & Dohnal, V. (2016). Effect of additives on volatility of aroma compounds from dilute aqueous solutions. *Fluid Phase Equilibria*, *407*, 217–223.

Barrios-González, J. (2012). Solid-state fermentation: Physiology of solid medium, its molecular basis and applications. *Process Biochemistry*, *47*(2), 175–185.

Bayramoglu, G., Celikbicak, O., Kilic, M., & Arica, M. Y. (2022). Immobilization of *Candida rugosa* lipase on magnetic chitosan beads and application in flavor esters synthesis. *Food Chemistry*, *366*, 130699.

Beli, C. M., Mageste, J. M., & Taketani, N. F. (2019). Bioprospecção de enzimas para cosmética: Seu impacto na biotecnologia. *Revista Ensaios Pioneiros*, *3*, 10–24.

Bharathi, D., & Rajalakshmi, G. (2019). Microbial lipases: An overview of screening, production and purification. *Biocatalysis and Agricultural Biotechnology*, *22*, 101368.

Bharathi, D., Rajalakshmi, G., & Komathi, S. (2018). Optimization and production of lipase enzyme from bacterial strains isolated from petrol spilled soil. *Journal of King Saud University–Science*, 1–4.

Bhardwaj, K. K., & Gupta, R. (2017). Synthesis of chirally pure enantiomers by lipase. *Journal of Oleo Science*, *66*, 1073–1084.

Bhosale, H., Shaheen, U., & Kadam, T. (2016). Characterization of a hyper thermostable alkaline lipase from *Bacillus sonorensis* 4R. *Enzyme Research*, *2016*, 4170684.

Bilal, M., Iqbal, H. M., Guo, S., Hu, H., Wang, W., & Zhang, X. (2018). State-of-the-art protein engineering approaches using biological macromolecules: A review from immobilization to implementation view point. *International Journal of Biological Macromolecules*, *108*, 893–901.

Bolina, I. C., Gomes, R. A., & Mendes, A. A. (2021). Biolubricant production from several oleaginous feedstocks using lipases as catalysts: Current scenario and future perspectives. *BioEnergy Research*, *14*(4), 1039–1057.

Cao, M., Fonseca, L. M., Schoenfuss, T. C., & Rankin, S. A. (2014). Homogenization and lipase treatment of milk and resulting methyl ketone generation in blue cheese. *Journal of Agricultural and Food Chemistry*, *62*, 5726–5733.

Carvalho, A. C., Fonseca, T. D., Mattos, M. C., Oliveira, M. D., Lemos, T. L., Molinari, F., et al. (2015). Recent advances in lipase-mediated preparation of pharmaceuticals and their intermediates. *International Journal of Molecular Sciences*, *16*, 29682–29716.

Castilla, A., Panizza, P., Rodríguez, D., Bonino, L., Díaz, P., Irazoqui, G., et al. (2016). A novel thermophilic and halophilic esterase from *Janibacter* sp. R02, the first member of a new lipase family (Family XVII). *Enzyme and Microbial Technology*, *98*, 86.

Chandra, P., Singh, R., & Arora, P. K. (2020). Microbial lipases and their industrial applications: A comprehensive review. *Microbial Cell Factories*, *19*(1), 1–42.

Choudhury, A. K. (2020). Enzyme applications in textile chemical processing. In *Sustainable Technologies for Fashion and Textiles* (pp. 91–115). Sawston: Woodhead Publishing.

Colla, L. M., Ficanha, A. M., Rizzardi, J., Bertolin, T. E., Reinehr, C. O., & Costa, J. A. V. (2015). Production and characterization of lipases by two new isolates of *Aspergillus* through solid-state and submerged fermentation. *BioMed Research International, 2015, 725959.*

Colla, L. M., Primaz, A. L., Benedetti, S., Loss, R. A., Lima, M. D., Reinehr, C. O., & Costa, J. A. V. (2016). Surface response methodology for the optimization of lipase production under submerged fermentation by filamentous fungi. *Brazilian Journal of Microbiology*, *47*(2), 461–467.

Colonia, B. S. O., Woiciechowski, A. L., Malanski, R., Letti, L. A. J., & Soccol, C. R. (2019). Pulp improvement of oil palm empty fruit bunches associated to solid-state bio pulping and biobleaching with xylanase and lignin peroxidase cocktail produced by *Aspergillus* sp. LPB-5. *Bioresource Technology*, *285*, 121361.

Cordova, J., & Baratti, J. (2006). Improving lipase production by nutrient source modification using *Rhizopus homothallicus* cultured in solid state fermentation. *Process Biochemistry*, *41*, 2264–2269.

Costa, M. J., Silva, M. R., Ferreira, E. E., Carvalho, A. K., Basso, R. C., Pereira, E. B., et al. (2020). Enzymatic biodiesel production by hydro esterification using waste cooking oil as feedstock. *Chemical Engineering and Processing*, *157*, 108131.

Costa, T. M., Hermann, K. L., Garcia-Roman, M., Valle, R. D. C. S. C., & Tavares, L. B. B. (2017). Lipase production by *Aspergillus niger* grown in different agro-industrial wastes by solid-state fermentation. *Brazilian Journal of Chemical Engineering*, *34*(2), 419–427.

Cui, J., Lin, T., Feng, Y., Tan, Z., & Jia, S. (2017). Preparation of spherical cross-linked lipase aggregates with improved activity, stability and reusability characteristic in water-in-ionic liquid microemulsion. *Journal of Chemical Technology and Biotechnology*, *92*, 1785–1793.

Darwish, S. S., Hassan, M. E., Ahmed, H. E., El Fadl, M. A., & El Bhery, M. B. (2020). Evaluation of effectiveness of covalently immobilized α-amylase and lipase in cleaning of historical textiles. *Bio Interface Research in Applied Chemistry*, *11*, 9952–9962.

Dayanandan, A., Rani, S., Shanmugavel, M., Gnanamani, A., & Rajakumar, G. S. (2013). Enhanced production of *Aspergillus tamarii* lipase for recovery of fat from tannery fleshing's. *Brazilian Journal of Microbiology*, *44*(4), 1089–1095.

De Jesus, M. V., de Oliveira, T. S., Ferreira, R. D., de Lima, A. M., da Silva Rodrigues, J. R., Silva, C. F., et al. (2016). Produção de lipase utilizando manipueira como fonte alternativa de carbono. *Scientia Plena*, *12*, 054208.

de Moura Barboza, A., da Silva, A. B., da Silva, E. M., de Souza, W. P., Soares, M. A., de Vasconcelos, L. G., et al. (2019). A biosensor based on microbial lipase immobilized on lamellar zinc hydroxide-decorated gold nanoparticles for carbendazim determination. *Analytical Methods*, *11*, 5388–5397.

De Souza, C. E., Ribeiro, B. D., & Coelho, M. A. (2019). Characterization and application of *Yarrowia lipolytica* lipase obtained by solid-state fermentation in the synthesis of different esters used in the food industry. *Applied Biochemistry and Biotechnology*, *189*, 933–959.

Dhiman, S., & Chapadgaonkar, S. S. (2013). Optimization of lipase production medium for a bacterial isolate. *International Journal of Chemical Technology Research*, *5*, 2837–2843.

Dias, R. F., & Carvalho, C. D. (2017). Bioeconomic no Brazil e no Mundo: Panorama actual e perspectives. *Revista Virtual de Química*, *9*, 410–430.

Ekinci, A. P., Dinçer, B., Baltaş, N., & Adıgüzel, A. (2016). Partial purification and characterization of lipase from *Geobacillus stearothermophilus* AH22. *Journal of Enzyme Inhibition and Medicinal Chemistry*, *31*, 325–331.

El-Shemy, N. S., El-Hawary, N. S., & El-Sayed, H. (2016). Basic and reactive-dyeable polyester fabrics using lipase enzymes. *Journal of Chemical Engineering & Process Technology*, *7*, 1.

Eş, I., Vieira, J. D., & Amaral, A. C. (2015). Principles, techniques, and applications of biocatalyst immobilization for industrial application. *Applied Microbiology and Biotechnology*, *99*, 2065–2082.

Facchini, F. D., Vici, A. C., Pereira, M. G., Jorge, J. A., & de Moraes, M. D. (2016). Enhanced lipase production of *Fusarium verticillioides* by using response surface methodology and wastewater pretreatment application. *Journal of Biochemical Technology*, *6*, 996–1002.

Fan, Y., Su, F., Li, K., Ke, C., & Yan, Y. (2017). Carbon nanotube filled with magnetic iron oxide and modified with polyamidation dendrimers for immobilizing lipase toward application in biodiesel production. *Scientific Reports*, *7*, 45643.

Ferraz, J. L., Souza, L. O., Silva, T. P., & Franco, M. (2018). Obtaining of microbial lipase: A brief review. *Recen*, *20*, 30–53.

Gao, J., Ou, X., Xu, P., Zong, M., & Lou, W. (2018). Cloning, overexpression, and characterization of a novel organic solvent-tolerant lipase from *Paenibacillus pasadenensis* CS0611. *Chinese Journal of Catalysis*, *39*, 937–945.

Gao, K., Wang, X., Jiang, H., Sun, J., & Mao, X. (2021). Identification of a GDSL lipase from *Streptomyces bacillaris* and its application in the preparation of free astaxanthin. *Journal of Biotechnology*, *325*, 280–287.

García-Silvera, E. E., Martínez-Morales, F., Bertrand, B., Morales-Guzmán, D., Rosas-Galván, N. S., León-Rodríguez, R., et al. (2018). Production and application of a thermostable lipase from *Serratia marcescens* in detergent formulation and biodiesel production. *Biotechnology and Applied Biochemistry*, *65*, 156–172.

Garrido, J. V., & Silva, C. F. (2016). Prospecção tecnológica e científica da utilização de lipases microbianas para tratamento de efluentes. *Cadernos de Prospecção*, *9*, 298–306.

Hasanah, U., Sani, N. D., Heng, L. Y., Idroes, R., & Safitri, E. (2019). Construction of a hydrogel pectin-based triglyceride optical biosensor with immobilized lipase enzymes. *Biosensors*, *9*, 135.

Hu, J., Cai, W., Wang, C., Du, X., Lin, J., & Cai, J. (2018). Purification and characterization of alkaline lipase production by *Pseudomonas aeruginosa* HFE733 and application for biodegradation in food wastewater treatment. *Biotechnology & Biotechnological Equipment*, *32*, 583–590.

Iuliano, M., Sarno, M., De Pasquale, S., & Ponticorvo, E. (2020). *Candida rugosa* lipase for the biodiesel production from renewable sources. *Renewable Energy*, *162*, 124–133.

Javed, S., Azeem, F., Hussain, S., Rasul, I., Siddique, M. H., Riaz, M., et al. (2018). Bacterial lipases: A review on purification and characterization. *Progress in Biophysics and Molecular Biology*, *132*, 23–34.

Jiaojiao, X., Yan, Y., Bin, Z., & Feng, L. (2022). Improved catalytic performance of carrier-free immobilized lipase by advanced cross-linked enzyme aggregates technology. *Bioprocess and Biosystems Engineering*, *45*, 147–158.

Kalantzi, S., Mamma, D., Kalogeris, E., & Kekos, D. (2010). Improved properties of cotton fabrics treated with lipase and its combination with pectinase. *Fibers & Textiles in Eastern Europe*, *18*, 86–92.

Kirana, S., Arshad, Z., Nosheen, S., Kamal, S., Gulzar, T., Majeed, M. S., et al. (2016). Microbial lipases: Production and applications: A review. *Journal of Biochemistry, Biotechnology and Biomaterials*, *1*, 7–20.

Kirsh, D. (1935). Lipase production by *Penicillium oxalicum* and *Aspergillus flavus*. *Botanical Gazette*, *97*, 321–333.

Ktata, A., Krayem, N., Aloulou, A., Bezzine, S., Sayari, A., Chamkha, M., et al. (2019). Purification, biochemical and molecular study of lipase producing from a newly thermoalkaliphilic *Aeribacillus pallidus* for oily wastewater treatment. *Journal of Biochemistry*, *167*, 89–99.

Ktata, A., Krayem, N., Aloulou, A., Bezzine, S., Sayari, A., Chamkha, M., et al. (2020). Purification, biochemical and molecular study of lipase producing from a newly thermoalkaliphilic *Aeribacillus pallidus* for oily wastewater treatment. *Journal of Biochemistry*, *167*, 89–99.

Kuepethkaew, S., Sangkharak, K., Benjakul, S., & Klomklao, S. (2017). Laundry detergent-stable lipase from Pacific white shrimp (*Litopenaeus vannamei*) hepatopancreas: Effect of extraction media and biochemical characterization. *International Journal of Food Properties*, *20*, 769–781.

Kumar, A., Gudiukaite, R., Gricajeva, A., Sadauskas, M., Malunavicius, V., Kamyab, H., et al. (2020). Microbial lipolytic enzymes—promising energy-efficient biocatalysts in bioremediation. *Energy*, *192*, 116674.

Kumar, A., Park, G. D., Patel, S. K. S., Kondaveeti, S., Otari, S., Anwar, M. Z., et al. (2019). $SiO_2$ microparticles with carbon nanotube-derived mesopores as an efficient support for enzyme immobilization. *Chemical Engineering Journal*, *359*, 1252–1264.

Kumar, J. A., & Kumar, M. S. (2020). A study on improving dyeability of polyester fabric using lipase enzyme. *Autex Research Journal*, *20*, 243–249.

Kumar, K., Usha, K. Y., Satyanarayana, S. V., & Sailaja, V. (2014). Characterization of partially purified lipase from *Saccharomyces cerevisiae*. *International Journal of Pharmacy and Pharmaceutical Sciences*, *6*, 514–517.

Kumar, K., Yadav, A. N., Kumar, V., Vyas, P., & Dhaliwal, H. S. (2017). Food waste: A potential bioresource for extraction of nutraceuticals and bioactive compounds. *Bioresources and Bioprocessing*, *4*, 18.

Lan, D., Qu, M., Yang, B., & Wang, Y. (2016). Enhancing production of lipase MAS1 from marine *Streptomyces* sp. strain in *Pichia pastoris* by chaperones co-expression. *Electronic Journal of Biotechnology*, *22*, 62–67.

Larik, I. A., Qazi, M. A., Phulpoto, A. H., Haleem, A., Ahmed, S., & Kanhar, N. A. (2019). *Stenotrophomonas maltophilia* strain 5DMD: An efficient biosurfactant-producing bacterium for biodegradation of diesel oil and used engine oil. *International Journal of Environmental Science and Technology*, *16*, 259–268.

Le, L. T. H. L., Yoo, W., Jeon, S., Lee, C., Kim, K. K., Lee, J. H., et al. (2020). Biodiesel and flavor compound production using a novel promiscuous cold-adapted SGNH-type lipase (HaSGNH1) from the psychrophilic bacterium *Halocynthiibacter arcticus*. *Biotechnology for Biofuels*, *13*, 55.

Lee, L. P., Karbul, H. M., Citartan, M., Gopinath, S. C., Lakshmipriya, T., & Tang, T. H. (2015). Lipase-secreting *Bacillus* species in an oil-contaminated habitat: Promising strains to alleviate oil pollution. *BioMed Research International*, 1–10.
Li, C. Y., Cheng, C. Y., & Chen, T. L. (2001). Production of *Acinetobacter radioresistens* lipase using Tween 80 as the carbon source. *Enzyme and Microbial Technology*, *29*, 258–263.
Liu, X., & Kokare, C. (2017). Microbial enzymes of use in industry. In *Biotechnology of Microbial Enzymes* (pp. 267–298). London: Academic Press.
Mateos-Díaz, E., Rodríguez, J. A., de los Ángeles Camacho-Ruiz, M., & Mateos-Díaz, J. C. (2012). High-throughput screening method for lipases/esterases. In *Lipases and Phospholipases* (pp. 89–100). Humana Press.
Melis, S., Pauly, A., Gerits, L. R., Pareyt, B., & Delcour, J. A. (2017). Lipases as processing aids in the separation of wheat flour into gluten and starch: Impact on the lipid population, gluten agglomeration, and yield. *Journal of Agricultural and Food Chemistry*, *65*, 1932–1940.
Memarpoor-Yazdi, M., Karbalaei-Heidari, H. R., & Doroodmand, M. M. (2018). Enantioselective hydrolysis of ibuprofen ethyl ester by a thermophilic immobilized lipase, ELT, from *Rhodothermus marinus*. *Biochemical Engineering Journal*, *130*, 55–65.
Memarpoor-Yazdi, M., Karbalaei-Heidari, H. R., & Khajeh, K. (2017). Production of the renewable extremophile lipase: Valuable biocatalyst with potential usage in food industry. *Food and Bioproducts Processing*, *102*, 153–166.
Messias, J. M., da Costa, B. Z., de Lima, V. M., Dekker, R. F., Rezende, M. I., Krieger, N., & Barbosa, A. M. (2009). Screening *Botryosphaeria* species for lipases: Production of lipase by *Botryosphaeria ribis* EC-01 grown on soybean oil and other carbon sources. *Enzyme and Microbial Technology*, *45*, 426–431.
Nguyen, H. H., Lee, S. H., Lee, U. J., Fermin, C. D., & Kim, M. (2019). Immobilized enzymes in biosensor applications. *Materials*, *12*, 121.
Nimkande, V. D., & Bafana, A. (2022). A review on the utility of microbial lipases in wastewater treatment. *Journal of Water Process Engineering*, *46*, 102591.
Niyonzima, F. N., & More, S. S. (2015). Microbial detergent compatible lipases. *Journal of Scientific and Industrial Research*, *74*, 105–113.
Özdemir, F. I., Tülek, A., & Erdoğan, D. (2021). Identification and heterologous production of a lipase from *Geobacillus kaustophilus* DSM 7263T and tailoring its N-terminal by a His-tag epitope. *Protein Journal*, *40*, 436–447.
Pasha, M. K., Dai, L., Liu, D., Du, W., & Guo, M. (2021). Biodiesel production with enzymatic technology: Progress and perspectives. *Biofuels, Bioproducts and Biorefining*, *15*, 1526–1548.
Pérez, M. M., Gonçalves, E. C., Vici, A. C., Salgado, J. C., & de Moraes Polizeli, M. D. (2019). Fungal lipases: Versatile tools for white biotechnology. In *Recent Advancement in White Biotechnology Through Fungi* (pp. 361–404). Cham: Springer.
Priyanka, P., Kinsella, G., Henehan, G. T., & Ryan, B. J. (2019). Isolation, purification and characterization of a novel solvent stable lipase from *Pseudomonas reinekei*. *Protein Expression and Purification*, *153*, 121–130.

Qian, J., Zhao, C., Ding, J., Chen, Y., & Guo, H. (2020). Preparation of nano-enzyme aggregates by crosslinking lipase with sodium tripolyphosphate. *Process Biochemistry*, *97*, 19–26.

Rahman, I. A., Rahman, R. N., Salleh, A. B., & Basri, M. (2013). Formulation and evaluation of an automatic dishwashing detergent containing T1 lipase. *Journal of Surfactants and Detergents*, *16*, 427–434.

Rajan, A., Kumar, D. S., & Nair, A. J. (2011). Isolation of a novel alkaline lipase producing fungus *Aspergillus fumigatus* MTCC 9657 from aged and crude rice bran oil and quantification by HPTLC. *International Journal of Biology and Chemistry*, *5*(11), 116–126.

Ray, A. (2012). Application of lipase in industry. *Asian Journal of Pharmaceutical Technology*, *2*, 33–37.

Rodriguez, J. A., Mateos, J. C., Nungaray, J., González, V., Bhagnagar, T., Roussos, S., Cordova, J., & Baratti, J. (2006). Improving lipase production by nutrient source modification using *Rhizopus homothallicus* cultured in solid state fermentation. *Process Biochemistry*, *41*, 2264–2269.

Romero, C. M., Pera, L. M., Loto, F., Vallejos, C., Castro, G., & Baigori, M. D. (2012). Purification of an organic solvent-tolerant lipase from *Aspergillus niger* MYA 135 and its application in ester synthesis. *Biocatalysis and Agricultural Biotechnology*, *1*(1), 25–31.

Sahoo, R. K., Sahu, A., & Subudhi, E. (2020). Bioremediation of hydrocarbon using bacterial lipase from waste biomass. *Iranian Journal of Science and Technology, Transactions A: Science*, *44*, 1287–1293.

Salihu, A., & Alam, M. Z. (2015). Solvent tolerant lipases: A review. *Process Biochemistry*, *50*, 86–96.

Salihu, A., Bala, M., & Alam, M. Z. (2016). Lipase production by *Aspergillus niger* using sheanut cake: An optimization study. *Journal of Taibah University for Science*, *10*, 850–859.

Samoylova, Y. V., Sorokina, K. N., Piligaev, A. V., & Parmon, V. N. (2018). Preparation of stable cross-linked enzyme aggregates (CLEAs) of a *Ureibacillus thermosphaericus* esterase for application in malathion removal from wastewater. *Catalysts*, *8*, 154–173.

Sandoval, G., Casas-Godoy, L., Bonet-Ragel, K., Rodrigues, J., Ferreira-Dias, S., & Valero, F. (2017). Enzyme catalyzed production of biodiesel as alternative to chemical-catalyzed processes: Advantages and constraints. *Current Biochemical Engineering*, *4*, 109–141.

Sankaran, R., Show, P. L., & Chang, J. S. (2016). Biodiesel production using immobilized lipase: Feasibility and challenges. *Biofuels, Bioproducts and Biorefining*, *10*, 896–916.

Saraswat, R., Verma, V., Sistla, S., & Bhushan, I. (2017). Evaluation of alkali and thermotolerant lipase from an indigenous isolated *Bacillus* strain for detergent formulation. *Electronic Journal of Biotechnology*, *30*, 33–38.

Sarmah, N., Revathi, D., Sheelu, G., Yamuna Rani, K., Sridhar, S., Mehtab, V., et al. (2018). Recent advances on sources and industrial applications of lipases. *Biotechnology Progress*, *34*, 5–28.

Sarmah, N., Revathi, G., Sheelu, G., Rani, Y. K., Sridhar, S., Mehtab, V., & Sumana, C. (2017). Recent advances on sources and industrial applications of lipases. *Biotechnology Progress*, *34*, 1.

Sawant, G., Ghosh, S., Banesh, S., Bhaumik, J., & Banerjee, U. C. (2016). *In silico* approach towards lipase mediated chemoenzymatic synthesis of (S)-ranolazine, as an anti-anginal drug. *RSC Advances*, *6*, 49150–49157.

Schaffarczyk, M., Østdal, H., & Koehler, P. (2014). Lipases in wheat breadmaking: Analysis and functional effects of lipid reaction products. *Journal of Agricultural and Food Chemistry*, *62*, 8229–8237.

Sethi, B. K., Rout, J. R., Das, R., Nanda, P. K., & Sahoo, S. L. (2013). Lipase production by *Aspergillus terreus* using mustard seed oil cake as a carbon source. *Annals of Microbiology*, *63*(1), 241–252.

Shalini, P., Deepanraj, B., Vijayalakshmi, S., & Ranjitha, J. (2021). Synthesis and characterization of lipase immobilized magnetic nanoparticles and its role as a catalyst in biodiesel production. *Materials Today: Proceedings*, *10*, 1016.

Sheldon, R. A. (2011). Cross-linked enzyme aggregates as industrial biocatalysts. *Organic Process Research & Development*, *15*, 213–223.

Shu, Z. Y., Yang, J. K., & Yan, Y. J. (2007). Purification and characterization of a lipase from *Aspergillus niger* F044. *Chinese Journal of Biotechnology*, *23*(1), 96–101.

Sikora, A., Chełminiak-Dudkiewicz, D., Ziegler-Borowska, M., & Marszałł, M. P. (2017). Enantioseparation of (RS)-atenolol with the use of lipases immobilized onto new-synthesized magnetic nanoparticles. *Tetrahedron: Asymmetry*, *28*, 374–380.

Sirisha, V. L., Jain, A., & Jain, A. (2016). Enzyme immobilization: An overview on methods, support material, and applications of immobilized enzymes. *Advances in Food and Nutrition Research*, *79*, 179–211.

Soares, J. L., Cammarota, M. C., Gutarra, M. L., & Volschan, I. (2019). Reduction of scum accumulation through the addition of low-cost enzymatic extract in the feeding of high-rate anaerobic reactor. *Water Science and Technology*, *80*, 67–74.

Sonawane, A., Manickam, P., & Bhansali, S. (2017). Stability of enzymatic biosensors for wearable applications. *IEEE Reviews in Biomedical Engineering*, *10*, 174–186.

Stauch, B., Fisher, S. J., & Cianci, M. (2015). Open and closed states of *Candida antarctica* lipase B: Protonation and the mechanism of interfacial activation. *Journal of Lipid Research*, *56*, 2348–2358.

Su, L., Hong, R., Guo, X., Wu, J., & Xia, Y. (2016). Short-chain aliphatic ester synthesis using *Thermobifida fusca* cutinase. *Food Chemistry*, *206*, 131–136.

Sun, H., Zhang, H., Ang, E. L., & Zhao, H. (2018). Biocatalysis for the synthesis of pharmaceuticals and pharmaceutical intermediates. *Bioorganic & Medicinal Chemistry*, *26*, 1275–1284.

Takó, M., Kotogán, A., Papp, T., Kadaikunnan, S., & Vágvölgyi, C. (2017). Purification and properties of extracellular lipases with transesterification activity and 1,3-regioselectivity from *Rhizomucor miehei* and *Rhizopus oryzae*. *Journal of Microbiology and Biotechnology*, *27*, 277–288.

Taskin, M., Ucar, M. H., Unver, Y., Kara, A. A., Ozdemir, M., & Ortucu, S. (2016). Lipase production with free and immobilized cells of cold-adapted yeast *Rhodotorula glutinis* HL25. *Biocatalysis and Agricultural Biotechnology*, *8*, 97–103.

Thapa, S., Li, H., O'Hair, J., Bhatti, S., Chen, F. C., Nasr, K. A., et al. (2019). Biochemical characteristics of microbial enzymes and their significance from industrial perspectives. *Molecular Biotechnology*, *61*, 579–601.

Turati, D. F. M., Almeida, A. F., Terrone, C. C., Nascimento, J. M., Terrasan, C. R., Fernandez-Lorente, G., & Carmona, E. C. (2019). Thermotolerant lipase from *Penicillium* sp. section *Gracilenta* CBMAI 1583: Effect of carbon sources on enzyme production, biochemical properties of crude and purified enzyme and substrate specificity. *Biocatalysis and Agricultural Biotechnology*, *17*, 15–24.

Unni, K. N., Priji, P., Sajith, S., Faisal, P. A., & Benjamin, S. (2016). *Pseudomonas aeruginosa* strain BUP2, a novel bacterium inhabiting the rumen of Malabari goat, produces an efficient lipase. *Biological (Bratislava)*, *71*, 378–387.

Xin, R., Khan, F. I., Zhao, Z., Zhang, Z., Yang, B., & Wang, Y. (2017). A comparative study on kinetics and substrate specificities of phospholipase A1 with *Thermomyces lanuginosus* lipase. *Journal of Colloid and Interface Science*, *488*, 149–154.

Xing, S., Zhu, R., Li, C., He, L., Zeng, X., & Zhang, Q. (2020). Gene cloning, expression, purification and characterization of a sn-1,3 extracellular lipase from *Aspergillus niger* GZUF36. *Journal of Food Science and Technology*, *57*, 2669–2680.

Yang, W., Cao, H., Xu, L., Zhang, H., & Yan, Y. (2015a). A novel eurythermic and thermostable lipase LipM from *Pseudomonas moraviensis* M9 and its application in the partial hydrolysis of algal oil. *BMC Biotechnology*, *15*, 94.

Yang, W., He, Y., Xu, L., Zhang, H., & Yan, Y. (2016). A new extracellular thermosolvent-stable lipase from *Burkholderia ubonensis* SL-4: Identification, characterization and application for biodiesel production. *Journal of Molecular Catalysis B: Enzymatic*, *126*, 76–89.

Zarevúcka, M. (2012). Olive oil as inductor of microbial lipase. In *Olive Oil—Constituents, Quality, Health Properties and Bioconversions* (pp. 457–470). InTech Europe, Rijeka, Croatia.

Zehani, N., Kherrat, R., Dzyadevych, S. V., & Jaffrezic-Renault, N. (2015). A micro conductometric biosensor based on lipase extracted from *Candida rugosa* for direct and rapid detection of organophosphate pesticides. *International Journal of Environmental Analytical Chemistry*, *95*, 466–479.

Zha, D., Xu, L., Zhang, H., & Yan, Y. (2014). Molecular identification of lipase LipA from *Pseudomonas protegens* Pf-5 and characterization of two whole-cell biocatalysts Pf-5 and Top10lipA. *Journal of Microbiology and Biotechnology*, *24*, 619.

Zhao, J., Liu, S., Gao, Y., Ma, M., Yan, X., Cheng, D., et al. (2021). Characterization of a novel lipase from *Bacillus licheniformis* NCU CS-5 for applications in detergent industry and biodegradation of 2,4-D butyl ester. *International Journal of Biological Macromolecules*, *176*, 126–136.

Zhou, J., Chen, W. W., Jia, Z. B., Huang, G. R., Hong, Y., Tao, J. J., & Luo, X. B. (2012). Purification and characterization of lipase produced by *Aspergillus oryzae* CJLU-31 isolated from waste cooking oily soil. *American Journal of Food Technology*, *7*(10), 596–608.

**CHAPTER 10**

# Microbial Production of Omega-3 Polyunsaturated Fatty Acids and Their Role in the Healthcare and Pharmaceutical Industry

PRITI PAL,[1] AKHILESH KUMAR SINGH,[2,*] BRIJESH PANDEY,[2]
ANAND PRAKASH,[2] PRAKASH KUMAR SARANGI,[3,*]
LAXUMAN SHARMA,[4] and RAJESH KUMAR SRIVASTAVA[5]

[1]*Amity Institute of Biotechnology, Amity University Uttar Pradesh, Lucknow Campus, Lucknow, India*

[2]*Department of Biotechnology, School of Life Sciences, Mahatma Gandhi Central University, Motihari, Bihar, India*

[3]*College of Agriculture, Central Agricultural University, Imphal, Manipur, India*

[4]*Department of Horticulture, Sikkim University, Gangtok, Sikkim, India*

[5]*Department of Biotechnology, School of Core Engineering, GITAM (Deemed to be University), Visakhapatnam, Andhra Pradesh, India*

*Corresponding author

## ABSTRACT

Microorganisms offer a sustainable alternative to fish for producing omega-3 fatty acids. They can grow in both autotrophic and heterotrophic modes, but heterotrophic microorganisms are preferred due to easier fermentation optimization and higher yields. Omega-3 polyunsaturated fatty acids (PUFAs), especially docosahexaenoic acid (DHA) and

Industrial Biotechnology: Current Progress and Novel Technologies.
Prakash Kumar Sarangi, Akhilesh Kumar Singh, Rajesh Kumar Srivastava, and Brijesh Pandey (Eds.)


DOI: 10.1201/9781779642233-10

eicosapentaenoic acid (EPA), have gained global attention for their essential roles in human health and nutrition, as well as concerns over declining marine sources. Microbial cell factories—including microalgae, thraustochytrids, fungi, and yeasts—are capable of synthesizing a wide range of fatty acids, from short-chain (C6) to long-chain (C36), encompassing saturated (SFA), monounsaturated (MUFA), and polyunsaturated (PUFA) types. Depending on their fatty acid composition, microbial oils serve as nutraceutical ingredients or as feedstocks for biodiesel production. Their ability to produce very long-chain omega-3 PUFAs makes them highly valuable for aquafeed, functional foods, and pharmaceutical applications. This chapter provides a critical overview of microbial sources of omega-3 PUFAs, their nutritional significance, commercial exploitation, and diverse applications. It highlights the growing importance of microbial production systems in meeting global omega-3 demands sustainably.

## 10.1 INTRODUCTION

Multiple double bonds are found in fatty acids, which are known as polyunsaturated fatty acids (PUFAs). They are divided into four families based on the position of the first double bond closest to the terminal methyl group: the omega-3 family, which is derived from α-linolenic acid (ALA, 18:3n-3), the omega-6 family, which is derived from linoleic acid (LA, 18:2n-6), the omega-7 family, which is derived from palmitoleic acid (PA, 16:1n-7), and the omega-9 family, which is derived from linoleic acid (OA, 18:1n-9). The only essential fatty acids (EFA) for humans are LA and ALA (Nagy and Tiuca, 2017). The maintenance of human health requires a variety of PUFAs, particularly those from the omega-6 and omega-3 families. Dihomo-γ-linolenic acid (DGLA), arachidonic acid (AA), and eicosapentaenoic acid (EPA) are the precursors of several eicosanoids, including prostaglandins, leukotrienes, and lipoxins, which are highly significant for the regular operation of many systems (Philpott et al., 2018). Osteoporosis, Alzheimer's disease (AD), Parkinson's disease, chronic inflammatory disease, and atherosclerosis can all be prevented or treated with omega-3 PUFAs, especially EPA and docosahexaenoic acid (DHA) (Dourou et al., 2018a). Omega-3 PUFAs have been used as dietary supplements for pregnant women and as components in infant formula food because they have positive effects on brain development during pregnancy and early life stages. More oil rich in omega-3 PUFAs is required due to the expanding markets for food, pharmaceuticals, personal care items, and nutritional supplements (Zárate et al., 2017). However, fish oil, the primary source of EPA and DHA, has seen a sharp decline in both quality and quantity Therefore, the enrichment of EPA and DHA in fish oil has been the subject of numerous studies. Fractional distillation, urea complexation, fractional crystallization, supercritical fluid extraction chromatography, metal ion extraction, and lipase catalysis are just a few of the methods that have been employed (Bellou et al., 2016). Lipase catalysis has been a promising technique among the enrichment methods because the enzymatic method is gentler and greener and can minimize oxidation, polymerization, and cis-trans isomerization of oil-containing PUFAs. Many research studies on the anti-cancer properties of GLA and EPA have demonstrated that amphiphilic preparations of these fatty acids make cancer cell lines like HL-60 and MCF-7 toxic to them (Sayegh et al., 2016). The main commercial source of omega-3 PUFAs is fish. Fish oil production does have some disadvantages, though, such as the risk of fish population extinction brought on by overfishing and the potential for contaminants like heavy metals to be present (Ryckebosch et al., 2012). The most reliable alternative method for producing omega-3 PUFAs is probably microorganisms. The primary producers of PUFAs are fungi and microalgae, while oleaginous yeasts can only produce omega-3 PUFAs after undergoing genetic modification (Bellou et al., 2016). Seasonal and climatic changes have no bearing on the production of microbial omega-3 PUFAs, which also don't need arable land. Additionally, microorganisms can produce oils of a high purity while growing at rapid rates in a variety of inexpensive substrates. Single-cell oil (SCO) production is inhibited by high production costs, which are partly due to high fermentation costs (Dourou et al., 2018a). One solution to this problem is to combine the production of SCO with other biotechnological applications, such as the biotreatment of various wastes and/or byproducts. Increased omega-3 PUFAs production has been advocated for using naturally occurring microbes, metabolically enhanced mutants derived from them, and strains based on popular microbial workhorses with heterologous expressed omega-3 PUFAs genes and pathways, among other approaches. When many microbial cell factories grow under heterotrophic conditions in the absence of light, it is advantageous to generate high-cell-density cultures on a large scale. In addition to single-cell production, recent attempts (not covered here) have also attempted omega-3 PUFAs overproduction in genetically modified (GM) fish and crops (Athenaki et al., 2018). There is no doubt that the industry has given biotechnological omega-3 PUFAs production a lot of attention. When compared to omega-3 PUFAs-enriched oils, meals, and other formulations, which are sold as food and feed supplements, purified omega-3 PUFAs are more expensive as the active ingredients in pharmaceuticals and medical treatments (Daskalaki et al., 2019). The focus of the current review is on the primary omega-3 PUFAs-producing microorganisms (fungi and microalgae), as well as recent initiatives to produce SCOs rich in omega-3 PUFAs from microorganisms grown on various kinds of organic residues.

## 10.2 OMEGA-3 FATTY ACID PRODUCTION BY MICROORGANISMS

Therefore, a more efficient, quicker, and environmentally friendly source of omega-3 PUFAs is required. Therefore, these strategies would require the industrial extraction of omega-3 PUFAs and essential microbial oils from microalgae and other potential microorganisms. These microbial oils are also referred to as single-cell oils because they are produced by single-celled microorganisms (SCOs) (Ratledgea, 2013). Ochsenreither et al. (2016) claim that SCOs are intracellular storage lipids that comprise 20–80% of dry biomass at the start of the stationary phase and rise when the organisms are grown at lower temperatures, which promotes the process of fatty acid synthesis.

The omega-3 PUFAs synthesis takes place in nutrient-limited situations (such as those lacking in nitrogen or phosphorus) under a constant supply of acetyl-CoA and NADPH, but preferably with a high amount of carbon sources to maintain the microorganism's constant growth rate (Ochsenreither et al., 2016). In nutrient-limited conditions, a series of enzymes are activated that contribute to citrate accumulation in the mitochondria and, ultimately, to the continual production of Acetyl-CoA in microorganisms. Studies indicate that oleaginous microorganisms are known to catalyze the oxidative decarboxylation of isocitrate by the action of AMP (adenosine monophosphate)-dependent isocitrate dehydrogenase enzyme, in contrast to many non-oleaginous microorganisms. This is a crucial stage in the TCA cycle that produces citrate. However, under nitrogen deficiency conditions, AMP deaminase is active and catalyzes the breakdown of AMP into IMP (inosine monophosphate/inosinic acid) and ammonia, which lowers the amount of AMP in the mitochondria. As a result, the aconitase enzyme that is involved in converting isocitrate into citrate is suppressed. This enables the transport of citrate into the cytosol, where it is cleaved into acetyl-CoA by ATP-citrate lyase. This continuous production of acetyl-CoA, combined with NADPH (possibly recovered by the pentose phosphate pathway), results in increased lipid accumulation. Elongation and desaturation reactions, which are triggered by the activity of the enzymes elongase and desaturase, respectively, are necessary for the production of EFAs like EPA and DHA shown in Table 10.1. Stearic and palmitic acid are produced as a result of these processes in the majority of organisms (Ochsenreither et al., 2016).

## 10.3 NATURAL ORGANISMS FOR ADVANCED PRODUCTION

### *10.3.1 MICROALGAE*

Microalgae are notable for their capacity to store significantly more PUFAs in neutral triacyl glycerides and cell membrane lipids (TAGs). *Schizochytrium*, *Aurantiochytrium*, and *Thraustochytrium* are unicellular thraustochytrids that contain significant amounts of DHA (Chen et al., 2020). Despite still being referred to as microalgae, these microbes only function as saprophytic decomposers in the marine environment (Khozin-Goldberg et al., 2016). EPA is primarily produced by photosynthetic microalgae, including *Phaeodactylum tricornutum* (Hamilton et al., 2016), *Nannochloropsis oceanica* (Sirisuk et al., 2018), and *Dunaliella salina* (Diao et al., 2020). Another species, primarily stored LA and ALA (Norashikin et al., 2018), is the green alga *Chlorella vulgaris*. They are recognized as a reliable source of essential oils and a renewable resource for the production of biofuels. Microalgae use both organic and inorganic carbon sources as substrates by using a variety of growth techniques, such as phototrophic (using carbon dioxide as a carbon source and sunlight as a source of energy), heterotrophic (using organic carbon sources), and mixotrophic cultivation. Both organic and inorganic carbon sources are used in photosynthesis. Numerous factors, such as light intensity, temperature, pH, dissolved oxygen levels, nutrient concentration, and the presence of carbon dioxide, affect the microalgae's rate of cellular growth and lipid accumulation (Bajpai and Bajpai, 1993). Therefore, to achieve

**TABLE 10.1** Various microbial species with their EPA and DHA concentrations

| Microorganisms | Substrate | DHA Concentration (%Total lipid) | EPA Concentration (% Total Lipid) | References |
|---|---|---|---|---|
| *Aurantiochytrium* sp. KRS101 | Modified basal medium glucose (60 g/L) | 19.88 | – | Hong et al. (2011) |
| *Aurantiochytrium* 4W-1b | Glucose (30 g/L) | 27.9 | – | Nakazawa et al. (2012) |
| *Alexandrium sanguinea*<br>*Chlorella ellipsoidea*<br>*Chlamydomonas* sp. | Photoautotrophic<br>Photoautotrophic<br>Photoautotrophic | 23.8<br>3.1<br>3.2 | 20.1<br>34.6<br>19.7 | Suh et al. (2015) |
| *Mortierella Alpina* ST1358* | GY medium (2% (*w/v*) glucose and 1% yeast extract) | – | 26.4 | Okuda et al. (2015) |
| *Aurantiochytrium* sp. ATCC PRA-276 | Glucose (30 g/L) | 12.5 | – | Furlan et al. (2017) |
| *Aurantiochytrium* sp. KRS101 | Orange peel extract glucose (5.9 g/L), fructose (5.6 g/L), organic acids | 14.31 | – | Park et al. (2018) |
| *Aurantiochytrium* SW1 | Fructose (70 g/L) | 25 | – | Nazir et al. (2018) |
| *Aurantiochytrium* sp. ATCC PRA-276 | Organosolv-pretreated birch hydrolysate (30 g/L glucose) | 35.76 | – | Patel et al. (2019) |
| *P. tricornutum* | Autotrophic<br>Mixotrophic, Glucose (2 g/L)<br>Mixotrophic, Birch hydrolysates<br>Mixotrophic, Spruce hydrolysates | 1.65<br>3.56<br>4.32<br>4.89 | 13.43<br>18.38<br>19.80<br>19.87 | Patel et al. (2019) |
| *Schizochytrium limacinum* SR21 | Organosolv-pretreated spruce hydrolysate (60 g/L glucose) | 66.72 | – | Patel et al. (2020) |

EPA, Eicosapentaenoic acid; DHA, Docosahexaenoic acid.

maximum productivity from the cultivation of each microalgal species, it is crucial to understand the ideal conditions for each species. Several enzymatic reactions that occur in the microalgae's ER and chloroplasts, respectively, result in the synthesis of TAGs and the assembly of glycolipids. In response to physical, chemical, and environmental stresses, it is thought that large amounts of lipids (particularly neutral lipids in the form of TAGs/oil bodies), which could be used as carbon and energy storage necessary for its survival, are produced (Patel et al., 2020). Microalgae are essential for the production of omega-3 PUFAs by oleaginous microbes (such as *Thraustochytrids*, *Schizochytrium*). The omega-3 PUFAs-rich edible oils produced by these microorganisms are thought to be superior to those produced by more conventional means. This includes the ease of cultivation, assuming no particular environmental conditions are needed for the process; the availability of specific enzymes that improve lipid accumulation; and the presence of antioxidants, such as carotenoids or tocopherols, which stop omega-3 PUFAs from auto-oxidation and lengthen the shelf-life of the substance (Patel et al., 2020). Increased omega-3 PUFAs production by microalgae may be achieved by altering culture conditions, such as lighting, photoperiod, temperature, pH, salinity, agitation speed, and carbon and nitrogen concentrations (Yin et al., 2019a), manipulating oxidative stress (Ren et al., 2017b), subjecting the organism to environmental stresses (such as nitrogen starvation and high salinity), or using adaptive evolution with high oxygen as a selection pressure (Sun et al., 2016). Additionally, genetic engineering has been used to improve lipid accumulation capacity and/or omega-3 PUFAs content. The long-chain fatty acid elongase genes of *Thalassiosira pseudonana* (Cook and Hildebrand, 2016) were overexpressed, as were the malic enzyme on *Phaeodactylum tricornutum* (Xue et al., 2015), and *Nannochloropsis*'s genome was edited using CRISPR/Cas9 technology (Wang et al., 2016). Eutrophic lakes in particular experience changes in many environmental factors, such as nutrient deficiency, salinity, temperature, light, UV rays, and others because of the growth-restraining stresses brought on by overcrowding (algal bloom formation) and an increase in organic matter. As a result, competition for food, light, and other vital resources for survival then develops. Thus, omega-3 PUFAs and other lipids can be easily extracted by altering the growth conditions of these microalgae. Some of the organisms that can produce omega-3 PUFAs include *Nannochloropsis* sp., *Dunaliella* sp. (by modifying temperature, salinity, and light intensity),

*Pavlova lutheri* (by lowering temperature), and *Crythecodinium cohnii* ATCC 30556. It was found that the DHA content of the total fatty acids increased by 569% when grown in 9 g l. Additionally, studies show that lipid peroxidation is found to boost the generation of omega-3 PUFAs and that changes in growth conditions may occasionally result in the production of ROS (Xie et al., 2017).

Several other methods could help to extract omega-3 PUFAs from organisms in addition to applying external stress conditions, possibly even resulting in a higher yield of the required substance. Mechanistic engineering of metabolism is one such strategy. Numerous organisms have been identified as having genes encoding crucial enzymes required for the biosynthesis of fatty acids, including the model organism *Chlamydomonas reinhardtii*, *P. tricornutum*, *Ostreococcus tauri*, and *Thalassiosira pseudonana*. With the aid of inducible promoters, it is possible to increase the production of EPA and DHA by overexpressing some of the most important omega-3 PUFAs-producing enzymes, such as desaturases and elongases. This is made possible by metabolically engineering a few specific strains that can accumulate a remarkable amount of lipids. Typically, long-chain omega-3 PUFAs with high TAG content are chosen for this purpose.

### 10.3.2 YEAST AND MOLDS

Yeasts with the capacity to grow in high cell densities can produce high lipid content on a variety of carbon sources (such as lignocellulose substrates). Lipids, which account for 20% of their dry cell biomass, are typically said to be present in them. This can be increased by up to 70% when grown in nutrient-limited conditions (for example, nitrogen or phosphorous) (Thevenieau and Nicaud, 2013), making industrial production possible. This typically occurs when a crucial nutrient other than the carbon source is removed. One such nutrient is nitrogen, which is crucial for the synthesis of many proteins and nucleic acids, causing the organisms to be forced to accumulate a lot of lipids. This affects the organism's C/N ratio, which affects its growth rate. It is discovered that this growth rate is slower than the rate of lipid accumulation as a result (Thevenieau and Nicaud, 2013). Filamentous fungi can be grown on a variety of affordable feedstock, including sewage sludge, glycerol, water molasses, and agricultural waste, making them a reliable source of biofuel production (Patel et al., 2020). The EFAs, including AA (α-linolenic acid), GLA, EPA, and DHA, are said to be synthesized by them (Thevenieau and Nicaud, 2013). Even though it has been reported that some eukaryotic fungi produce high levels of omega-3 PUFAs, to achieve optimized fatty acid profiles and a higher yield of the lipids on a larger scale, more research is needed to fully understand the intricate mechanisms and various production techniques. Dimorphic yeasts and fungi, such as *Yarrowia lipolytica*, *Mortierella alpina*, and *Mucor circinelloides*, have defense mechanisms that are already present to protect them from the negative effects of omega-3 PUFAs biosynthesis and their highly effective lipid metabolism. It follows that the fact that these microbes are among the top omega-3 PUFAs producers in the world is not surprising. Even better, the number of producers keeps expanding. For instance, recent research on oleaginous yeasts such as *Ashbya gossypii* (Ledesma-Amaro et al., 2018), *Rhodosporidium toruloides* (Arbter et al., 2019), and others has shown promising potential.

### 10.3.3 FUNGI

Numerous fungi from the phylum Mucoromycete (previously categorized as Zygomycota; Spatafora et al., 2016) are known to accumulate significant amounts of storage lipids rich in omega-3 PUFAs when grown in nitrogen-limited environments. These organisms, which have 6 and 5 desaturases, can add numerous double bonds to the acyl chains of membrane phospholipids that are positioned beta for esterification (Bellou et al., 2016). Respective yeast species can build up significant amounts of storage lipids, but they are unable to synthesize omega-3 PUFAs because they lack the aforementioned membrane-bound desaturases. Fatty acids with more than one double bond, such as LA and ALA, are not of commercial importance because they are prevalent in plants and fungi and can be generated by some yeast species (Klug and Daum, 2014). However, filamentous fungi are not as well suited for industrial applications as oleaginous yeasts, which is why they are used in the omega-3 PUFAs manufacturing phase after genetic modification. Yeasts from the *Candida*, *Yarrowia*, *Rhodosporidium*, *Cryptococcus*, and *Lipomyces* genera could be genetically altered to produce omega-3 PUFAs (Qin et al., 2017). On an industrial scale, GLA, EPA, and DHA are produced using strains of the well-studied oleaginous yeast *Y. lipolytica* that have already undergone genetic engineering (Xie et al., 2015). Multiple copies of various chimeric genes were put together from different omega-3 PUFAs producing organisms, and *Y. lipolytica* was further altered by losing its fatty acid degradation pathway. Around 41 copies of 19 different genes were present in the engineered strain (Xie et al., 2015). In the near future, adaptive laboratory evolution techniques can be used to improve *Y. lipolytica*'s capacity for lipid accumulation (Daskalaki et al., 2019). Several strains of *Cunninghamella echinulata*, *Mucor circinelloides*, *Umbellopsis isabellina*, *Umbellopsis ramanniana*, *Thamnidium elegans*, and *Zygorhynchus moelleri* produce GLA, with *M. circinelloides* having the ability to synthesize GLA at a percentage of 25% weight or more, in total lipids. Although *Umbellopsis isabellina* can accumulate large amounts of lipids, these lipids only contain GLA in small amounts (Papanikolaou and Aggelis, 2019). *Mortierella alpina* strains are renowned for their ability to synthesize AA up to 44% of the total lipids and EPA at significant percentages when grown at lower temperatures (Kikukawa et al., 2018). EPA can also be made from the lipids of Pythium species, formerly thought of as fungi (Liang et al., 2012). Except for the heterotrophic, fungoid-like marine protists known as Thraustochytrids, fungi cannot synthesize DHA (Marchan et al., 2018). DHA makes up to 80% of the total lipids in thraustochytrids like *Thraustochytrium* sp., *Schizochytrium* sp., and *Labyrinthula* sp. (Li et al., 2015).

### 10.3.4 BACTERIAL SPECIES AS PATHWAY DONORS DESPITE LIMITED OMEGA-3 PUFA PRODUCTION

Certain bacteria synthesize omega-3 PUFAs without oxygen. Similar to this, various cyanobacteria produce a range of omega-3 PUFAs (Poole et al., 2020). Recent advancements include the discovery of new species and early attempts to boost omega-3 PUFAs production, which, it must be said, are still in the proof-of-concept stage. *Colwellia* strains can make up to 17% of TFAs (DHA) (Kusube et al., 2017). *Cerulenin*, a FAS inhibitor, increased the levels of DHA in *Colwellia psychrerythraea* 34H (Wan et al., 2016). *Shewanella* sp., a different deep-sea bacterium, accumulated enough EPA to be responsible for up to 36% of TFAs (Zhang and Burgess, 2017). *Cerulenin* increased EPA generation in *Shewanella electrodiphila* MAR441, and chemical mutagenesis increased efficiency at low temperatures (Zhang and Burgess, 2017). The ability to produce EPA varied among genetically closely related *Vibrio* spp. strains, showing that the gene cluster was spread by horizontal gene transfer (Estupinan et al., 2020).

Since there have not been many studies in recent years, it's possible that other marine psychrophiles that have previously been reported to naturally accumulate high levels of omega-3 PUFAs have not undergone any further development (Moi et al., 2018). All significant omega-3 PUFAs in terrestrial myxobacteria were produced by *Arthrobacter* species (Garcia et al., 2016), whereas *Sorangium cellulosum* only produced LA (Yoshida et al., 2016), and *Phaselicystis flava* was enriched in ARA (Garcia et al., 2009).

## 10.4 BIOSYNTHETIC PATHWAY FOR THE PRODUCTION OF OMEGA—3FAS: ALA, EPA, DHA

The majority of living things do not naturally produce omega-3 PUFAs (Kabeya et al., 2018). For the cell membrane to remain fluid and respond to stresses, such as temperature, UV light, and osmotic pressure, omega-3 PUFAs incorporation is essential (Adarme-Vega et al., 2012). Omega-3 PUFAs have a high degree of unsaturation, which makes them easily oxidized. This peroxidation is undesirable because it lowers product titer and produces ROS, which severely oxidize the cells that produce it (Morabito et al., 2019). Through a series of reactions involving the catalytic enzymes desaturases and elongates (alpha-linolenic) ALA is converted into DHA and EPA (Li et al., 2018). The two main pathways that the sequential steps evolved through are referred to as the aerobic pathway and involve desaturase and elongates, respectively. In bacteria, the latter pathway, known as the anaerobic pathway, polyketide synthase (PKS) enzymes are involved. The percentage purity/yield of specific microalgal by-products purified using different purification methods, such as acid digestion, Soxhlet extraction, urea, and saponification, are displayed (Diao et al., 2018). The HPLC method was used to determine the omega-3 PUFAs' purity, and the results showed that EPA and DHA were 95% and 99% pure, respectively (Liu et al., 2018).

## 10.5 DESATURATION AND ELONGATION REACTIONS IN ALTERNATION DURING THE BIOSYNTHESIS OF AEROBIC OMEGA-3 PUFAS

The aerobic omega-3 PUFAs biosynthetic pathway is found in all eukaryotic organisms, including animals, some plants, and bacteria (at least in part) (Qiu et al., 2020). The final category is quite varied and consists of PUFAs ALA and LA, different kinds of 16-carbon fatty acids, and dimorphic fungi (Khan et al., 2019). Desaturases and elongates work in tandem to lengthen and modify the backbones of ALA and LA, producing the omega-3 derivatives EPA and DHA (for ALA) and the omega-6 derivative ARA (for LA) (Li-Beisson et al., 2019). There are alternate pathways for the first two conversions: the D6 pathway (Mao et al., 2017) and the alternate D8 pathway (Monroig and Kabeya, 2018). The inability of mammalian cells to incorporate double bonds into the v3 and v6 positions on the fatty acid backbone prevents them from producing LA and ALA. From that point on in the pathway, they have all the enzymes required to produce longer and more unsaturated omega-3 PUFAs, including DHA, EPA, and ARA. However, this ability is extremely limited in humans and is deemed insufficient from a medical perspective (Kabeya et al., 2018). Even high dietary ALA intake does not affect plasma DHA, and dietary LA has little impact on plasma ARA (Plourde and Cunnane, 2007).

## 10.6 ANAEROBIC OMEGA-3 PUFAS BIOSYNTHESIS USING POLYKETIDE SYNTHASES-LIKE ENZYMES

The common aerobic pathway has long been thought to be the mechanism by which marine bacteria synthesize EPA and DHA, even though this has been known since the 1980s. Therefore, the efforts to clone the genes responsible for EPA biosynthesis (Yazawa, 1996) and the subsequent identification of a novel anaerobic pathway for the synthesis of omega-3 PUFAs in bacteria (Metz et al., 2001) were major achievements in omega-3 PUFAs research. The aerobic pathway and the anaerobic route are fundamentally dissimilar. It does not interact with FAS but instead creates omega-3 PUFAs from scratch using an enzyme complex resembling polyketide synthase, a PUFA synthase. Condensation, dehydration, and keto-reduction occur repeatedly along the pathway (Harwood, 2019), and a tiny regulator known as the chain length factor (Hayashi et al., 2020) also controls length. It has been found that bacteria (Gemperlein et al., 2018) and unicellular microalgae (Allemann and Allen, 2018) can synthesize anaerobic omega-3 PUFAs. It has an advantage over the aerobic method for producing excess omega-3 PUFAs because it uses almost 50% less NAD(P)H (Gemperlein et al., 2019). The pfa gene clusters encode the various domains of PUFA synthase. These groups typically contain three to five genes, such as *pfa123* in *Schizochytrium* species and myxobacteria (Garcia et al., 2016) and *pfaABCDE* in *Shewanella* species (Hayashi et al., 2020).

## 10.7 MICROBIAL CULTURE AND PRODUCTION

Numerous bioactive molecules are thought to receive some of their nutrition from microorganisms. Microbe cultivation can occasionally be challenging to attempt for commercial production. It is influenced by many factors, including the culture chosen, the type of bioreactors used, pH, light, temperature, water, dietary needs, and energy sources. The best selection of strains and the appropriate culture medium serve as crucial feed-stock for channeling microbial production for industrial acceptance to overcome the drawbacks.

## 10.8 STRATEGIES FOR ENHANCING PRODUCTION OF OMEGA-3 FATTY ACIDS

Salinity, temperature, pH, nutrients, type of species and duration of intense light, and others all have an impact on the production of omega-3 PUFAs by microbes. Omega-3 PUFAs are primarily produced by phytoplankton and algae and are passed along the food chain to marine fishes. Micro-algae can quickly adapt to changing environmental conditions such as light, temperature, salinity, pH, nutrients, and culture duration due to their metabolic plasticity, which influences both growth and the biochemical makeup of the algae's lipid content (Pal et al., 2011). Therefore, specific abiotic stress exposures could be used as a powerful tool to trigger a metabolic reorientation and boost the production of particular bioactive substances, like the long-chain PUFAs (Tatsuzawa and Takizawa, 1995). The production of omega-3 PUFAs and lipid is increased when two micro-algae, *Chlorella vulgaris* (a freshwater microalga) and *D. salina* (a halo-tolerant microalga), are repeatedly exposed to varying intensities of salt stress. However, *C. vulgaris* produces fewer omega-3 PUFAs and lipids than *D. salina* because it lacks the cell wall, which is thought to be crucial for lipid extraction and omega-3 formation under salt stress (Rismani and Shariati, 2017). When the temperature was lowered to up to 15°C,

*Pavlova Lutheri* revealed an elevated EPA amount of 30.3%. Similar to this, *P. cornutum*'s increased EPA content indicated a temperature change of 12 hours from 25°C to 10°C (Paliwal et al., 2017). With the cultivation of *C. cohnii* algae in sodium chloride (9000 mg/l), increasing total DHA amount to 56.9% of total fatty acids, an increase in omega-3 PUFAs level as fatty acids was anticipated. Omega-3 PUFAs have good flow behavior and were traditionally used in the cell membrane in regulating fluidity at low temperatures. The production of peroxides and ROS can also be explained by the increase in omega-3 PUFAs content (Singh et al., 2018). In comparison to *Chlorella* sp., which showed an increased lipid content under low light conditions, *P. Consortium's* EPA content increased up to 19.84% under UV stress. As a result, altering abiotic stress is a crucial tool for raising the content of lipids and fatty acids in different microalgae (Adarme-Vega et al., 2012).

## 10.9 FERMENTATION BIOTECHNOLOGY RESPONSIBLE FOR INCREASING PRODUCTION OF OMEGA-3 PUFAS

Bioactive compounds are formed using the fermentation process during the sequential steps of culture, harvesting, lipid extraction, byproduct formation, and the production of omega-3 PUFAs in microbes, as shown in Figure 10.1. Producing food items enriched in omega-3 PUFAs is sustainable, safe, and economical due to the abundance of omega-3 PUFAs and their health benefits. Since they contain a double bond, which makes them chemically unstable and susceptible to oxidation, it is necessary to formulate omega-3 PUFAs through a fermentation process to increase the product yield. One such instance is the production of ALA and GLA from omega-3 PUFAs by filamentous fungi (Kikukawa et al., 2018). Time restrictions are a problem with this process. Thus, the repeated fed fermentation method increases the productivity of omega-3 PUFAs, which are then further balanced by agitation and aeration rate. *Mortierella alpine* is another example of a fungus that produces ARA; by simply altering the fermentation process, the dry cell weight, lipid content, and percentage yield of ARA were increased by 14.8%, 25.8%, and 7.8%, respectively. The productivity of non-filamentous fungi EPA and DHA were increased by using kinetic modeling in conjunction with a multistage continuous fermentation technique. In EPA-producing *Y. lipolytica*, the two-stage fermentation process increases EPA productivity by 8% and EPA concentration by 40%. In real-time analysis, the omega-3 PUFAs fermentation process is a useful tool for determining oxygen uptake, $CO_2$ evolution, and ROS (Zhao and Qiu, 2019).

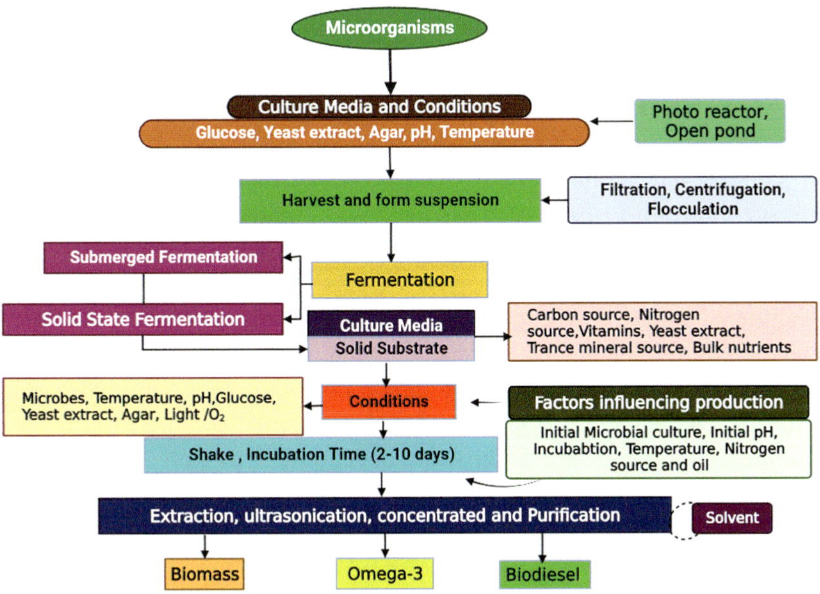


**FIGURE 10.1** The fermentation process used to produce omega-3 fatty acids from microorganisms is shown schematically.

## 10.10 OMEGA-3 FATTY ACID PRODUCTION FOR COMMERCIAL PURPOSES

In open ponds, hybrid systems, photo-bioreactors, or even raceways/flow-through systems, the procedure should first be used to successfully increase the micro-algal cellular density for large-scale production. The algal cells are completely separated from the media by simple procedures like centrifugation, filtration, or flocculation. For better lipid extraction using organic solvents (typically "hexane"), they are further dried. Other techniques for enriching omega-3 PUFAs include PUFA transformation (esterification of PUFA), supercritical fluid extraction (fractionation in supercritical $CO_2$), urea complexation (fatty acid solubilization with the addition of urea and ethanol under the application of heat), vacuum-based/

temperature-based molecular/fraction distillation, and winterization (reduction in temperature). Additionally, by further processing the micro-algal products, this process has been crucial in the production of biodiesel, biochar, high-value bioactive compounds, and non-natural esters, which are all used in many pharmaceutical and nutraceutical products.

Diatoms, specifically *P. tricornutum*, are a significant source of omega-3 PUFAs production. Because *P. tricornutum* is not a naturally abundant producer of EPA and DHA, metabolic engineering is used to make it industrially relevant by over-expressing heterologous genes encoding enzymes involved in the synthesis of omega-3 PUFAs. This was shown by contrasting the amounts of DHA produced by the wild type and the transgenic strain Pt Elo5 of *P. tricornutum* (Tocher et al., 2019). Studies have also suggested that a *P. tricornutum* strain with altered metabolism makes a huge amount of omega-3 PUFAs. This organism was chosen because of its genome sequencing, capacity to produce high-value lipids, and quick growth cycle.

For the fermentation-based production of omega-3 PUFAs, the metabolically engineered *Y. lipolytica* strain is regarded as a trustworthy and commercially secure strain (for strain development as well as commercial production). For use in industrial food processing, this organism is regarded as GRAS. Additionally, it has been used to produce single cells quickly and inexpensively. It produces both AA and LA. However, to meet commercial demands, they are genetically altered by increasing the copy number of the genes that code for the enzymes that catalyze their biosynthesis (AA). The fermentation procedure used here employs a two-stage fed-batch method to boost the production of both biomass and EPA. Both nitrogen and carbohydrate sources are present in the first stage, which is referred to as the "growth phase," but these sources are scarce in the second stage, which is referred to as the "production phase," which metabolically promotes a significant buildup of EPA-rich lipids. It helps to produce better results to test this technique in various ways. It is well known that this process yields wholesome EPA that can be synthetically altered and tailored to any desired composition. By using GC analysis, further quantification is accomplished. This can be used as a crucial source of omega-3 PUFAs that finds use in a variety of contexts, including functional and infant foods, dietary supplements, animal feeds, and the pharmaceutical industry. This biotechnological approach assists in the synthesis of novel sustainable products to replace conventional non-sustainable sources.

## 10.11 MICROBIAL OMEGA-3 FATTY ACID APPLICATIONS

### 10.11.1 THERAPEUTIC IMPORTANCE

Omega-3 PUFAs are essential to humans in many ways, but their pathological effects, which impact human health conditions and slow the progression of some diseases, are particularly significant. They are known to play a major role in the prevention of a variety of diseases, and their anti-arrhythmic, anti-inflammatory, anti-thrombotic, anti-atherosclerotic, anti-fibrotic, and endothelial relaxation characteristics do indeed work to their benefit, especially in the case of cardiovascular dysfunctions (CVDs).

Omega-3 PUFAs are thought to be crucially significant for mental well-being and have a range of therapeutic advantages, especially when given along with antidepressant therapy. This is because it monitors depression when there are high levels of omega-3 PUFAs in the blood. Additionally, there is a link between the levels of omega-3 PUFAs in the body and the rates of homicide and mental disorders (Radcliffe et al., 2016).

Studies show that giving omega-3 PUFA-rich supplements to young children with attention deficit hyperactivity disorder (ADHD) or any other related developmental disorders results in appreciable improvements. According to Messamore and McNamara (2016), serious problems like bipolar disorder, schizophrenia, and other psychiatric illnesses have been linked to low EPA and DHA levels in erythrocytes. Any area of the body benefits physiologically from omega-3 PUFAs that are inflammatory, including those related to psoriasis, migraine, lupus erythematosus, diabetes, atherosclerosis, hypertriglyceridemia, and high blood pressure (Bajpai and Bajpai, 1993).

### 10.11.2 FETAL DEVELOPMENT

Due to recent research, omega-3 PUFAs have also taken center stage in the maternal diet, which has always been centered on being highly nutrient-dense, with adequate protein and calorie intake. This is because omega-3 PUFAs have numerous advantages for the development of the fetus. Pregnant or nursing women are advised to consume 8 to 12 ounces of seafood per week, which is equivalent to 300 to 900 mg of EPA and DHA daily, an essential component of the daily recommended intake of nutrients. The fetal brain and eye are effectively developed as a result. In addition, EPA and DHA both focus on preventing preterm birth, which is the primary cause of numerous infant casualties. They do this by inhibiting the activity of certain prostaglandins, such as PTLA2 and PTLF2a, which helps prolong the gestation period by reducing the rate of uterine inflammation, which is frequently associated with premature birth. Pregnant women who consume EPA and DHA help shield their unborn children from allergies (Swanson et al., 2012).

### *10.11.3 CARDIOVASCULAR DISEASES*

It is a circulatory condition that is primarily determined by plaque (a buildup of cholesterol or calcium in the arteries), which causes atherosclerosis and increases the risk of the formation of blood clots. This is a result of the heart muscle being inflamed (myocarditis), which is known to promote the development of such artery plaques and cause blood clots, which cause heart attacks and strokes. Inflammation's primary protective function is the repair of any damaged tissue and the defense against infections. When it is sustained at low levels within the blood vessels, though, it can occasionally become lethal, causing chronic inflammation that encourages the development of other chronic diseases, especially those connected to the heart and blood vessels, like coronary vascular diseases.

Due to their carcinogenic effects, smoking, and obesity, the two main risk-building factors that lead to CVDs, are easily predisposed to in our current way of life. In the case of smoking, the toxicants in the smoke that are released over time are the primary cause of immune and CVDs. Additionally, it decreases the amount of EFAs in the brain's adipose tissues, which has an impact on certain regions of the brain that deal with pressure and satisfaction, particularly the area of the brain responsible for decision-making due to the disruption of neurotransmission brought on by the decline in the amount of Omega-3 PUFAs. According to studies, regular Omega-3 PUFAs supplementation may help smokers with their intense nicotine cravings. These supplements have many benefits, including being readily available, and affordable, and lowering the risk of side effects that would otherwise be the case when using medications instead (Domenichiello et al., 2014).

### 10.11.4 NEURODEGENERATIVE DISORDERS

Omega-3 PUFAs are well known for their enhancing effect in neurodegenerative diseases because of the high concentration of omega-3 PUFAs in synaptic neuronal membranes, which helps in modulating vascular and immune functions and directly influences the health of the central nervous system (CNS). Omega-3 PUFAs are known to be crucial for neuronal differentiation and cell proliferation during the embryonic stage. Studies imply that apoptosis and lower omega-3 PUFAs concentrations are related. The brain is enriched in all of the major lipid and fatty acid classes, with n-3 and n-6 fatty acids accounting for 30 to 35% of these, which is important for neurotransmitter signaling. Since omega-3 PUFAs influence cognitive functions, a deficiency in them may increase the risk of memory loss, distorted thinking, speech difficulties, mental retardation, stroke, trauma, and other serious neurodegenerative diseases like Alzheimer disease and dementia, among others. Furthermore, it has been established that altered lipid metabolism pathways frequently occur in people with neurodegenerative diseases (Nagy and Tiuca, 2017). According to Genevieve et al. (2004), dietary EPA and DHA consumption lowers the risk of neuropsychiatric diseases. Fatty acids help to improve the elasticity, ion permeability, membrane organization, and all biological membranes have both structural and functional components. This enhances neuronal function by facilitating glucose uptake into the brain more easily. Omega-3 PUFAs, a phospholipid ester discovered in the basal membrane, contribute to neurotransmission and neurogenesis by enhancing synaptic transmission and improving cellular flexibility and integrity. They are also known to protect the brain from the harmful effects of oxidative stress (Nagy and Tiuca, 2017). DHA is currently a crucial ingredient of preference in a variety of food products because of its importance in enhancing brain development, particularly in the neonatal brain, when consumed during pregnancy as they protect against apoptotic cell death. Increased DHA intake helps lower the risk of dementia (Dyall and Michael-Titus, 2017). Contrarily, EPA has anti-inflammatory, anti-oxidative, and neuroprotective properties. The risk of neurological disorders like ADHD, bipolar disorder, depression, and schizophrenia is therefore reduced when EPA and DHA are combined (chronic mental disorder dealing with a combination of hallucinations). Omega-3 PUFAs and vitamin B12 together in the diet have been shown to reduce the risk of neurodevelopmental disorders (Rathod et al., 2016).

Additionally, studies show that an imbalance in the levels of omega-3 PUFAs in the brain has an effect on mental health conditions like pressure, stress, and depression. Several studies using commercial omega-3 PUFA capsules and placebos were carried out to balance human mental health shown in Figure 10.2.

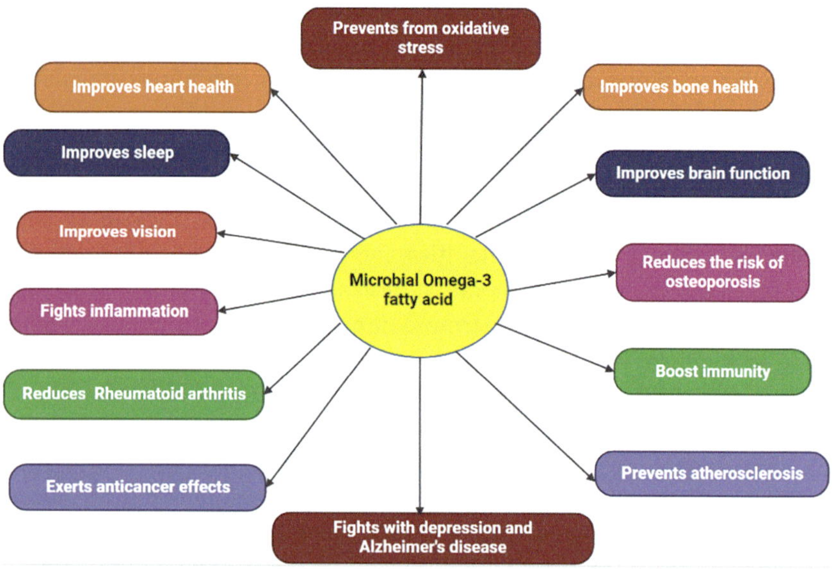


**FIGURE 10.2** Application of microbial Omega-3 fatty acids in healthcare industry.

### *10.11.5 DEPRESSION*

It is a mental health disorder that shows up as a lack of interest in daily activities or as poor performance and reduced motivation for work. These emotions are often expressed as anger, melancholy, or a sense of loss. Studies show that glycolipids, glycerophospholipids, and sphingolipids, in addition to omega-3 PUFAs, are essential in managing depression. When clinical reports showing low levels of erythrocyte ALA in depressed patients were analyzed, this was confirmed. Inflammatory diseases and depression are both brought on by high n-6/n-3 ratios. When the brain tissues of people with long-term depression were examined during autopsies, very little DHA was found there. Consequently, a high concentration of AA/DHA creates a useful human depression biomarker (Wysoczański et al., 2016).

### 10.11.6 HYPERTENSION

Normal definitions of hypertension include raised artery blood pressure brought on by improved endothelial, peripheral vascular, and insulin resistance. Therefore, it is crucial to take the right steps to manage and prevent it. It is known that consuming ALA from a variety of sources can effectively lower blood pressure (Das, 2010).

### 10.11.7 ATTENTION DEFICIT HYPERACTIVITY DISORDER

The behavioral and learning disorders associated with ADHD in both adults and children are significantly impacted by the loss of a few essential Omega-3 PUFAs from a person's diet. Improvements in the behavioral patterns of those with ADHD were observed after a consistent Omega-3 PUFAs body supplementation, particularly about controlling anxiety, anger, shyness, self-control, impulsivity, restlessness, and other recognizable changes in symptoms (Wysoczański et al., 2016).

### 10.11.8 ALZHEIMER'S DISEASE (AD)

AD is a common form of dementia, especially in elderly people, according to reports. The extracellular deposition of amyloid peptides and the coexistence of intracellular neurofibrillary tangles in the brain serve as distinguishing features. Due to this, a person's behavior and mood occasionally experience extreme variations (Dyall and Michael-Titus, 2017). Synaptosomes function as vesicles containing neurotransmitters, essential for effective neurotransmission, and This function is shared by plasmogens, an essential class of neuronal lipids, and DHA. In the hippocampus of AD patients, lower concentrations of plasmogen and DHA are found, which affects the neurotransmission process. As a result, synapses and efficient cognitive function are lost, which eventually leads to higher levels of AD. Because they are well known for their neuronal protective and restorative abilities against a variety of CNS disorders, omega-3 PUFAs are a well-liked treatment option for AD (Wysoczański et al., 2016).

### 10.11.9 AMELIORATION OF SEVERAL SKIN-RELATED DISORDERS

Improvement of some skin-related conditions, including allergies, dermatitis, photoaging, and skin cancer. Skin defense, homeostasis, and omega-3 PUFAs, particularly EPA and DHA, have a well-synchronized relationship. According to some reports, the omega-3 PUFAs in fish oil control cytokines activity by regulating their production, which reduces skin inflammation and speeds up wound healing. Fish oils and essential omega-3 PUFAs were applied topically using a variety of experimental techniques on cell-based and animal models, which resulted in the development of cosmetic and dermatological applications for omega-3 PUFAs (Huang et al., 2018). Tropical skin creams are produced commercially using hyper-oxygenated fatty acids (HOFA). Processing for the aforementioned is done in a controlled environment using UV light and gaseous oxygen bubbling, which transforms peroxides into fatty acid esters. LAs are thought to maintain the skin's ability to retain moisture, which helps to prevent dehydration. In addition to being used as detergents, artificial lubricants, and even surfactants in the form of fatty acids, alcohols, or amines, fatty acids are primarily used in the production of soap.

### 10.11.10 PROBIOTICS

Healthy probiotics and omega-3 PUFAs together: Studies have shown that by retaining high levels of omega-3 PUFAs in the digestive system, co-microencapsulating probiotic bacteria with omega-3 PUFAs rich tuna oil can improve the probiotic bacteria's survival and ability to adhere to the intestines. Omega-3 PUFA-supplemented probiotics have been shown to have favorable effects on inflammation, adipose tissue function, and hepatic lipid metabolism, all of which help to prevent the onset of hepatic sclerosis (Hibbelna and Gowb, 2015).

### 10.11.11 BIOMARKERS

Omega-3 PUFAs are also found to be a useful biomarker for many diseases, helping us to understand the biological function or dysfunction in response to the progression of a particular disease or concerning any available therapeutics. Different levels of omega-3 PUFAs, which are modified in a variety of disease conditions, have been linked to a number of physiological and pathological consequences in the normal operation of the human body. As a result, these biomarkers aid in the identification of various diseases, the assessment of their risks, and the beginning of an appropriate diagnosis. Due to its high specificity, moderate sensitivity, and affordable price, this aspect also aids in simple biomarker screening (Nagy and Tiuca, 2017). Omega-3 PUFAs are therefore thought to be valuable biomarkers for detecting diseases like CVDs, rheumatoid arthritis, atherosclerosis, and even depression. It also helps to highlight the various microbes' distinctive fatty acid profiles, which vary from one organism to another.

### *10.11.12 BIODIESEL*

Beneficial sources of biodiesel produced through a process that is unaffected by environmental variables like weather, season, or location. Due to the short lifespan of microbes, this process is also quicker than that used to make biodiesel from other sources (Yangi and Zhang, 2016). There is speculation that several oleaginous yeasts, molds, and microalgae are used in the production of commercial biodiesel. Microbes that do not produce much biodiesel have their metabolisms changed so they can produce more lipids. Through metabolic engineering, an organism's entire genome, lipidome, metabolome, proteome, and transcriptome can be changed as well as specific subsets of these components. Therefore, a thorough understanding of these concepts helps in the development of a modified strain of organism that efficiently produces omega-3 PUFAs (Patel et al., 2020). The aforementioned studies thus demonstrate the therapeutic value of Omega-3 PUFAs in its broadest sense. In addition to their powerful therapeutic effects, omega-3 PUFAs have a number of other uses, including:

- **Antibacterial Activity:** Both EPA and DHA are known for their antimicrobial qualities. Studies indicate that they also start antibacterial, antiviral, and antifungal activity because they are known to start bactericidal and fungicidal activities, increase *Plasmodium* sp. mortality, fight viral infections by inhibiting viral replication, and induce anti-hepatitis C virus activity. Additionally, pathogens cannot easily evade host defense mechanisms through the activation of resistance genes, the development of virulence factors, the creation of biofilms to withstand hostile environments, and other mechanisms. Additionally, studies indicate that omega-3 PUFAs can prevent virulent pathogens from producing cytotoxins, maintaining antibacterial activity. Because it is unclear whether antioxidant effectiveness is directly correlated with antimicrobial activity, omega-3 PUFAs have chosen a variety of mechanisms, including intracellular protein leakage, inhibiting yeast growth, and competing with other electron donors within the cell. According to Hamilton et al. (2015), omega-3 PUFAs also block or interfere with cell-to-cell communication, interfere with the maintenance of membrane hydrophobicity, slow ATP synthesis, interfere with the electron transport system, cause cellular leakage, and even stop FA synthesis by inhibiting the activity of FsbI enzymes. These facts open the door for numerous researchers to take these substances into account as potential adjutants or different antimicrobial therapeutic agents (Chanda et al., 2018). A number of bacterial species, whose capacity for survival depends on the appropriate maintenance of the membrane viscosity by controlling the structure of fatty acids by their environmental requirements, are said to be affected by omega-3 PUFAs in terms of the hydrophobicity and integrity of the membrane as well as the cell surface charge that results in electron leakage and cell death. The maintenance of membrane viscosity is necessary because it is essential for many cellular processes, including the passive permeability of hydrophobic molecules, the transport of active solutes, and protein-protein interactions (Chanda et al., 2018).

- **Use of Omega-3 PUFAs in Aquaculture:** Research with Australian sea foods to determine the foundations of maximizing their advantages: According to Nichols et al. (2014), adding omega-3 PUFAs to aqua feeds is said to improve the healthiness of Australian seafood. As a result, many consumable products containing omega-3 PUFAs that offer numerous health advantages are developed. In addition to these, omega-3 PUFAs applications are found in agriculture and aquaculture, where they aid in reducing microbial development and growth (Chanda et al., 2018).

## 10.12 CONCLUSIONS

The main producers of omega-3 PUFAs are microbes, which are regarded as sustainable, eco-friendly, powerful, and safe. Due to the significant impact omega-3 PUFAs have on human health and the anticipated supply/demand imbalance in the near future, a lucrative market has emerged.

Omega-3 PUFAs-producing microbes currently have a lot of potential for industrial use. Nutraceuticals work to improve human health. It is now known that microalgae may serve as a direct source of fatty acids, which is encouraging large-scale production of omega-3 PUFAs supplements that contain omega-3 PUFAs and their use as bio lipids. The production, sustainability, availability, and effective extraction of omega-3 PUFAs from microorganisms will all need to be improved in the future. It will also be necessary to identify the number of microbial species with the greatest potential to produce EFAs. We can anticipate custom-made strains that surpass commercially available isolates and may even approach theoretical limits based on recent trends. The operation of bioprocesses must be further optimized for industrial implementation to lower costs and boost sustainability, for instance by using waste streams and non-food renewables. Finally, to advance this field, we should keep looking for fresh, omega-3 PUFAs-rich microbes in nature.

## KEYWORDS

- **docosahexaenoic acid**
- **eicosapentaenoic acid**
- **microbial cell factories**
- **omega-3 fatty acids**
- **polyunsaturated fatty acids**
- **single-cell oils**

## REFERENCES

Adarme-Vega, T. C., Lim, D. K., Timmins, M., Vernen, F., Li, Y., & Schenk, P. M. (2012). Microalgal bio factories: A promising approach towards sustainable omega-3 fatty acid production. *Microbial Cell Factories*, *11*, 96.

Allemann, M. N., & Allen, E. E. (2018). Characterization and application of marine microbial omega-3 polyunsaturated fatty acid synthesis. *Methods in Enzymology*, *605*, 3–32.

Arbter, P., Sinha, A., Troesch, J., Utesch, T., & Zeng, A. P. (2019). Redox governed electro-fermentation improves lipid production by the oleaginous yeast *Rhodosporidium toruloides*. *Bioresource Technology*, *294*, 122122.

Athenaki, M., Gardeli, C., Diamantopoulou, P., et al. (2018). Lipids from yeasts and fungi: Physiology, production and analytical considerations. *Journal of Applied Microbiology, 124*, 336–367.

Bajpai, P., & Bajpai, P. K. (1993). Eicosatetraenoic acid (EPA) production from microorganisms: A review. *Journal of Biotechnology, 30*, 161–183.

Bellou, S., Triantaphyllidou, I. E., Aggeli, D., et al. (2016). Microbial oils as food additives: Recent approaches for improving microbial oil production and its polyunsaturated fatty acid content. *Current Opinion in Biotechnology, 37*, 24–35.

Chanda, W., Joseph, T. P., Guo, X. F., Wang, W. D., Liu, M., Vuai, M. S., Padhiar, A. A., & Zhong, M. T. (2018). Effectiveness of omega-3 polyunsaturated fatty acids against microbial pathogens. *Biomedicine and Biotechnology, 19*, 253–262.

Chen, C. Y., Lee, M. H., Dong, C. D., Leong, Y. K., & Chang, J. S. (2020). Enhanced production of microalgal lipids using a heterotrophic marine microalga *Thraustochytrium* sp. BM2. *Biochemical Engineering Journal, 154*.

Cook, O., & Hildebrand, M. (2016). Enhancing LC-PUFA production in *Thalassiosira pseudonana* by overexpressing the endogenous fatty acid elongate genes. *Journal of Applied Phycology, 28*, 897–905.

Das, U. N. (2010). Essential fatty acids and their metabolites in the context of hypertension. *Hypertension Research, 33*, 782–785.

Daskalaki, A., Perdikouli, N., Aggeli, D., et al. (2019). Laboratory evolution strategies for improving lipid accumulation in *Yarrowia lipolytica. Applied Microbiology and Biotechnology, 103*, 8585–8596.

Diao, J., Li, X., Pei, G., Liu, L., & Chen, L. (2018). Comparative metabolomic analysis of *Crypthecodinium cohnii* in response to different dissolved oxygen levels during docosahexaenoic acid fermentation. *Biochemical and Biophysical Research Communications, 499*, 941–947.

Diao, J., Song, X., Guo, T., Wang, F., Chen, L., & Zhang, W. (2020). Cellular engineering strategies toward sustainable omega-3 long chain polyunsaturated fatty acids production: State of the art and perspectives. *Biotechnology Advances, 40*, 107497.

Domenichiello, A. F., Kitson, A. P., & Bazinet, R. P. (2014). Is docosahexaenoic acid synthesis from α-linolenic acid sufficient to supply the adult brain? *Progress in Lipid Research, 59*, 54–66.

Dourou, M., Aggeli, D., Papanikolaou, S., et al. (2018a). Critical steps in carbon metabolism affecting lipid accumulation and their regulation in oleaginous microorganisms. *Applied Microbiology and Biotechnology, 102*, 2509–2523.

Dyall, S. C., & Michael-Titus, A. T. (2017). Neurological benefits of omega-3 fatty acids. *NeuroMolecular Medicine, 10*, 219–235.

Estupinan, M., Hernandez, I., Saitua, E., Bilbao, M. E., Mendibil, I., Ferrer, J., & Alonso-Saez, L. (2020). Novel *Vibrio* spp. strains producing omega-3 fatty acids isolated from coastal seawater. *Marine Drugs, 18*.

Furlan, V. J. M., Maus, V., Batista, I., & Bandarra, N. M. (2017). Production of docosahexaenoic acid by *Aurantiochytrium* sp. ATCC PRA-276. *Brazilian Journal of Microbiology, 48*, 359–365.

Garcia, R. O., Reichenbach, H., Ring, M. W., & Müller, R. (2009). *Phaselicystis flava* gen. nov., sp. nov., an arachidonic acid-containing soil myxobacterium, and the description of *Phaselicystidaceae* fam. nov. *International Journal of Systematic and Evolutionary Microbiology*, *59*, 1524–1530.

Garcia, R., Stadler, M., Gemperlein, K., & Müller, R. (2016). *Aetherobacter fasciculatus* gen. nov., sp. nov. and *Aetherobacter rufus* sp. nov., novel myxobacteria with promising biotechnological applications. *International Journal of Systematic and Evolutionary Microbiology*, *66*, 928–938.

Gemperlein, K., Dietrich, D., Kohlstedt, M., Zipf, G., Bernauer, H. S., Wittmann, C., Wenzel, S. C., & Müller, R. (2019). Polyunsaturated fatty acid production by *Yarrowia lipolytica* employing designed mycobacterial PUFA synthases. *Nature Communications*, *10*, 4055.

Gemperlein, K., Zaburannyi, N., Garcia, R., La Clair, J. J., & Müller, R. (2018). Metabolic and biosynthetic diversity in marine myxobacteria. *Marine Drugs*, *16*.

Genevieve, Y., & Julie, C. (2004). Omega-3 fatty acids and neuropsychiatric disorders. *Reproduction Nutrition Development*, *45*, 1–28.

Hamilton, M. L., Powers, S., Napier, J. A., & Sayanova, O. (2016). Heterotrophic production of omega-3 long-chain polyunsaturated fatty acids by tropically converted marine diatom *Phaeodactylum tricornutum*. *Marine Drugs*, *14*.

Hamilton, M. L., Warwick, J., Terry, A., Allen, M. J., Napier, J. A., & Sayanova, O. (2015). Towards the industrial production of omega-3 long chain polyunsaturated fatty acids from a genetically modified diatom *Phaeodactylum tricornutum*. *PLoS One*, *10*, e0144054.

Harwood, J. L. (2019). Algae: Critical sources of very long-chain polyunsaturated fatty acids. *Biomolecules*, *9*.

Hayashi, S., Satoh, Y., Ogasawara, Y., & Dairi, T. (2020). Recent advances in functional analysis of polyunsaturated fatty acid synthases. *Current Opinion in Chemical Biology*, *59*, 30–36.

Hibbeln, J. R., & Gow, R. V. (2015). Omega-3 fatty acid and nutrient deficits in adverse neurodevelopment and childhood behaviors. *Child and Adolescent Psychiatric Clinics of North America*, *23*, 555–590.

Hong, W. K., Rairakhwada, D., Seo, P. S., Park, S. Y., Hur, B. K., Kim, C. H., & Seo, J. W. (2011). Production of lipids containing high levels of docosahexaenoic acid by a newly isolated microalga, *Aurantiochytrium* sp. KRS101. *Applied Biochemistry and Biotechnology*, *164*, 1468–1480.

Huang, T. H., Wang, P. W., Yang, S. C., Chou, W. L., & Fang, J. Y. (2018). Cosmetic and therapeutic applications of fish oil's fatty acids on the skin. *Marine Drugs*, *16*, 256.

Kabeya, N., Fonseca, M. M., Ferrier, D. E. K., Navarro, J. C., Bay, L. K., Francis, D. S., Tocher, D. R., Castro, L. F. C., & Monroig, O. (2018). Genes for de novo biosynthesis of omega-3 polyunsaturated fatty acids are widespread in animals. *Science Advances*, *4*, eaar6849.

Khan, M. A. K., Yang, J., Hussain, S. A., Zhang, H., Liang, L., Garre, V., & Song, Y. (2019). Construction of DGLA producing cell factory by genetic modification of *Mucor circinelloides*. *Microbial Cell Factories*, *18*, 64.

Khozin-Goldberg, I., Leu, S., & Boussiba, S. (2016). Microalgae as a source for VLC-PUFA production. *Subcellular Biochemistry*, *86*, 471–510.

Kikukawa, H., Sakuradani, E., Ando, A., et al. (2018). Arachidonic acid production by the oleaginous fungus *Mortierella alpina* 1S-4: A review. *Journal of Advanced Research*, *11*, 15–22.

Klug, L., & Daum, G. (2014). Yeast lipid metabolism at a glance. *FEMS Yeast Research, 14*, 369–388.

Kusube, M., Kyaw, T. S., Tanikawa, K., Chastain, R. A., Hardy, K. M., Cameron, J., & Bartlett, D. H. (2017). *Colwellia marinimaniae* sp. nov., a hyperpiezophilic species isolated from an amphipod within the Challenger Deep, Mariana Trench. *International Journal of Systematic and Evolutionary Microbiology*, *67*, 824–831.

Ledesma-Amaro, R., Jimenez, A., & Revuelta, J. L. (2018). Pathway grafting for polyunsaturated fatty acids production in *Ashbya gossypii* through golden gate rapid assembly. *ACS Synthetic Biology*, *7*, 2340–2347.

Li, J., Liu, R., Chang, G., et al. (2015). A strategy for the highly efficient production of docosahexaenoic acid by *Aurantiochytrium limacinum* SR21 using glucose and glycerol as the mixed carbon sources. *Bioresource Technology*, *177*, 51–57.

Li, Z., Meng, T., Ling, X., Li, J., Zheng, C., Shi, Y., Chen, Z., Li, Q., Lu, Y., & He, N. (2018). Overexpression of malonyl-CoA: ACP trans acylase in *Schizochytrium* sp. to improve polyunsaturated fatty acid production. *Journal of Agricultural and Food Chemistry*, *66*, 5382–5391.

Liang, Y., Zhao, X., Strait, M., et al. (2012). Use of dry-milling derived thin stillage for producing eicosatetraenoic acid (EPA) by the fungus *Pythium irregulare*. *Bioresource Technology*, *111*, 404–409.

Li-Beisson, Y., Thelen, J. J., Fedosejevs, E., & Harwood, J. L. (2019). The lipid biochemistry of eukaryotic algae. *Progress in Lipid Research*, *74*, 31–68.

Liu, L., Wang, F., Yang, J., Li, X., Cui, J., Liu, J., Shi, M., Wang, K., Chen, L., & Zhang, W. (2018). Nitrogen feeding strategies and metabolomic analysis to alleviate high nitrogen inhibition on docosahexaenoic acid production in *Crypthecodinium cohnii*. *Journal of Agricultural and Food Chemistry*, *66*, 10640–10650.

Mao, X., Liu, Z., Sun, J., & Lee, S. Y. (2017). Metabolic engineering for the microbial production of marine bioactive compounds. *Biotechnology Advances*, *35*, 1004–1021.

Marchan, F. L., Chang, K. J. L., Nichols, P. D., et al. (2018). Taxonomy, ecology and biotechnological applications of thraustochytrids: A review. *Biotechnology Advances*, *36*, 26–46.

Messamore, E., & McNamara, R. K. (2016). Detection and treatment of omega-3 fatty acid deficiency in psychiatric practice: Rationale and implementation. *Lipids in Health and Disease*, *15*, 25.

Metz, J. G., Roessler, P., Facciotti, D., Levering, C., Dittrich, F., Lassner, M., Valentine, R., Lardizabal, K., Domergue, F., Yamada, A., et al. (2001). Production of polyunsaturated fatty acids by polyketide synthases in both prokaryotes and eukaryotes. *Science*, *293*, 290–293.

Moi, I. M., Leow, A. T. C., Ali, M. S. M., Rahman, R., Salleh, A. B., & Sabri, S. (2018). Polyunsaturated fatty acids in marine bacteria and strategies to enhance their production. *Applied Microbiology and Biotechnology*, *102*, 5811–5826.

Monroig, O., & Kabeya, N. (2018). Desaturases and elongates involved in polyunsaturated fatty acid biosynthesis in aquatic invertebrates: A comprehensive review. *Fisheries Science*, *84*, 911–928.

Morabito, C., Bournaud, C., Maes, C., Schuler, M., Aiese Cigliano, R., Dellero, Y., Maréchal, E., Amato, A., & Rébeillé, F. (2019). The lipid metabolism in thraustochytrids. *Progress in Lipid Research*, *76*, 101007.

Nagy, K., & Tiuca, I. D. (2017). Importance of fatty acids in physiopathology of human body. *Corpus ID: 54513514*.

Nakazawa, A., Matsuura, H., Kose, R., Ito, K., Ueda, M., Honda, D., Inouye, I., Kaya, K., & Watanabe, M. M. (2012). Optimization of biomass and fatty acid production by *Aurantiochytrium* sp. strain 4W-1b. *Procedia Environmental Sciences*, *15*, 27–33.

Nazir, Y., Shuib, S., Kalil, M. S., Song, Y., & Hamıd, A. A. (2018). Optimization of culture conditions for enhanced growth, lipid and docosahexaenoic acid (DHA) production of *Aurantiochytrium* SW1 by response surface methodology. *Scientific Reports*, *8*, 1–12.

Nichols, P. D., McManus, A., Krail, K., Sinclair, A. J., & Miller, M. (2014). Recent advances in omega-3: Health benefits, sources, products and bioavailability. *Nutrients*, *6*, 3727–3733.

Norashikin, M. N., Loh, S. H., Aziz, A., & Cha, T. S. (2018). Metabolic engineering of fatty acid biosynthesis in *Chlorella vulgaris* using an endogenous omega-3 fatty acid desaturase gene with its promoter. *Algal Research*, *31*, 262–275.

Ochsenreither, K., Glück, C., Stressler, T., Fischer, L., & Syldatk, C. (2016). Production strategies and applications of microbial single cell oils. *Frontiers in Microbiology*, *7*, 1539.

Okuda, T., Ando, A., Negoro, H., Muratsubaki, T., Kikukawa, H., Sakamoto, T., Sakuradani, E., Shimizu, S., & Ogawa, J. (2015). Eicosatetraenoic acid (EPA) production by an oleaginous fungus *Mortierella alpina* expressing the Δ17 desaturase gene under ordinary temperature. *European Journal of Lipid Science and Technology*, *117*, 1919–1927.

Pal, D., Khozin-Goldberg, I., Cohen, Z., & Boussiba, S. (2011). The effect of light, salinity, and nitrogen availability on lipid production by *Nannochloropsis* sp. *Applied Microbiology and Biotechnology*, *90*(4), 1429–1441.

Paliwal, C., Mitra, M., Bhayani, K., Bharadwaj, S. V. V., Ghosh, T., Dubey, S., & Mishra, S. (2017). Abiotic stresses as tools for metabolites in microalgae. *Bioresource Technology*, *244*, 1216–1226.

Papanikolaou, S., & Aggelis, G. (2019). Sources of microbial oils with emphasis to *Mortierella (Umbelopsis) isabellina* fungus. *World Journal of Microbiology and Biotechnology*, *35*, 1–19.

Park, W. K., Moon, M., Shin, S. E., Cho, J. M., Suh, W. I., Chang, Y. K., & Lee, B. (2018). Economical DHA (docosahexaenoic acid) production from *Aurantiochytrium* sp. KRS101 using orange peel extract and low-cost nitrogen sources. *Algal Research*, *29*, 71–79.

Patel, A., Karageorgou, D., Rova, E., Katapodis, P., Rova, U., Christakopoulos, P., & Matsakas, L. (2020). An overview of potential oleaginous microorganisms and their role in biodiesel and omega-3 fatty acid-based industries. *Journal of Biomedical Science*, *8*, 434.

Patel, A., Liefeldt, S., Rova, U., Christakopoulos, P., & Matsakas, L. (2020). Coproduction of DHA and squalene by thraustochytrid from forest biomass. *Scientific Reports*, *10*, 1–12.

Patel, A., Matsakas, L., Hrůzová, K., Rova, U., & Christakopoulos, P. (2019). Biosynthesis of nutraceutical fatty acids by the oleaginous marine microalgae *Phaeodactylum tricornutum* utilizing hydrolysates from organosolv-pretreated birch and spruce biomass. *Marine Drugs*, *17*, 119.

Patel, A., Rova, U., Christakopoulos, P., & Matsakas, L. (2019). Simultaneous production of DHA and squalene from *Aurantiochytrium* sp. grown on forest biomass hydrolysates. *Biotechnology for Biofuels*, *12*, 1–12.

Philpott, J. D., Witard, O., & Galloway, S. D. R. (2018). Applications of omega-3 polyunsaturated fatty acid supplementation for sport performance. *Research in Sports Medicine: An International Journal*, *27*, 219–237.

Plourde, M., & Cunnane, S. C. (2007). Extremely limited synthesis of long chain polyunsaturates in adults: Implications for their dietary essentiality and use as supplements. *Applied Physiology, Nutrition, and Metabolism*, *32*, 619–634.

Poole, L. B., Parsonage, D., Sergeant, S., Miller, L. R., Lee, J., Furdui, C. M., & Chilton, F. H. (2020). Acyl-lipid desaturases and Vipp1 cooperate in cyanobacteria to produce novel omega-3 PUFA-containing glycolipids. *Biotechnology for Biofuels*, *13*, 83.

Qin, L., Liu, L., Zeng, A. P., et al. (2017). From low-cost substrates to single cell oils synthesized by oleaginous yeasts. *Bioresource Technology*, *245*, 1507–1519.

Qiu, X., Xie, X., & Meesapyodsuk, D. (2020). Molecular mechanisms for biosynthesis and assembly of nutritionally important very long chain polyunsaturated fatty acids in microorganisms. *Progress in Lipid Research*, *79*, 101047.

Radcliffe, J. E., Thomas, J., Bramley, A. L., Radford, B. E., Scholey, A. B., Pipingas, A., Thomas, C. J., & Itsiopoulos, C. (2016). Controversies in omega-3 efficacy and novel concepts for application. *Journal of Nutritional Intermediary Metabolism*, *5*, 11–22.

Rathod, R., Kale, A., & Joshi, S. (2016). Novel insights into the effect of vitamin B12. *Journal of Biomedical Science*, *25*, 17.

Ratledge, C. (2013). Microbial oils: An introductory overview of current status and future prospects. *OCL Journal*, *20*, D602.

Ren, L. J., Sun, X. M., Ji, X. J., et al. (2017). Enhancement of docosahexaenoic acid synthesis by manipulation of antioxidant capacity and prevention of oxidative damage in *Schizochytrium* sp. *Bioresource Technology*, *223*, 141–148.

Rismani, S., & Shariati, M. (2017). Changes of the total lipid and omega-3 fatty acid contents in two microalgae *Dunaliella salina* and *Chlorella vulgaris* under salt stress. *Brazilian Archives of Biology and Technology*, *60*, 1–11.

Ryckebosch, E., Bruneel, C., Muylaert, K., et al. (2012). Microalgae as an alternative source of omega-3 long chain polyunsaturated fatty acids. *Lipid Technology*, *24*, 128–130.

Sakayu, S., Shinmen, Y., Kawashima, H., Akimoto, K., & Yamada, H. (1988). Fungal mycelia as a novel source of eicosatetraenoic acid: Activation of enzyme(s) involved in eicosatetraenoic acid production at low temperature. *Biochemical and Biophysical Research Communications*, *150*, 335–341.

Sayegh, F., Elazzazy, A., Bellou, S., et al. (2016). Production of polyunsaturated single cell oils possessing antimicrobial and anticancer properties. *Annals of Microbiology*, *66*, 937–948.

Singh, R., Upadhyay, A. K., Chandra, P., & Singh, D. P. (2018). Sodium chloride incites reactive oxygen species in green algae *Chlorococcum humicola* and *Chlorella vulgaris*: Implication on lipid synthesis, mineral nutrients and antioxidant system. *Bioresource Technology*, *270*, 489–497.

Sirisuk, P., Sunwoo, I., Kim, S. H., Awah, C. C., Ra, H., Kim, J. M., Jeong, G. T., & Kim, S. K. (2018). Enhancement of biomass, lipids, and polyunsaturated fatty acid (PUFA) production in *Nannochloropsis oceanica* with a combination of single wavelength light emitting diodes (LEDs) and low temperature in a three-phase culture system. *Bioresource Technology*, *270*, 504–511.

Spatafora, J. W., Chang, Y., Benny, G. L., et al. (2016). A phylum-level phylogenetic classification of zygomycete fungi based on genome-scale data. *Mycologic*, *108*, 1028–1046.

Suh, S. S., Kim, S. J., Hwang, J., Park, M., Lee, T. K., Kil, E. J., & Lee, S. (2015). Fatty acid methyl ester profiles and nutritive values of 20 marine microalgae in Korea. *Asian Pacific Journal of Tropical Medicine*, *8*, 191–196.

Sun, X. M., Ren, L. J., Ji, X. J., et al. (2016). Adaptive evolution of *Schizochytrium* sp. by continuous high oxygen stimulations to enhance docosahexaenoic acid synthesis. *Bioresource Technology*, *211*, 374–381.

Swanson, D., Block, R., & Mousa, S. A. (2012). Omega-3 fatty acids EPA and DHA: Health benefits throughout life. *Advances in Nutrition*, *3*, 1–7.

Tatsuzawa, H., & Takizawa, E. (1995). Changes in lipid and fatty acid composition of *Pavlova lutheri*. *Phytochemistry*, *40*(2), 397–400.

Techtmann, S. M., Fitzgerald, K. S., Stelling, S. C., Joyner, D. C., Uttukar, S. M., Harris, A. P., Alshibli, N. K., Brown, S. D., & Hazen, T. C. (2016). *Colwellia psychrerythraea* strains from distant deep-sea basins show adaptation to local conditions. *Frontiers in Environmental Science*, *4*.

Thevenieau, F., & Nicaud, J. M. (2013). Microorganisms as sources of oils. *OCL Journal*, *20*, D603.

Tocher, D. R., Betancor, M. B., Sprague, M., Olsen, R. E., & Napier, J. A. (2019). Omega-3 long-chain polyunsaturated fatty acids, EPA and DHA: Bridging the gap between supply and demand. *Nutrients*, *11*, 89.

Wan, X., Peng, Y. F., Zhou, X. R., Gong, Y. M., Huang, F. H., & Moncalian, G. (2016). Effect of cerulenin on fatty acid composition and gene expression pattern of DHA-producing strain *Colwellia psychrerythraea* strain 34H. *Microbial Cell Factories*, *15*, 30.

Wang, Q., Lu, Y., Xin, Y., et al. (2016). Genome editing of model oleaginous microalgae *Nannochloropsis* spp. by CRISPR/Cas9. *The Plant Journal*, *88*, 1071–1081.

Wysoczanski, T., Sokoła-Wysoczanska, E., Pezkala, J., Lochynski, S., Czyż, K., Bodkowski, R., Herbinger, G., & Patkowska-Sokoła, B. (2016). Omega-3 fatty acids and their role in central nervous system – A review. *Current Medicinal Chemistry*, *23*, 816–831.

Xie, D., Jackson, E. N., & Zhu, Q. (2015). Sustainable source of omega-3 eicosapentaenoic acid from metabolically engineered *Yarrowia lipolytica*: From fundamental research to commercial production. *Applied Microbiology and Biotechnology*, *99*, 1599–1610.

Xie, D., Miller, E., Tyreus, B., Jackson, E. N., & Zhu, Q. (2017). Sustainable production of omega-3 eicosapentaenoic acid by fermentation of metabolically engineered *Yarrowia lipolytica*. In *Green Chemistry and Sustainable Technology: Quality Living Through Chemurgy and Green Chemistry* (pp. 17–33). Berlin, Heidelberg: Springer.

Xue, J., Niu, Y. F., Huang, T., et al. (2015). Genetic improvement of the microalga *Phaeodactylum tricornutum* for boosting neutral lipid accumulation. *Metabolic Engineering*, *27*, 1–9.

Yangi, S., & Zhang, H. (2016). Enhanced polyunsaturated fatty acids production in *Mortierella alpina* by SSF and the enrichment in chicken breasts. *Food & Nutrition Research*, *60*.

Yazawa, K. (1996). Production of eicosapentaenoic acid from marine bacteria. *Lipids*, *31*(Suppl), S297–S300.

Yin, F. W., Zhang, Y. T., Jiang, J. Y., et al. (2019a). Efficient docosahexaenoic acid production by *Schizochytrium* sp. via a two-phase pH control strategy using ammonia and citric acid as pH regulators. *Process Biochemistry*, *77*, 1–7.
Yoshida, K., Hashimoto, M., Hori, R., Adachi, T., Okuyama, H., Orikasa, Y., Nagamine, T., Shimizu, S., Ueno, A., & Morita, N. (2016). Bacterial long-chain polyunsaturated fatty acids: Their biosynthetic genes, functions, and practical use. *Marine Drugs*, *14*.
Zárate, R., El Jaber-Vazdekis, N., Tejera, N., et al. (2017). Significance of long chain polyunsaturated fatty acids in human health. *Clinical and Translational Medicine*, *6*, 25.
Zhang, J., & Burgess, J. G. (2017). Enhanced eicosatetraenoic acid production by a new deep-sea marine bacterium *Shewanella electrodiphila* MAR441T. *PLoS One*, *12*, e0188081.
Zhao, X. M., & Qiu, X. (2019). Very long chain polyunsaturated fatty acids accumulated in triacylglycerol are channeled from phosphatidylcholine in *Thraustochytrium*. *Frontiers in Microbiology*, *10*.

CHAPTER 11

# Industrial Importance of Bacterial Protein Production

PRADEEP KUMAR* and VIRENDRA KUMAR

*Department of NMR and MRI Facility, All India Institute of Medical Sciences, New Delhi, Delhi, India*

*Corresponding author

## ABSTRACT

Genetic methods are often used to identify high-yielding bacterial variants among industrial microorganisms and to boost product yield for commercially viable production. Bacteria are preferred over non-microbial proteins for large-scale production of recombinant proteins due to their higher yields, economic viability, consistency, ease of modification, and optimization, among other advantages. Bacteria with the greatest industrial importance are particularly *E. coli, Streptomyces, Bacillus subtilis, and Pseudomonas*. Somatostatin, human insulin, interferon, growth hormone (GH), and enzymes are a few of the significant pharmacological proteins being produced via genetic engineering. Due to the rapid advancement of microbial technology, bacterial proteins or enzymes are currently receiving a lot of attention. These substances may be used as food additives, vitamins, antibodies, antibiotics, vaccines, and a variety of other products to improve people's everyday lives. In the pharmaceutical and enzyme industries, both native and recombinant proteins are utilized for various applications. Milk, food, polymers, textiles, paper, pulp, detergents, and plastics are increasingly used in various industries. This chapter focuses on the fundamentals and composition of bacterial proteins, as well as on the application-based kinds and subgroups of these proteins, as well as

Industrial Biotechnology: Current Progress and Novel Technologies.
Prakash Kumar Sarangi, Akhilesh Kumar Singh, Rajesh Kumar Srivastava, and Brijesh Pandey (Eds.)


DOI: 10.1201/9781779642233-11

on genetic engineering and developmental strategies and the mechanisms necessary for elevated protein synthesis.

## 11.1 INTRODUCTION

Proteins are the macromolecules required for all the many biological processes that make life possible. Proteins include nitrogen and vital amino acids that are required for survival by both humans and animals (Hou et al., 2018; Wu, 2009). New structural and functional proteins (enzymes and hormones) are made from these amino acids. Around 20 amino acids make up dietary proteins, of which many are essential and must be taken from food (Hou et al., 2018; Wu, 2009). Proteins can get denatured by a variety of factors, such as pH, temperature, salt concentration, shearing, surface, and interface contact including the formation of protein aggregates, organic solvents, lyophilization, moisture content, and protein concentration (Chen et al., 2021). The fast advancement of microbial technology, which may readily provide support in daily life in the shape of enzymes, dietary supplements, antibiotics, vitamins, antibodies, vaccines, and many other forms, is currently drawing a lot of attention to bacterial proteins (Vitorino et al., 2017). Bacterial proteins are preferred for the production of recombinant proteins on a huge scale due to their high yields, commercial feasibility, uniformity, simplicity of modification and optimization, continuous supply due to seasonal rise and fall, higher catalytic activity, and a host of other benefits over nonbacterial proteins (Gupta et al., 2016; Rosano et al., 2014). Recombinant protein manufacturing methods that are effective are becoming more and more valued above conventional methods that need a large number of high-quality proteins to be commercially successful. These approaches include molecular biology methods, advances in proteomic technology, and simple culture environment modification (Gopal et al., 2013; Tripathi et al., 2019). The present chapter is on the fundamentals and a brief overview of bacterial proteins with their application founded types and parts, developmental methodologies including genetic production, and systems necessary for increased recombinant protein expansion (Kamionka et al., 2011; Rosano et al., 2014). Due to the low cost and simplicity of bacterial culture, the expression method is a better option for the production of therapeutic proteins both on a scale and in the industry. Using recombinant DNA technology, it is also possible to make protein molecules with different properties.

In some conditions, protein engineering can be utilized to compensate for bacterial cells' lack of post-translational modification processes including maturation, glycosylation, proteolytic protein, and constricted potential for the synthesis of disulfide bridges (Kamionka et al., 2011; Rosano et al., 2014). Protein engineering is frequently used to modify a protein's biological activity or to enhance protein stability. Genetic fusions of two proteins can provide more complex changes. This chapter provides several instances of therapeutic proteins that have been genetically altered. It highlights how crucial it is to create a build without any extraneous amino acid residues (Kamionka et al., 2011; Rosano et al., 2014).

More and more proteins that are crucial to the industry are produced by bacteria. These cells may be used in an inclusive variety of applications depending upon expression of additional genes by bacteria. The influence of recombinant proteins on therapeutic applications is particularly impressive (Huang et al., 2012). Bacteria are used in the construction of several medicinal proteins, including hormones, interleukin, and insulin. *Escherichia coli* has acted as the host for the creation of viral proteins and virus-like nanoparticles, specifically for the purpose of producing vaccines (Chou et al., 2007). Recombinant proteins made from Bacillus and Pseudomonas have been employed in bioremediation, soil cleaning, and oil recovery in addition to medicinal uses (Fenibo et al., 2019). The generation of biofuel from energy sources, where bacterial cellulases and hemicelluloses play crucial roles in the breakdown of polymeric lignocellulosic biomass to fermentable sugars, is one significant application that is seeing growing interest. Consequently, xylanases from *Klebsiella* and *Lysinibacillus strains* and cellulase enzymes from cellulosic bacteria such as *Clostridium* and *Saccharophagus* strains have been created by recombinant means (Kim et al., 2012). Extracellular secretion of proteins is required while complete bacterial cells producing recombinant proteins are utilized to interact with a polymeric substance, such as polypeptides because cells are unable to take up polymer substrates (Lynd et al., 2002). Secretion of these proteins extracellularly might considerably simplify the complexity of a production process in cases where pure recombinant proteins are employed directly. This is because it would eliminate the necessity for cell lysis and ease the load of removing host proteins (Wingfield, 2015). Additionally, the release of highly expressed proteins decreases the development of inclusion bodies, facilitates folding, permits the creation of disulfide bonds, lowers the negative effects of cytotoxic proteins, and reduces the effects of intracellular protein degradation (Kleiner-Grote et al., 2018).

In terms of industrial application, bacteria production is an important part of the synthesis of the variability of proteins that are beneficial to humans and have significantly altered our quality of life and lifespan. Beverages, food additives, healthcare items, and pharmaceuticals are some of these products. Industrial microbiology and protein purification advancements have made it possible to isolate enzymes in commercially viable amounts. Today, their utilization is typical throughout numerous industries, including winemaking. Enzymes are used in a variety of industrial processes, such as the production of detergents, baked products, beverages, pharmaceuticals, textiles, fermented dairy products, and leather goods (Richardson et al., 2018; Singh et al., 2016).

## 11.2 SOME IMPORTANT BACTERIA AND BACTERIAL SPECIES

### 11.2.1 *ESCHERICHIA COLI*

*Escherichia coli* has been used for the production of recombinant proteins ever since the first recombinant DNA methods were developed using its genetic material and bacteriophage infection (Rosano et al., 2014). As a result of the acquired information on *E. coli* genetics and physiology, as well as the growing number of genetic engineering techniques that have been tailored to this bacterium, *E. coli* is selected as a host when trying to produce a novel protein. Additionally, given its quick growth and straightforward culture techniques, it is the preferred host for producing a significant quantity of proteins both in laboratories and on an industrial scale (Rosano et al., 2014). The main challenges encountered during protein construction in *E. coli* include plasmid loss and antibiotic-based preservation, unexpected chemical inducers of gene expression, recombinant plasmid or protein-mediated metabolic cargo and stress responses, absence of post-translational modifications (inability to form disulfide linkage), proteolytic and aggregation digestion, and complex downstream (Rosano et al., 2014).

### 11.2.2 *STREPTOMYCES* GENUS

The genus *Streptomyces* contains gram-positive bacteria that live in soil. These actinobacteria have similar complex morphologies and high GC contents (70%) (Barka et al., 2015). Numerous secondary metabolites with antibacterial, anticancer, and antiparasitic activities are produced by the whole *Streptomyces* genus. Several extracellular enzymes, including lipases, nucleases, cellulases, and amylases (Shivlata et al., 2015). These bacteria produce secreted enzymes that have a variety of uses in biotechnology, including biocatalysts and bioremediation, to maintain their intricate life cycles. There are significant economic and environmental advantages to using enzymes as biocatalysts to manufacture compounds in a variety of areas like food, medicines, and fuels. Most antibiotics are obtained from *Streptomyces*, including lactams, macrolides, glycopeptides, and tetracyclines (de Carvalho et al., 2017). The first antibiotic to be extracted from *Streptomyces* was actinomycin (de Carvalho et al., 2017). The efficiency of antibiotics has been threatened by a rise in antibiotic resistance among pathogenic bacteria, which may bring an end to the golden age of antibiotic discovery (Adrio et al., 2014). However, the fusion of genome mining with next-generation sequencing might change the study of antibiotics. Analysis of the genetic potential of antibiotic manufacturers shows >10% usage, which infers that there is a vast, pure genetic pool ready to be used to find new medications (Adrio et al., 2014). Because *Streptomyces* can synthesize a variety of proteins and enzymes, it has developed into an actinobacterium that is appealing to industry. *Streptomyces* genus strains produce more than 80% of the physiologically active chemicals with medicinal characteristics (De Simeis et al., 2021). It is hypothesized that advancements in production techniques, knowledge of the synthesis of proteins and peptides, and physiological characteristics of streptomyces growth may aid in the identification of certain proteins and boost the production of already-known proteins and enzymes. However, advances in synthetic biology and genetic production are enhancing *Streptomyces* strains, which is expected to increase recombinant protein output (De Simeis et al., 2021).

### 11.2.3 BACILLUS SUBTILIS

*Bacillus subtilis*, the most widely known gram-positive bacterium, has a variety of significant characteristics, including the capacity to thrive on cheap carbon sources, having obvious genetic backgrounds, and having created genetic modification techniques (Gu et al., 2018). It has been shown that the bacterium subtilis is an ideal host for the creation of recombinant proteins and other substances. Several systems and synthetic biology techniques were used to identify the productive features of *B. subtilis*. It is possible to examine *B. subtilis* thoroughly and further enhance it through metabolic engineering (Gu et al., 2018). The main organism exploited in industrial applications and metabolic engineering is *B. subtilis*. It is now possible to effectively cultivate *B. subtilis* as bacterial cell factories (Gu et al., 2018).

### *11.2.4 PSEUDOMONAS SPECIES*

The gram-negative, polar flagellated, rod-shaped bacterium *Pseudomonas* is one of the most studied prokaryote genera (Diggle et al., 2020). In order to correctly identify *Pseudomonas* species, it is vital to keep in mind that these bacterium's morphological traits are shared by a variety of bacteria genera (Scales et al., 2014). These bacteria are easily distinguished from genera that are identical to them using advanced nucleic acid-based methods, revealing the taxonomic relationships between many bacterial species, including the genus *Pseudomonas*. *Pseudomonas aeruginosa* has practical uses in several sectors of commerce and industry all over the world. Several proteins (enzymes), including lipase, protease, and others, are produced in the industries using strains of *Pseudomonas aeruginosa* (Scales et al., 2014).

## 11.3 BACTERIAL PROTEIN SYNTHESIS AND THEIR COMPONENT

In general, transcription, which creates an intermediate messenger RNA or mRNA using one strand of the duplex DNA as a template, and translation are the two steps involved in the creation of proteins in bacteria (the process of translating mRNA data into linear model linear models of amino acids to create a polypeptide). The DNA strand with the same sequence as the mRNA template (and to which it is complementary) but with uracil in lieu of thymine is referred to as the coding strand. Anticoding or template strands are the names given to these two DNA strands collectively. Transcription is the method through which DNA is converted into RNA. The process is carried out by the enzyme RNA polymerase. The same enzyme is responsible for carrying out the transcription of each gene in a bacterial cell, together with mRNA, rRNA, and transfer RNA or tRNA. At certain places in the DNA, RNA polymerase initiates and terminates transcription. Transcription begins at promoter sites, which are recognized and occupied by RNA polymerase. There are several stages that makeup transcription, including template recognition, initiation, elongation, and termination. The linear mRNA nucleotide sequence is translated into the matching protein as a linear sequence of peptide bond-linked amino acids.

### 11.3.1 RECOMBINANT PROTEINS

Proteins that have been synthesized using recombinant DNA technology are known as recombinant proteins. Proteins are used in a variety of products, such as feed, vaccinations, medications, detergents, and cosmetics (Adrio et al., 2010). Simply taking proteins out of their natural sources will not be enough to meet the increased demand for them. Recombinant DNA technology provides a more efficient means to generate large amounts of proteins (Adrio et al., 2010). There are advantages and disadvantages to this strategy. For instance, insulin, a hormone whose production is restricted in diabetes patients and which saves many lives, has previously been produced using recombinant DNA technology (Gupta et al., 2016). The target protein's properties can also be changed using the recombinant DNA approach. However, there are still concerns about the safety and ethics of recombinant DNA technology (Gupta et al., 2016). Significant bacteria used in the construction and synthesizing of recombinant proteins such as *Caulobacter crescentus, Pseudoalteromonas haloplanktis, Pseudomonas fluorescens, Pseudomonas putida, Streptomyces lividans, Streptomyces griseus, Mycobacterium smegmatis, Lactococcus lactis, Lactobacillus casei, Lactobacillus reuteri, Bacillus licheniformis, Lactobacillus gasseri,* and so forth (Table 11.1) (Ferrer-Miralles et al., 2013).

### 11.3.2 RECOMBINANT PROTEINS EXPRESSED IN BACTERIA SYSTEM

The bacterial approach for producing therapeutic recombinant proteins is thought to be appealing due to its low costs, fast bacterial growth, and average productivity (Owczarek et al., 2019; Rosano et al., 2014). Since *E. coli* is a model organism with well-known genetics and biology, it is not unexpected that the bulk of bacterial expression platforms uses it as the host (such as the *Pseudomonas* or *Streptomyces* system) (Owczarek et al., 2019; Rosano et al., 2014). The *Lactococcus lactis* system is frequently taken into consideration while producing recombinant therapies that deal with membrane proteins. Human insulin (Humulin), which was manufactured in *E. coli* and was the first designed biopharmaceutical for the treatment of diabetes, initially appeared in the early 1980s. It was authorized by the Food and Drug Administration or FDA in 1982. The *E. coli* system now generates a wide range of proteins, such as interleukins, GH, tumor necrosis factor (TNF), and interferons (Owczarek et al., 2019). Fusion proteins constructed from cytosolic proteins and polypeptides with less than 100 nucleotides in their sequence function maximally. Because *E. coli* is so simple to utilize with many common plasmid vectors, it often allows the optimization stage to be bypassed in the production of protein therapeutics. A common method of expression in *E. coli* using bacteriophage T7 RNA polymerase, which some structural genomics associations even recommend as a "what-to-try-first" strategy (Francis et al., 2010). Since the method greatly increases the level of protein synthesis, it was suggested to produce globular prokaryotic and soluble eukaryotic proteins. *E. coli* produces chemicals as opposed to eukaryotic cells, which produce proteins. Although the plasmid that transports a target protein to the periplasmic membrane may form disulfide bonds, *E. coli* does not carry out posttranslational modifications (PTMs) such as proteolytic, disulfide linkage, phosphorylation, and glycosylation processing (Francis et al., 2010). Because PMTs are crucial for biological activity, stability, and folding processes, a recombinant protein made from bacteria could not work. However, attaching synthetic PTSs could be the solution to this problem. Another problem with the bacterial expression system is the presence of genes with atypical codons, such as those that are widespread in the human genome but rare in that particular bacterium. A protein biomolecule's synthesis is usually prematurely stopped due to its commonly inadequate expression. For rare codon site-directed replacement or unusual codon codons, it can be recommended to use *E. coli* plasmids (Gasser et al., 2008). Finally, bacteria that overproduce recombinant proteins are susceptible to stresses that affect protein solubility due to metabolic or structural factors. When converting a protein biomolecule into a soluble form, the following factors should be taken into account: the ideal temperature, the composition of the medium, the number of plasmid copies, or the potency of the promoter's real activity (Figure 11.1).

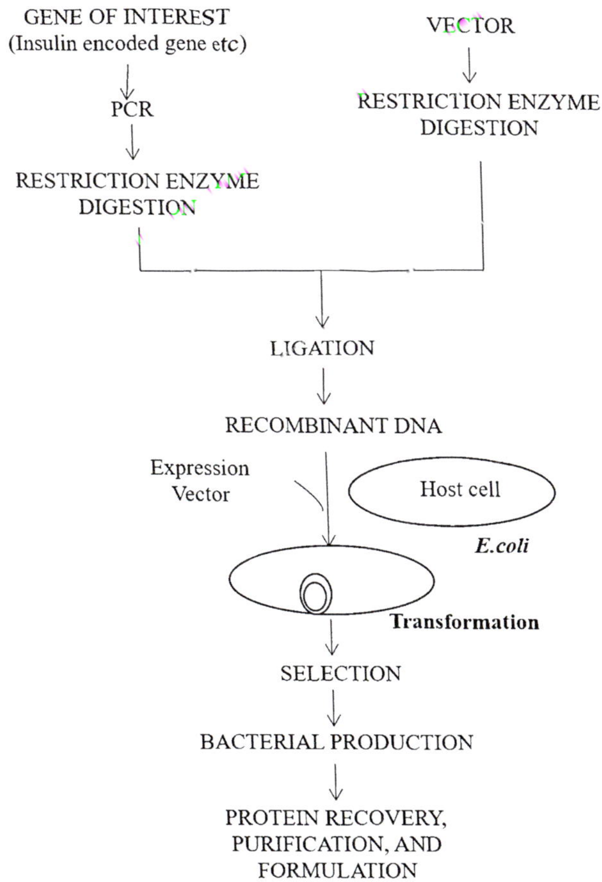


**FIGURE 11.1** Simple presentation of recombinant protein steps and process.

## 11.4 ISOLATION OF MICROORGANISMS ESPECIALLY BACTERIA

The harmful bacteria must first be eliminated from their native settings before a producer strain may be created. As an alternative, organizations that maintain culture collections might be contacted for pure cultures of microorganisms. The most common microorganisms that are important for the industry include bacteria, actinomycetes, fungi, and algae. These microbes are present almost everywhere, including in the soil, water, air, and tissues of both plants and animals (Bonnet et al., 2019). However, soils, lakes, and river muck are the most typical sources of industrial microorganisms. Frequently, the biological environment where the desired microorganism is more likely to be isolated will be determined by the characteristics of the product that will be created from the desired microbe and the process of development. For instance, if the objective is to locate a source of enzymes that can withstand high temperatures, hot water springs are the appropriate location to go (Sharma et al., 2014). Numerous intricate isolation techniques have been created; however, no one technique can identify every bacterium present in a sample. Numerous techniques can be used to isolate different bacteria, including UV radiation, air drying, or heating at 120°C, continuous percolation and filtration, washings from root systems, treatment with detergents or alcohols, pre-inoculation with toxic agents, selective inhibitors (antimetabolites and antibiotics, etc.), nutritional (certain C and N sources), nutritional changes, pH and temperature changes, as well as aeration (Bonnet et al., 2019). A fraction of the microorganisms present in a sample is intended to be selectively multiplied using enrichment techniques. The main isolation methods routinely used for soil samples are dilution, gradient plate, aerosol dilution, flotation, and variable centrifugation (Bonnet et al., 2019).

## 11.5 SCREENING OF MICROORGANISMS FOR PROTEINS

Following the isolation of bacteria, their screening follows next. Primary screening is a collection of extremely advanced methods that enables the identification and isolation of microorganisms generating the necessary peptide or polypeptide (proteins and enzymes). The ideal primary screening procedure should be rapid, inexpensive, predictive, specific but effective for a wide range of peptides and polypeptides, and usable on a large scale (Singh et al., 2016). Since many isolates should be screened in order to find a small number of suitable ones, primary screening takes a lot of time and effort. For a range of bacterial proteins, quick and efficient screening methods have been developed that use either a protein's characteristic or that of its peptides or polypeptides to identify promising isolates. Some of the screening methods, such as those for extracellular enzymes and enzyme inhibitors, are rather straightforward (Singh et al., 2016). The screening is typically difficult and time-consuming for the majority of valuable bacterial products, and it frequently necessitates two or more procedures. In some circumstances, focusing on a particular bacterial group that is predicted to produce protein may be useful. For instance, *Actinomycetes* that do not belong to the *genus Streptomyces* are the focus of the current quest for novel proteins. Using appropriately created, specialized screening approaches, it is possible to find proteins that have pharmacological effects other than those of antibiotics (Singh et al., 2016).

Proteins, which can either be intracellular or extracellular, must be isolated from bacteria. Recombinant biomolecules must first be released in a soluble fraction after disrupting cells to extract intracellular proteins (Wingfield, 2015). Due to their multiple classes and varied natures, an appropriate detergent should be selected, unique to a certain protein, in a way to maximize protein constancy and extraction effectiveness. As a result, a detergent component utilized for protein extraction ought to be both highly effective and less disruptive to protein structure. Bacterial cells can be lysed by a variety of methods, including chemical and mechanical ones such as osmotic shock lysis and enzyme digestion (Wingfield, 2015) (Figure 11.2).

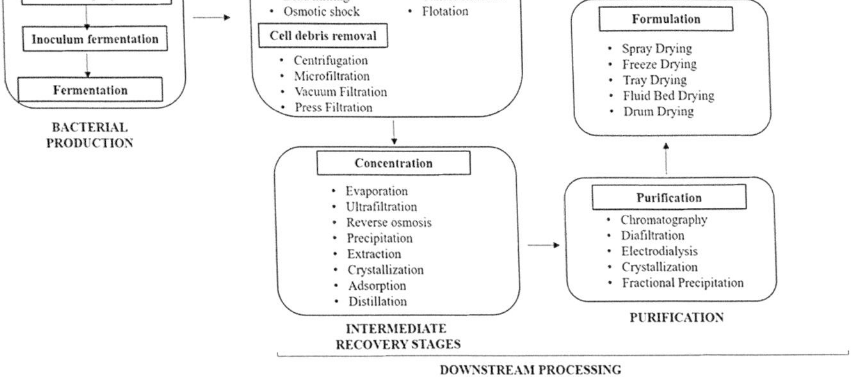


**FIGURE 11.2** Outline of bacterial culture, extraction purification process, and involved techniques.

Recombinant protein manufacturing is possible on a variety of platforms, and each of these systems has a wealth of features (Owczarek et al., 2019). Recombinant biopharmaceuticals can be created using both prokaryotic and eukaryotic cells, including those found in bacteria, filamentous fungi, yeasts, microalgae, insect cells, mammalian cells, and transgenic or GM organisms (animal and plant species) (Owczarek et al., 2019). The choice of the production platform is determined by the target protein's characteristics, including its structure and biological activity. The easier it is to extract and purify a protein of interest, the more desirable it is. The anatomy of a cell is reflected in the primary distinction between the many expression systems that may be used. A nucleus, endoplasmic reticulum (ER), and Golgi apparatus, which are crucial for transport and PTM, are absent from bacterial cells (Francis et al., 2010; Owczarek et al., 2019). Mammalian or insect cells often give the splicing of mRNA that is similar to that of humans. However, maintaining these hosts could be excessively time- and money-consuming. Other systems may thus prove to be more effective and cost-effective. In order to achieve scalability and high yield, special consideration should be given to the selection of a platform for recombinant pharmaceutical manufacture (Owczarek et al., 2019).

## 11.6 EXTRACTION

Cells must first be broken up in order to extract intracellular proteins, and then recombinant protein molecules must be released in a soluble fraction (Owczarek et al., 2019; Tripathi et al., 2019). Due to their multiple classes and varied natures, an appropriate detergent should be selected, unique to a certain protein, in instruction to maximize protein constancy and extraction effectiveness. When recovering membrane proteins or cytosolic proteins from tissues rich in lipids, carbohydrates, and other nonprotein components, for instance, appropriate procedures should be used (Owczarek et al., 2019; Tripathi et al., 2019). Cell lysis can be accomplished using a variety of techniques, such as chemical and mechanical ones including osmotic shock lysis, enzyme digestion, sonication, or homogenization. The "ultimate" but most difficult recovery phase purification can begin after the proteins have been eliminated (Owczarek et al., 2019; Tripathi et al., 2019).

## 11.7 PURIFICATION TECHNIQUES

Even though technology has evolved since the invention of heterologous synthesis, researchers still regard purification as the greatest difficulty in the production of biotherapeutics (Kamionka, 2011). Extraneous proteins, endotoxins, or contaminants are not permitted in biopharmaceutical proteins or other proteins used in human medicine. The target protein is separated throughout the purification process while maintaining its chemical makeup and biological activity (Owczarek et al., 2019). Purification procedures account for between about 45 and 92% of the overall costs involved in manufacturing recombinant proteins. As a result, the purification strategy is crucial throughout the whole production process. Considerations for big recovery, simplicity, cost, and laboratory repeatability should all be taken into account. To fulfill the mandatory strictness of purity, which occasionally reaches 99% in the biopharmaceutical business, a chromatography technique is often necessary. The purification procedure is very important since it certifies the protein drug's purity beyond a shadow of a doubt. Important factors include the development of the host cell, cell culture, cell bank building, protein biosynthesis, purification process, and subsequent protein analysis, formulation, handling, and storage, as well as ensuring the purity, activity, and safety of the finished protein products (Owczarek et al., 2019).

Each method of protein purification uses a different protein characteristic, such as size exclusion. Proteins with a range in size are separated using chromatography, while proteins with a range in charge are separated using ion exchange chromatography, proteins with a range in hydrophobic interaction are separated using reverse-phase chromatography, and proteins with a range in ligand specificity are separated using affinity chromatography (Hong et al., 2012; Owczarek et al., 2019).

Upstream and downstream sequences make up the bioprocess for producing recombinant proteins. Before and during the creation of protein, the cells are fermented, including in the upstream process, and the finished protein is either expelled from the cells into the culture media, or the cells are lysed and the cell lysates are processed, including in the downstream process (Baumann et al., 2016). Examples of downstream processes include protein purification, protein formulation (notably concentration), bioconjugation, protein bioconjugate purification, and protein folding. Separating soluble and insoluble cell debris and medium components are further operations. Only one downstream step may be required depending on the protein and its particular requirements (Gupta et al., 2016; Richardson et al., 2018; Tripathi et al., 2019;).

## 11.8 QUANTIFICATION OF PROTEIN YIELDS

After density gradient centrifugation or filtration, relative quantitation can be used to determine which fractions are proteins and should be mixed for further processing. Either measurements of proteins or lipids serve as the basis for the quantitation. When comparing relative concentrations, dry weights of lyophilized extracellular quantifiable are occasionally employed; however, it should be noted that this procedure also quantifies the materials. A reference point for protein yields in comparison studies should be the volume of the original bacterial culture, as measured by optical density (OD), CFU, CFU/mL, protein, and bacterial pellet wet and dry weight (Azatian et al., 2019).

## 11.9 PROTEIN QUANTIFICATION

Several well-known techniques, including the Lowry (Lowry et al., 1951), Bradford (Bradford, 1976), and bicinchoninic acid test (Brown et al., 1989) assays, as well as image analysis of stained and immunodetected gel-separated materials, are used to quantify proteins. *P. aeruginosa* entire cell lysates and isolated proteins from matching culture supernatants are immunoblotted and densitometrically assessed (Goldring, 2019; Redmile-Gordon et al., 2013). The share of proteins in cell-free supernatants is then used to proportionally reflect the quantity of protein. Protein preparation samples from *Salmonella* and *E. coli* are separated using SDS-PAGE, stained with Coomassie Blue, and the densitometric measurements of the bands corresponding to the required proteins are performed. In a manner similar to this, a sample of bacterial protein is separated on a gel, stained with Coomassie Blue, and its relative quantity is calculated as a percentage of the overall protein production (Goldring, 2019; Redmile-Gordon et al., 2013).

## 11.10 THERAPEUTIC PEPTIDES AND PROTEINS AND BACTERIAL SOURCES

Therapeutic proteins and peptides like human insulin and somatostatin (Asadi et al., 2015; Baeshen et al., 2014; Rezaei et al., 2012). The GH,

-interferon, and other recent genetic engineering milestones include. Other significant recombinant proteins include the capsid proteins of the hematopoietic necrosis virus, Fab fragments, human nerve growth factor, human granulocyte colony-stimulating factor, single chain Fv fragments, and M. Table 11.1 lists the bacterial sources and applications for TB antigens, trypsin, Hsp65-hIL-2 fusion protein, fibronectin-binding protein A, a VP2-VP3 fusion protein of infectious pancreatic necrosis virus, pediocin PA-1, subtilisin, and CC chemokines (Ayala et al., 2013; Chi et al., 2009; Damelin et al., 2010; Dammeyer et al., 2011; Datta, 2021; Eom et al., 2010; Guo et al., 2012; Innocentin et al., 2009; Jin et al., 2011; Rippa et al., 2012; Simon et al., 2001; Toyokawa et al., 2010; Vigentini et al., 2006; Zhao et al., 2012).

### 11.10.1 HUMAN INSULIN

Due to the continuously increasing number of diabetes patients worldwide and the research into other insulin delivery methods, such as the oral route or inhalation, that need higher dosages, the demand for recombinant insulin is anticipated to increase in the near future (Baeshen et al., 2014). An appropriate host organism with efficient PTMs and protein folding machinery is required for the production of therapeutic recombinant proteins. Recombinant human insulin for therapeutic use in humans has mostly been produced using *E. coli* (Baeshen et al., 2014). Several recombinant protein-based drugs created utilizing various expression strategies have received FDA approval (Baeshen et al., 2014). The FDA has authorized a number of recombinant protein-based medications made using different expression techniques (Baeshen et al., 2014). In order to maintain glucose homeostasis, insulin is crucial. The two protein chains that make up insulin have a combined amino acid content of 51, with 21 amino acids each making up the A and B chains, which are connected by disulfide bridges (Baeshen et al., 2014). The precursor hormone proinsulin, which is converted into insulin, has a molecular mass of 5802 Da, an isoelectric point of 5.5, and 74 amino acids. Pro-insulin produced by beta cells is relatively inactive under biological conditions, but after being cleaved twice, the two chains (B and A) of the active hormone insulin and the physiologically inert C peptide are created. Disulfide bonds provide an antiparallel connection that connects the B (helical center segment) and A chains on the C-terminal helix (Asadi et al., 2015). The center terminals of the C- and N-terminal helices of A and B are joined to the A and B chains via a disulfide bridge. In response to stimulation, pro-insulin, insulin, and the C-peptide-containing granules in the beta cells release insulin into the capillaries of the islet cells. These capillaries empty into the portal vein, which carries blood from the intestines and stomach to the liver. After being exposed to hyperglycemia for 30 minutes, the blood's level of insulin will increase. Healthy adults have a pancreas storage of 200 units on average, and they produce around a tablespoon of insulin into their circulation each day (Asadi et al., 2015).

### 11.10.2 HUMAN GROWTH HORMONE

Human growth hormone (rGH) is a single-chain polypeptide that plays a part in many biological processes, such as the metabolism of proteins, lipids, and carbohydrates, as well as in growth, immunity, and development. Both children and adults' humans can lack GH (Rezaei et al., 2012). Recombinant human GH produced by prokaryotes is typically administered as a therapy for this illness. It is recommended to produce human GH using prokaryotic expression methods since no glycosylated form of the hormone is a physiologically active protein. This has removed the need for pituitary-derived preparation. The ability to express proteins in host cells like *E. coli* has been made possible by advancements in recombinant DNA technology. Recombinant *E. coli* is used in high cell-density fermentation to produce excessive amounts of recombinant proteins. Strong, inducible promoter systems, such as lPL, lPR, and T7, were often used by *E. coli* (Rezaei et al., 2012; Rosano et al., 2014).

### 11.10.3 INTERFERON

Natural glycoproteins called interferons are created by eukaryotic cells that are infected with viruses and serve to protect host cells against viral infection. Enzymatic synthesis of a human leukocyte interferon cDNA was carried out, and the vector pBR322 was then introduced into *Escherichia coli* (Goeddel et al., 1980; Swiecki et al., 2011). An interferon polypeptide with 165 amino acids is followed by a signal peptide with 23 amino acids in the DNA sequence. The fact that interferons target host cells rather than particular viruses is a standout property of these proteins (Goeddel et al., 1980; Swiecki et al., 2011).

## 11.11 IMPORTANCE OF MICROBIAL ENZYMES IN BIOTECHNOLOGY

Industrial enzymes are mostly produced by bacteria. Researchers were able to safely transfer genes that code for a certain feature from one organism to another because of innovative technological advancements. Additionally, this enhances the creation of enzymes and ensures a sufficient supply. In many aspects, the quality and output of bacteria enzymes have improved because of biotechnological technologies (Adrio et al., 2014). There are several benefits to using biotechnology instead of more conventional techniques for producing bacterial enzymes. By avoiding other undesirable qualities, the genetic alteration of a bacterium is directed to assure the transmission of the desired phenotype. Enzyme synthesis requires extremely little energy and raw resources, and the products made possible by biotechnological methods will have little effect on the environment. It has been determined that using enzymes made from bacterial sources is safe, and they substitute chemical processes that burn energy and harm the environmental (Adrio et al., 2014). Microorganisms offer an amazing variety of catalysts in a wide number of sectors, like pharmaceuticals, specialty chemicals, food, domestic care, animal feed, and scientific industries. Due to the unique properties of enzymes, such as their high selectivity, quick action, and biodegradability, industrial advances backed by enzymes can function under gentler reaction conditions, resulting in more yields and less waste creation (Adrio et al., 2014).

## 11.12 SOME IMPORTANT ENZYMES AND BACTERIAL SPECIES

### *11.12.1 PROTEASES*

*Pseudomonas aeruginosa* is known to produce proteases and peptidyl peptide hydrolases, which are helpful in businesses that denature amino acids by adding water across peptide initiation and catalyze peptide synthesis in organic solvents and cleansers with limited water content (Akbarian et al., 2022). Proteolytic enzymes are present in the majority of living organisms and are crucial for cell differentiation and growth. *Pseudomonas aeruginosa* produces extracellular protease, which has the most protease activity at pH 9.5, at 37°C, and 48 hours of incubation, primarily from maltose (Akbarian et al., 2022).

### 11.12.2 LIPASE

Glycerol ester hydrolases called lipases hydrolyze the ester links in glycerides at the water-oil line. According to current studies, *Pseudomonas aeruginosa* is the most widely used bacteria for the production of lipases, which have found application in various fields of commercial importance (Chandra et al., 2020). In recent decades, the production of microbial lipase has become more significant. These enzymes consume specific biotechnological requirements in a variety of industrial fields, such as environmental waste management, cosmetology, and food, thanks to their biomolecular structure and catalytic possessions. In particular, lipase performance is a catalyst for the combination of esters and for the transesterification of the oil to produce biodiesel (Adrio et al., 2014).

### 11.12.3 A-AMYLASE

Different types of bacteria can generate amylase; however, for commercial purposes, α-amylase is mostly obtained from the *genus Bacillus* (de Souza et al., 2010). It is possible to use the amylases produced by the bacteria *Bacillus licheniformis*, *Bacillus amyloliquefaciens*, and *Bacillus stearothermophilus* in a diversity of industrial progressions, together with those in the food, fermentation, textiles, and paper sectors (de Souza et al., 2010).

### 11.12.4 GLUCOSE ISOMERASE

*Bacillus* offers a spectacular and various species of bacteria, among others, that can manufacture glucose isomerase. Glucose and xylose are reversibly isomerized into fructose and xylulose, individually, by the enzyme glucose isomerase (Bhosale et al., 1996). The enzyme is used in the manufacturing of high-fructose corn syrup, which gives it the greatest market in the food industry. Diabetes sufferers can utilize high-fructose corn syrup, asymmetry blend of glucose and fructose that is 1.3 times sweetened than sucrose. In addition to being a necessary component of bacterial nutrition, glucose isomerase's interconversion of xylose to xylulose has potential use in the bio-conversion of hemicellulose to ethanol (Bhosale et al., 1996).

### 11.12.5 CELLULASES

When growing on cellulosic materials, a wide variety of microorganisms, including fungi and bacteria, also produce cellulases. These microbes might be mesophilic, thermophilic, aerobic, or anaerobic. The most well-researched cellulase producers among them are those belonging to the genera *Clostridium, Cellulomonas*, and *Thermomonospora* (Ejaz et al., 2021; Kuhad et al., 2011). These organisms have sophisticated enzyme machinery for cellulose destruction that consists of three different types of enzymatic components, allowing them to use cellulose as their primary food supply. Cellulases are now employed in the nutrition, animal feed, pharmaceutical formulation, laundry, paper and pulp, detergent production, agricultural, textile, and research industries. The creation of potent expression systems for industrial enzymes and their engineering for increased performance has been made possible by the advancement of molecular biotechnology (Ejaz et al., 2021; Kuhad et al., 2011).

### 11.12.6 B-GALACTOSIDASE

A β-galactosidase from the *thermophilic Thermus sp.* hydrolyzes lactose. The food industry has been working to create products with minimal or no lactose. As a result, the main biotechnological process that produces glucose and galactose monosaccharides from sugar enzymatic hydrolysis from the β-galactosidase enzyme emerges as having applications in the dairy business (Nakkharat et al., 2006; Saqib et al., 2017). Initially, milk used to make sweets and fermented dairy items underwent preliminary treatment with β-galactosidase. The sensory and technical qualities of the finished goods are improved as a result of this application, including increased sweetness, increased solubility, and a shorter fermentation time (Nakkharat et al., 2006; Saqib et al., 2017).

**TABLE 11.1** A List of Applications for Bacteria and Recombinant Proteins in Medical and Therapeutic

| Bacteria | Recombinant Proteins | Application | References |
|---|---|---|---|
| *Caulobacter crescentus* | Hematopoietic necrosis virus capsid proteins | Its straightforward composition, symmetrical structure, and conscience make it an effective instrument for a compound delivery system. | Simon et al. (2001) |
| | | Physical resistance to many unfavorable conditions guarantees oral delivery and long-term preservation. | |
| *Pseudoalteromonas Haloplanktis* | 3H6 Fab fragments | Anti-idiotypic antibody against the 2F5 anti-HIV-1 monoclonal antibody, which has a broad neutralizing spectrum. | Rippa et al. (2012) |
| *Pseudoalteromonas haloplanktis* | Human nerve growth factor | A very promising treatment for a number of immune-related pathologies, in addition to dementia of the central and peripheral nervous systems. | Vigentini et al. (2006) |
| *Pseudomonas Fluorescens* | Granulocyte colony-stimulating factor | Utilized in patients with certain malignancies and neutropenia brought on by particular forms of chemotherapy. | Datta (2021); Jin et al. (2011) |
| *Pseudomonas putida* | Single chain Fv fragments | Fragments are essential instruments for analysis, diagnosis, and treatment. | Dammeyer et al. (2011) |
| *Streptomyces lividans* | M. tuberculosis antigens | The development of diagnostic tools that can identify HIV-positive patients who are at a high risk of acquiring clinical TB will benefit from the use of these antigens. | Ayala et al. (2013) |
| *Streptomyces griseus* | Trypsin | These enzymatic characteristics were very comparable to those of actual eukaryotic trypsin that had been isolated from the pancreas of a cow. | Chi et al. (2009) |
| *Mycobacterium smegmatis* | Hsp65-hIL-2 fusion protein | The performance of lymphocytes is considerably improved by Hsp65/IL-2. As a result, the fusion protein created by Hsp65/IL-2 may one day be used to create a TB vaccine. | Guo et al. (2012) |

**TABLE 11.1** *(Continued)*

| Bacteria | Recombinant Proteins | Application | References |
|---|---|---|---|
| *Lactococcus lactis* | Fibronectin-binding protein A | The control of cell migration, tissue healing, and adhesion are all significantly influenced by human fibronectin. In the digestive system, bacterial adhesins frequently target fibronectin. | Innocentin et al. (2009) |
| *Lactobacillus casei* | Infectious pancreatic necrosis virus VP2-VP3 fusion protein | Using multivalent vaccinations for viral infections. | Zhao et al. (2012) |
| *Lactobacillus reuteri* | Pediocin PA-1 | The antimicrobial peptide pediocin PA-1, a class IIa bacteriocin, inhibits the clinically significant pathogens Listeria species and other pathogens. | Eom et al. (2010) |
| *Bacillus licheniformis* | Subtilisin | skincare products, eyeglass cleaners, and synthetic organic chemistry study. | Tcyokawa et al. (2010) |
| *Lactobacillus gasseri* | CC chemokines | A novel approach to preventing HIV transmission across mucosal membranes may include transduction in vaginal Lactobacillus species. | Damelin et al. (2010) |

### 11.12.7 SINGLE-CELL PROTEIN FROM BACTERIA

In general, microbial protein is known as single-cell protein, also called SCP, even if approximately of the generating microorganisms, including microalgae, fungus, bacteria, and maybe multicellular organisms, may also produce SCP. Bacteria contributed to protein requests when they are utilized to improve the protein content and quality of fermented meals, in addition to their direct usage as SCP (Ritala et al., 2017; Sasikala et al., 1995). Even though microbial protein only makes up a minor fraction of the present human diet, SCP is anticipated to become more significant as the world's demand for protein rises. Processes that offer substantially better efficiency and/or sustainability than traditional agriculture are made possible by fast growth rates or the capacity to use special substrates, such as $CO_2$ or methane (Matassa, 2016). When it comes to human consumption, just a few bacteria species are being used to make SCP. The variety of SCP sources utilized in animal feed is growing and is wider than those permitted for human consumption (Ritala et al., 2017). Nutritional medium, maybe from waste (a) growing, including solid state fermentation; (b) isolating and concentrating SCP, possibly drying it; and (c) lastly processing SCP into components and products. As SCP for human consumption is frequently created from food-grade substrates, there is confidence that techniques will be developed to make SCP from competitively cost waste materials from the food and beverage processing industries, as well as directly from forestry and agricultural sources. With the inclusion of algae to microbial protein suppliers, production from $CO_2$ has become feasible, and the greenhouse gas methane is providing a special source of carbon for SCP from bacteria (Ritala et al., 2017; Sasikala et al., 1995).

Furthermore, bacteria have a long history of use as SCP, particularly in animal feed. Bacterial SCP generally contains 50–80 percent protein on a dry weight basis, and the crucial amino acid concentration is predicted to be higher than the FAO criteria. Methionine concentrations of up to 3.0% have been seen, which is higher than what is generally found in algal or fungal SCP (Zamani et al., 2020). Bacteria that thrive in methanol and methane have comparable amino acid profiles. Due to its high nucleic acid content (8–12%), notably RNA, bacterial SCP, like fungus, needs to be processed before being utilized as feed or food. Along with protein and nucleic acid, bacterial SCP also supplies a few lipids and vitamins from the B group. Industries produced an SCP (Pruteen) from methanol using the microorganisms *Methylophilus methylotrophs* for animal feed. Pruteen, which contains up to 70% protein, was utilized in pig feed. Pruteen's production, however, was stopped because it was unable to compete with the more affordable animal feeds that were becoming available by the end of the 1970s (Patthawaro et al., 2019; Zamani et al., 2020). Originally produced from methanol, pruteen is now being produced from methane, which is gaining interest as a possible SCP substrate. The U-loop fermenter enhances the quantity of methane that is available to the bacteria by boosting the mass transfer rates of methane from the gas to the liquid phase. The fact that methane is a large by-product of producing pigs and cattle as well as being produced as biogas in areas like landfills and garbage cans makes it an interesting substrate (Ritala et al., 2017). The reactor design and selections for integrating flaring methanotrophic bacteria such as *Methylococcus capsulatus, Methylocystis parvus*, and *Methylosinus trichosporium* with the production of microbial oil and feed protein.

Further improvements in the production of bacterial SCP focus on enhancing various waste substrates and wastewater treatment by vaporization, much as how fungi make SCP (Ritala et al., 2017). As in the two-step treatment of potato starch production waste, *Aspergillus niger* is used to break down the fibers in the residual potato material, and *Bacillus licheniformis* is utilized to produce a protein. Another case of concurrently regulating wastewater and making SCP from waste from the manufacture of rubber sheets (Ritala et al., 2017). They demonstrated that the wastewater's chemical oxygen demand (COD), suspended solids, and total sulphones were reduced to levels compliant with Thailand's standards for use as irrigation water, and that the biomass produced was suitable for SCP by the purple no sulfur bacterium *Rhodopseudomonas palustris*. Soybean husk that had been fermented with *B. subtilis* to boost its nutritional value as a feed for monogastric animals was characterized as a distinctive secondary product that was co-produced with bacterial SCP. *Cupriavidus necator* cultivation on a large scale was done to produce biomass that was high in protein and polyhydroxyalkanoate (PHA) (Ritala et al., 2017).

## 11.13 APPLICATION OF BACTERIAL PROTEINS OR ENZYMES

Industrially manufactured proteins and enzymes are synthesized from bacterial sources and are widely employed in the medical and pharmaceutical industries. According to Singh et al. (2016), bacterial proteins or enzymes are also employed in the food, environment, leather, cosmetics, textiles, and detergent industries. Figure 11.3 provides a brief summary of these applications.

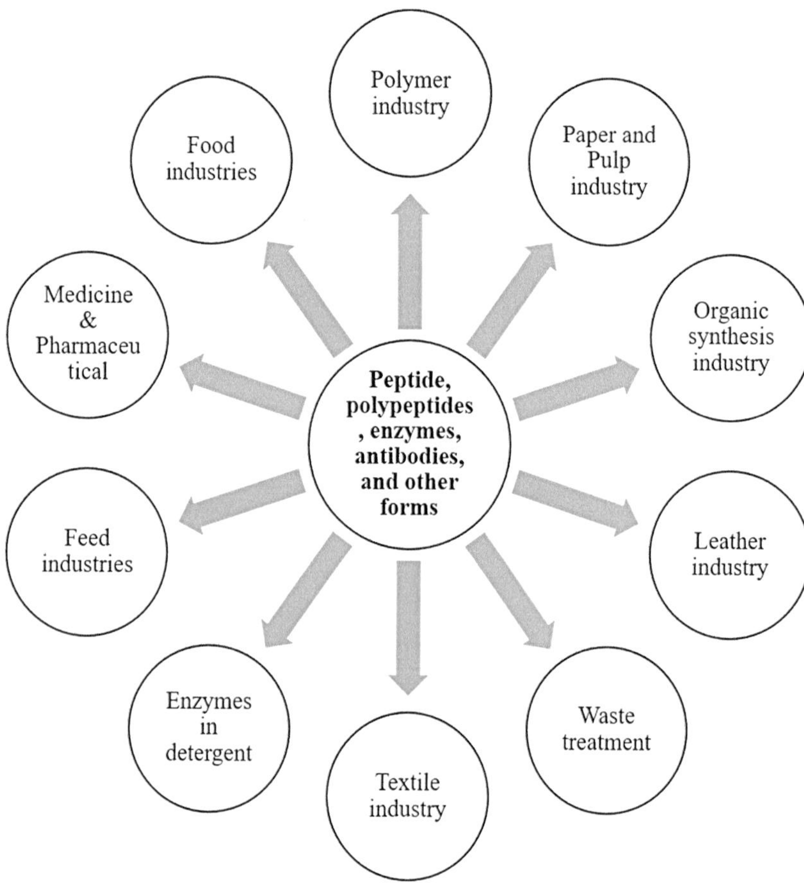


**FIGURE 11.3** Application of protein and polypeptide or enzyme in different industries.

### *11.13.1 MEDICINE AND PHARMACEUTICAL*

Enzymes serve a number of significant and essential functions in the pharmaceutical and analytical industries. These are broadly applied in diagnostic processes like ELISA and diabetes testing kits, as well as therapeutic medications for conditions including enzymatic deficiency and digestive problems (de la Fuente et al., 2021). The broad usage of enzymes for technical and systematic reasons is utilized to evaluate the catalytic activity of enzymes present in biological samples, as well as the concentration of substrates. Enzyme technology advancements have decreased or eliminated the requirement for hazardous radioactive elements in a range of immunoassays, which are used to assess a range of varieties of proteins (hormone and enzyme) (Singh et al., 2016). Enzymes are necessary for nucleic acid manipulation in genetic engineering research and development because they allow for site-specific DNA cleavage for molecular cloning and DNA polymerases for PCR-based DNA amplification (Singh et al., 2016). The following is a list of medicinal and therapeutic uses for bacteria and recombinant proteins shown in Table 11.1. Some significant bacteria, including *Clostridium perfringens, Lactobacillus plantarum, Bacillus subtilis, Pseudomonas acidovorans*, and derived proteins and enzymes, are used in health issues shown (Singh et al., 2016) in Table 11.2.

### 11.13.2 FOOD INDUSTRY

The usage of enzymes in the food area may assist in solving the problems with the quality of the food supply. These biomolecules effectively contribute to enhancing the creation of food and its many elements, including flavor, fragrance, color, texture, appearance, and nutritional value (Raveendran et al., 2018). The fundamental procedures have been modified to supply due to its direct with safer and higher-quality goods as a result of the comprehensive thoughtful of the role of enzymes in the food production and constituents' industry.

Furthermore, new fields like fat modification and sweetener technology attracted attention to enzymes. The food and beverage industry now dominates the market for industrial enzymes, and this trend is estimated to remain. To produce more juice with better color and flavor, regulate the brewing process to produce consistently high-quality beer, and improve the functional and nutritional characteristics of animal and plant proteins through enzymatic hydrolysis, enzymes are utilized in the beverage and food sectors. The food sector uses enzymes in a variety of areas, including brewing, juice production, dairy production, and baking (Singh et al., 2016). The primary application industry for microbial enzymes in the food sector, bakeries, employ them successfully all over the world

**TABLE 11.2** Different Protein or Enzyme Types are Used in Various Industrial Uses and Applications

| Bacteria | Proteins or Enzymes | Industrial Uses | |
|---|---|---|---|
| *Escherichia coli* | Asparaginase | Medicine and therapeutics | Anticancer activity |
| *Pseudomonas acidovorans* | Glutaminase | | Anticancer activity |
| *Lactobacillus plantarum* | Superoxide dismutase | | Anti-inflammatory activity |
| *Bacillus subtilis* | urokinase | | Anticoagulants activity |
| *Clostridium perfringens* | Collagenase | | Skin ulcers |
| *Bacillus subtilis* | Neutral proteinase | Dairy | Faster debittering and ripening of cheese |
| *Escherichia coli* | Lactase (β-galactosidase) | | Milk and whey products with decreased lactose |
| *Lactobacillus* sp. | Aminopeptidase | | Faster ripening of cheese |
| *Streptomyces* sp. | Transglutaminase | | Cross-linking of proteins |
| *Bacillus* sp. | Amylase | Baking | Bread softness, flour adjustments |
| *Bacillus stearothermophilus* | Maltogenic α-Amylase | | Lengthen the bread's shelf life |
| *Streptoverticillium* sp., *streptomyces* sp. | Transglutaminase | | Layered dough toughness |
| *Bacillus* | α-Amylase | Beverages | Starch hydrolysis |
| *Bacillus, Streptomyces* | β-Amylase | | Starch hydrolysis |
| *Bacillus subtilis* | β-Glucanase | | Restrict the growth of haze |
| *Bacillus* sp., *Klebsiella* sp. | Pullulanase | | Starch saccharification |
| *Lactobacillus brevis, L. plantarum* | Aminopeptidases | | During mashing, proteins are broken down |
| *Bacillus sp.* | Xylanase | Animal Feed | Enhanced starch digestibility |
| *Bacillus subtilis* | Protease | Pulp and Paper | Removing biofilm |
| *Bacillus licheniformis* | Amylase | | Improved drainage and decontamination |
| *Bacillus subtilis* | Laccase | | Bleaching without chlorine and delignification |
| *Bacillus* sp. | Cellulase | | Improved drainage and decontamination |
| *Streptomyces mobaraensis* | Transglutaminase | Polymer | Protein crosslinking |

**TABLE 11.2** *(Continued)*

| Bacteria | Proteins or Enzymes | Industrial Uses | |
|---|---|---|---|
| *Bacillus subtilis* | Amylase | Detergent | Removal of carbohydrate stains |
| *Bacillus subtilis* | Protease | | Removing protein stains |
| *Bacillus* sp. | Cellulase | | Clarification of colors |
| *Bacillus* sp. | Mannanase | | Mannan spot elimination |
| *Alcaligenes faecalis* | Alkaline protease | Leather | Removing hair, bating |
| *Bacillus subtilis* | Neutral Protease | | Removing hair, soaking |
| *Bacillus subtilis* | Amylase | | Fiber fracturing |
| *Corynebacterium glutamicum, Lactobacillus plantarum* | Superoxide dismutase | Cosmetics | Skincare, scavenging free radicals |
| *Bacillus subtilis* | Protease | | Getting rid of dead skin |
| *Bacillus subtilis,* | Laccase | | Hair dye |
| *Bacillus sp.* | Glycosyl transferase | Organic Acids | Synthesizing oligosaccharides |
| *Rhodococcus rhodochrous, Bacillus* sp. | Nitrile hydratase | | Nicotinamide, butyramide, and acrylamide are biosynthetic products. |
| *Corynebacterium* sp., *streptomyces murinus* | Glucose isomerase | | High fructose corn syrup production |
| *Bacillus* sp. | Acyltransferase | | Synthesizing of hydroxamic acids |
| *Bacillus subtilis* | Laccase | | Production of insecticides, flavoring agents, cosmetic pigments, and textile colors |
| *Rhodococcus erythropolis* | Amidase | Waste management | Destruction of wastes containing nitriles |
| *B. licheniformis* | Amylase | | Vegetable waste bioremediation |
| *Rhodococcus* sp. | Nitrile hydratase | | Destruction of wastes containing nitriles |
| *Pseudomonas* sp., *Rhodococcus sp* | Oxygenase | | Halogenated contaminants degradation |

*Source:* Khan et al. (2012); Raveendran et al. (2018); Singh et al. (2016).

to extend product shelf life, improve crumb softness and structure, and maintain dough stability. The growth in the use of microbial enzymes in cheese manufacturing is largely responsible for the increase in enzyme consumption in the dairy sector, which is the second-largest application business after the beverages industry (Singh et al., 2016). As demonstrated in Table 11.2, the dairy, baking, and beverage industries utilize *Bacillus subtilis, Escherichia coli, Lactobacillus* sp., *Streptomyces* sp., *Bacillus* sp., *Bacillus stearothermophilus*, *Streptoverticillium* sp., *Klebsiella* sp., *Lactobacillus brevis*, and *L. plantarum* (Khan et al., 2012; Raveendran et al., 2018; Singh et al., 2016).

### 11.13.3 FEED INDUSTRY

The production of feed enzymes has steadily increased as milk and meat consumption have increased around the globe. Feed enzymes are gaining importance due to their capacity to enhance nutrient digestion and encourage animal feed intake. Feed enzymes may be used in the production of an animal's food to break down specific feed components that could otherwise be poisonous or innutritious, for example (Golder et al., 2019; Matthews et al., 2019). Additionally, the addition of feed enzymes may enhance the protein nutritional content of the meals made accessible. These feed enzymes are playing a larger role in lowering feed costs and enhancing the quality of the meat, in addition to boosting the nutritional value of feed for improved feed conversion by the animals (Golder et al., 2019; Matthews et al., 2019). These enzymes are added to their meals because xylanase totally digests and breaks down large amounts of starch. *Bacillus* sp. is the most frequently used in the feed industry (Golder et al., 2019; Matthews et al., 2019).

### 11.13.4 PAPER AND PULP INDUSTRY

The paper and pulp industry has increasingly increased the usage of microbial enzymes as awareness of environmental problems has grown. This has helped to reduce the industry's harmful effects on the environment (Li et al., 2012). Utilizing enzymes reduces the number of chemicals processed, the energy required, and the processing time. Enzymes are also utilized to raise biological oxygen demand (BOD) and COD in order to improve drinking water, bleach in the paper and pulp industries, and waste treatment (Singh et al., 2016). Along with *Bacillus licheniformis* and other *Bacillus* species, *Bacillus subtilis* is one of the bacteria used in the paper and pulp industries (Singh et al., 2016) (Table 11.2).

### 11.13.5 POLYMER INDUSTRY

Utilizing microbial enzymes to create a biodegradable polymer has become necessary due to the rising demand for polymers and developing environmental safety concerns. Environmentally responsible procedures with a variety of advantages over conventional chemical processes include *in vitro* enzyme, catalysis, and polymer synthesis (Vroman et al., 2009). Because they are produced from renewable carbon sources through biological processes, biopolymers are materials that are healthy for the environment because they degrade after use through biological processes and release renewable resources like $CO_2$ and biomass back into the environment. Adhesion barriers, tissue engineering, orthopedic devices, and drug delivery control using polyesters, polycarbonates, and polyphosphates are a few examples of biopolymers employed in a variety of biomedical applications. The polymer industry makes use of *Streptomyces mobaraensis* (Manavitehrani et al., 2016). In order to enable *in situ* polymerization of materials, the biopolymer industry uses the enzyme transglutaminase to create cross-links in biopolymers (Manavitehrani et al., 2016).

### 11.13.6 LEATHER INDUSTRY

Biodegradable enzymes are a useful replacement to improve leather quality and decrease waste (Singh et al., 2016). The first attempt at employing enzymes in the leather industry was done during the dehairing process, which is the first stage in leather preparation and requires a large number of enzymes, including proteases, lipases, and amylases. Enzymatic dehairing applications are desirable because they may preserve hair while minimizing the amount of organic load emitted into the effluent. Enzymatic dehairing techniques reduce or do away with the need for hazardous chemicals like sulfide, lime, and amines (Singh et al., 2016). During several steps of the leather-processing process, including soaking, curing, liming, dehairing, bating, plucking, tanning, and degreasing, enzymes are used to expedite procedures and improve leather quality. *Alcaligenes faecalis* and *Bacillus subtilis* are mostly used in the leather industry.

### 11.13.7 COSMETICS INDUSTRY

Nowadays, enzymes are employed increasingly frequently in cosmetics. In toothpaste, mouthwash, hair color, and sunscreen lotion, enzymes act as free radical scavengers. Superoxide dismutase (SOD) is used to fight free radicals, heal skin damage brought on by germs, air pollution, and other hazardous agents, and prevent more skin damage (Jeeva et al., 2015; Singh et al., 2016). Together, the antioxidants SOD, peroxidases, and sunscreen lotion lessen erythema. By removing damaged or dead skin, proteases are utilized in skin treatments to clean and smooth the skin. Another enzyme that is typically present in toothpaste and mouthwash is endoglycosidase (Jeeva et al., 2015; Singh et al., 2016). It is used to whiten teeth, get rid of plaque, and eliminate deposits on gum tissue and teeth that cause odors. Laccase is used in hair coloring. Table 11.2 shows that the cosmetics industry frequently uses *Corynebacterium glutamicum, Lactobacillus plantarum*, and *Bacillus subtilis* (Jeeva et al., 2015; Singh et al., 2016).

### 11.13.8 DETERGENTS INDUSTRY

The growth and development of enzymes have had a significant positive impact on industrial detergents, one of the main application areas for enzymes today. Enzymes are present in detergent products to aid in their more effective removal of protein, carbohydrate, oil, and fat stains. Laundry detergents include weight-effective enzymes that improve whiteness, color, and fabric care while removing frayed cotton strands (Li et al., 2012). The hydrolase group enzymes that are used most frequently in detergent solutions include amylase and protease. Proteases, amylases, and cellulases may occasionally be used in concert for better stain removal and fabric maintenance. It is preferable to employ enzymes in detergent products since they have a good effect on public and environmental health due to the fact that they include fewer phosphates and bleaching agents (Singh et al., 2016). Other Bacillus species, such as *Bacillus subtilis*

(Singh et al., 2016), are extensively employed in the detergent industry; more information is provided in Table 11.2.

### 11.13.9 ORGANIC SYNTHESIS INDUSTRY

Enzymes are more selective than conventional methods used in commercial chemical synthesis because they are positional, chiral, and functional group-specific (Singh et al., 2016). Achieving such high selectivity during chemical synthesis is particularly beneficial as it may lead to fewer environmental concerns, easier separation, and little to no by-product formation (Singh et al., 2016). Additional advantages of enzyme-mediated commercial applications include high catalytic efficiency and comfortable working circumstances. Industrial synthetic chemistry has been making cheese and alcohol utilizing bacteria's catalytic capabilities for hundreds of years. Since they are necessary for cellular identification and communication processes, glycosyltransferases with high region and stereoselectivity are used to create oligosaccharides and polysaccharides in the industrial setting (Singh et al., 2016). Nitrile hydratase is responsible for the production of acrylamide. High fructose corn syrup, a substitute for sucrose in the food and beverage industry, is commercially produced in excess of a million metric tons per year (Singh et al., 2016). Numerous *Bacillus species*, including *Bacillus subtilis, Streptomyces murinus, Corynebacterium species, Rhodococcus rhodochrous*, and others, have uses, which are presented in Table 11.2.

### 11.13.10 WASTE TREATMENT

Enzymes are widely used for waste management, and many of them are involved in the breakdown of toxic pollutants. Various chemical compounds that are hazardous or dangerous to ecosystems and living creatures are found in both household and industrial waste (Thompson et al., 2009). Industrial effluents including phenols, aromatic amines, nitriles, and so forth, are treated using microbial enzymes by converting harmful chemical molecules into harmless ones through biodegradation or other means (Mohanan et al., 2020). Information on the waste treatment and application using *Rhodococcus erythropolis, B. licheniformis*, and *Pseudomonas* sp. (Mohanan et al., 2020) (Table 11.2).

## 11.14 CONCLUSION AND FUTURE DIRECTION

Because proteins offer enormous potential for many sectors to meet the needs of a rapidly expanding population and deal with the depletion of natural resources, the potential for using bacterial proteins (is promising). Three key requirements, including microbial sources, strain enhancement, and techniques for recovering enzymes in increasing quantities with excellent quality, underpin the production of microbial enzymes in industry. Traditional methods were replaced by membrane filtering technology enhanced with downstream processing to raise the proportion of enzyme recovery and also to enhance enzyme activity. This chapter has shown the potential of proteins in a number of industrial domains, together with medicine, food, feed, beverages, detergents, paper and pulp, and leather processing. The use of genetic engineering techniques in combination with a membrane filtering approach and a downstream process, which is thought to be a replacement for chemical methods, is where contemporary biotechnology will go in the future. Instead, frequent usage of these biomolecules might help to fulfill the growing need for food around the globe. Microorganism-produced enzymes offer enormous promise for waste management and, as a result, for the creation of a greener planet. Many industries take advantage of the usage of enzymes because they produce higher-quality products more quickly and with less pollution.

## KEYWORDS

- **bacillus subtilis**
- ***E. coli***
- **enzymes**
- **genetic engineering**
- **pseudomonas**
- **recombinant proteins**

## REFERENCES

Adrio, J. L., & Demain, A. L. (2010). Recombinant organisms for production of industrial products. *Bioengineered Bugs*, *1*, 116–131.

Adrio, J. L., & Demain, A. L. (2014). Microbial enzymes: Tools for biotechnological processes. *Biomolecules*, *4*, 117–139.

Akbarian, M., Khani, A., Eghbalpour, S., & Uversky, V. N. (2022). Bioactive peptides: Synthesis, sources, applications, and proposed mechanisms of action. *International Journal of Molecular Sciences*, *23*, 1445.

Asadi, A., Bruin, J. E., & Kieffer, T. J. (2015). Characterization of antibodies to products of proinsulin processing using immunofluorescence staining of pancreas in multiple species. *Journal of Histochemistry & Cytochemistry*, *63*, 646–662.

Ayala, J. C., Pimienta, E., Rodríguez, C., et al. (2013). Use of Strep-tag II for rapid detection and purification of *Mycobacterium tuberculosis* recombinant antigens secreted by *Streptomyces lividans*. *Journal of Microbiological Methods*, *94*, 192–198.

Azatian, S. B., Kaur, N., & Latham, M. P. (2019). Increasing the buffering capacity of minimal media leads to higher protein yield. *Journal of Biomolecular NMR*, *73*, 11–17.

Baeshen, N. A., Baeshen, M. N., Sheikh, A., et al. (2014). Cell factories for insulin production. *Microbial Cell Factories*, *13*, 141.

Barka, E. A., Vatsa, P., Sanchez, L., Gaveau-Vaillant, N., Jacquard, C., Meier-Kolthoff, J. P., Klenk, H. P., Clément, C., Ouhdouch, Y., & van Wezel, G. P. (2015). Taxonomy, physiology, and natural products of Actinobacteria. *Microbiology and Molecular Biology Reviews*, *80*, 1–43.

Baumann, P., & Hubbuch, J. (2016). Downstream process development strategies for effective bioprocesses: Trends, progress, and combinatorial approaches. *Engineering in Life Sciences*, *17*, 1142–1158.

Bhosale, S. H., Rao, M. B., & Deshpande, V. V. (1996). Molecular and industrial aspects of glucose isomerase. *Microbiological Reviews*, *60*, 280–300.

Bonnet, M., Lagier, J. C., Raoult, D., & Khelaifia, S. (2019). Bacterial culture through selective and non-selective conditions: The evolution of culture media in clinical microbiology. *New Microbes and New Infections*, *34*, 100622.

Chandra, P., Enespa, Singh, R., & Arora, P. K. (2020). Microbial lipases and their industrial applications: A comprehensive review. *Microbial Cell Factories*, *19*, 169.

Chen, Y., Mutukuri, T. T., Wilson, N. E., & Zhou, Q. T. (2021). Pharmaceutical protein solids: Drying technology, solid-state characterization and stability. *Advanced Drug Delivery Reviews*, *172*, 211–233.

Chi, W. J., Song, J. H., Oh, E. A., et al. (2009). Medium optimization and application of an affinity column chromatography for *Streptomyces griseus* trypsin production from the recombinant *Streptomyces griseus*. *Journal of Microbiology and Biotechnology*, *19*, 1191–1196.

Chou, C. P. (2007). Engineering cell physiology to enhance recombinant protein production in *Escherichia coli*. *Applied Microbiology and Biotechnology*, *76*, 521–532.

Damelin, L. H., Mavri-Damelin, D., Klaenhammer, T. R., & Tiemessen, C. T. (2010). Plasmid transduction using bacteriophage Phi(adh) for expression of CC chemokines by *Lactobacillus gasseri* ADH. *Applied and Environmental Microbiology*, *76*, 3878–3885.

Dammeyer, T., Steinwand, M., Krüger, S. C., Dübel, S., Hust, M., & Timmis, K. N. (2011). Efficient production of soluble recombinant single chain Fv fragments by a *Pseudomonas putida* strain KT2440 cell factory. *Microbial Cell Factories*, *10*, 11.

Datta, S. (2021). Optimizing granulocyte colony-stimulating factor transcript for enhanced expression in *Escherichia coli*. *Frontiers in Bioengineering and Biotechnology*, *9*, 630367.

De Carvalho, C. C. (2017). Whole cell biocatalysts: Essential workers from nature to the industry. *Microbial Biotechnology*, *10*, 250–263.

De la Fuente, M., Lombardero, L., Gómez-González, A., Solari, C., Angulo-Barturen, I., Acera, A., Vecino, E., Astigarraga, E., & Barreda-Gómez, G. (2021). Enzyme therapy: Current challenges and future perspectives. *International Journal of Molecular Sciences*, *22*, 9181.

De Simeis, D., & Serra, S. (2021). Actinomycetes: A never-ending source of bioactive compounds—An overview on antibiotics production. *Antibiotics (Basel)*, *10*, 483.

De Souza, P. M., & de Oliveira Magalhães, P. (2010). Application of microbial α-amylase in industry—A review. *Brazilian Journal of Microbiology*, *41*, 850–861.

Diggle, S. P., & Whiteley, M. (2020). Microbe profile: *Pseudomonas aeruginosa*: opportunistic pathogen and lab rat. *Microbiology (Reading)*, *166*, 30–33.

Ejaz, U., Sohail, M., & Ghanemi, A. (2021). Cellulases: from bioactivity to a variety of industrial applications. *Biomimetics (Basel)*, *6*, 44.

Eom, J. E., Moon, S. K., & Moon, G. S. (2010). Heterologous production of pediocin PA-1 in *Lactobacillus reuteri*. *Journal of Microbiology and Biotechnology*, *20*, 1215–1218.

Fenibo, E. O., Ijoma, G. N., Selvarajan, R., & Chikere, C. B. (2019). Microbial surfactants: the next generation multifunctional biomolecules for applications in the petroleum industry and its associated environmental remediation. *Microorganisms*, *7*, 581.

Ferrer-Miralles, N., & Villaverde, A. (2013). Bacterial cell factories for recombinant protein production; expanding the catalogue. *Microbial Cell Factories*, *12*, 113.

Francis, D. M., & Page, R. (2010). Strategies to optimize protein expression in *E. coli*. *Current Protocols in Protein Science*, *Chapter 5*(1): Unit 5.24, 1–29.

Gasser, B., Saloheimo, M., Rinas, U., Dragosits, M., Rodríguez-Carmona, E., Baumann, K., Giuliani, M., Parrilli, E., Branduardi, P., Lang, C., Porro, D., Ferrer, P., Tutino, M. L., Mattanovich, D., & Villaverde, A. (2008). Protein folding and conformational stress in microbial cells producing recombinant proteins: a host comparative overview. *Microbial Cell Factories*, *7*, 11.

Goeddel, D. V., Yelverton, E., Ullrich, A., et al. (1980). Human leukocyte interferon produced by *E. coli* is biologically active. *Nature*, *287*, 411–416.

Golder, H. M., Rossow, H. A., & Lean, I. J. (2019). Effects of in-feed enzymes on milk production and components, reproduction, and health in dairy cows. *Journal of Dairy Science*, *102*, 8011–8026.

Goldring, J. P. D. (2019). Measuring protein concentration with absorbance, Lowry, Bradford Coomassie Blue, or the Smith bicinchoninic acid assay before electrophoresis. *Methods in Molecular Biology*, *1855*, 31–39.

Gopal, G. J., & Kumar, A. (2013). Strategies for the production of recombinant protein in *Escherichia coli*. *Protein Journal*, *32*, 419–425.

Gu, Y., Xu, X., Wu, Y., et al. (2018). Advances and prospects of *Bacillus subtilis* cellular factories: from rational design to industrial applications. *Metabolic Engineering*, *50*, 109–121.

Guo, X. Q., Wei, Y. M., & Yu, B. (2012). Recombinant *Mycobacterium smegmatis* expressing Hsp65-hIL-2 fusion protein and its influence on lymphocyte function in mice. *Asian Pacific Journal of Tropical Medicine*, *5*, 347–351.

Gupta, V., Sengupta, M., Prakash, J., & Tripathy, B. C. (2016). Production of recombinant pharmaceutical proteins. In *Basic and Applied Aspects of Biotechnology* (pp. 77–101).

Hong, P., Koza, S., & Bouvier, E. S. (2012). Size-exclusion chromatography for the analysis of protein biotherapeutics and their aggregates. *Journal of Liquid Chromatography & Related Technologies*, *35*, 2923–2950.

Hou, Y., & Wu, G. (2018). Nutritionally essential amino acids. *Advances in Nutrition*, *9*, 849–851.

Huang, C. J., Lin, H., & Yang, X. (2012). Industrial production of recombinant therapeutics in *Escherichia coli* and its recent advancements. *Journal of Industrial Microbiology & Biotechnology*, *39*, 383–399.

Innocentin, S., Guimarães, V., Miyoshi, A., et al. (2009). *Lactococcus lactis* expressing either *Staphylococcus aureus* fibronectin-binding protein A or *Listeria monocytogenes* internalin A can efficiently internalize and deliver DNA in human epithelial cells. *Applied and Environmental Microbiology*, *75*, 4870–4878.

Jeeva, J. S., Sunitha, J., Ananthalakshmi, R., Rajkumari, S., Ramesh, M., & Krishnan, R. (2015). Enzymatic antioxidants and its role in oral diseases. *Journal of Pharmacy & Bioallied Sciences*, *7*(Suppl 1), S331–S333.

Jin, H., Cantin, G. T., Maki, S., et al. (2011). Soluble periplasmic production of human granulocyte colony-stimulating factor (G-CSF) in *Pseudomonas fluorescens*. *Protein Expression and Purification*, *78*, 69–77.

Kamionka, M. (2011). Engineering of therapeutic proteins production in *Escherichia coli*. *Current Pharmaceutical Biotechnology*, *12*, 268–274.

Khan, U., & Selamoglu, Z. (2020). Use of enzymes in dairy industry: a review of current progress. *Archives of Razi Institute*, *75*, 131–136.

Kim, Y. K., Lee, S. C., Cho, Y. Y., Oh, H. J., & Ko, Y. H. (2012). Isolation of cellulolytic *Bacillus subtilis* strains from agricultural environments. *ISRN Microbiology*, *2012*, 650563.

Kleiner-Grote, G. R. M., Risse, J. M., & Friehs, K. (2018). Secretion of recombinant proteins from *E. coli*. *Engineering in Life Sciences*, *18*, 532–550.

Kuhad, R. C., Gupta, R., & Singh, A. (2011). Microbial cellulases and their industrial applications. *Enzyme Research*, *2011*, 280696.

Lalucat, J., Bennasar, A., Bosch, R., García-Valdés, E., & Palleroni, N. J. (2006). Biology of *Pseudomonas stutzeri*. *Microbiology and Molecular Biology Reviews*, *70*, 510–547.

Li, S., Yang, X., Yang, S., Zhu, M., & Wang, X. (2012). Technology prospecting on enzymes: application, marketing and engineering. *Computational and Structural Biotechnology Journal*, *2*, e201209017.

Lynd, L. R., Weimer, P. J., van Zyl, W. H., & Pretorius, I. S. (2002). Microbial cellulose utilization: fundamentals and biotechnology. *Microbiology and Molecular Biology Reviews*, *66*, 506–577.

Manavitehrani, I., Fathi, A., Badr, H., Daly, S., Negahi Shirazi, A., & Dehghani, F. (2016). Biomedical applications of biodegradable polyesters. *Polymers (Basel)*, *8*, 20.

Matassa, S., Boon, N., Pikaar, I., & Verstraete, W. (2016). Microbial protein: future sustainable food supply route with low environmental footprint. *Microbial Biotechnology*, *9*, 568–575.

Matthews, C., Crispie, F., Lewis, E., Reid, M., O'Toole, P. W., & Cotter, P. D. (2019). The rumen microbiome: a crucial consideration when optimising milk and meat production and nitrogen utilisation efficiency. *Gut Microbes*, *10*, 115–132.

Mohanan, N., Montazer, Z., Sharma, P. K., & Levin, D. B. (2020). Microbial and enzymatic degradation of synthetic plastics. *Frontiers in Microbiology*, *11*, 580709.

Nakkharat, P., & Haltrich, D. (2006). Lactose hydrolysis and formation of galactooligosaccharides by a novel immobilized beta-galactosidase from the thermophilic fungus *Talaromyces thermophilus*. *Applied Biochemistry and Biotechnology*, *129–132*, 215–225.

Owczarek, B., Gerszberg, A., & Hnatuszko-Konka, K. (2019). A brief reminder of systems of production and chromatography-based recovery of recombinant protein biopharmaceuticals. *BioMed Research International*, *2019*, 4216060.

Patthawaro, S., & Saejung, C. (2019). Production of single cell protein from manure as animal feed by using photosynthetic bacteria. *Microbiology Open*, *8*, e913.

Raveendran, S., Parameswaran, B., Ummalyma, S. B., Abraham, A., Mathew, A. K., Madhavan, A., Rebello, S., & Pandey, A. (2018). Applications of microbial enzymes in food industry. *Food Technology and Biotechnology*, *56*, 16–30.

Redmile-Gordon, M. A., Armenise, E., White, R. P., Hirsch, P. R., & Goulding, K. W. (2013). A comparison of two colorimetric assays, based upon Lowry and Bradford techniques, to estimate total protein in soil extracts. *Soil Biology and Biochemistry*, *67*, 166–173.

Rezaei, M., & Zarkesh-Esfahani, S. H. (2012). Optimization of production of recombinant human growth hormone in *Escherichia coli*. *Journal of Research in Medical Sciences*, *17*, 681–685.

Richardson, D., Itkonen, J., Nievas, J., Urtti, A., & Casteleijn, M. G. (2018). Accelerated pharmaceutical protein development with integrated cell free expression, purification, and bioconjugation. *Scientific Reports*, *8*, 11967.

Rippa, V., Papa, R., Giuliani, M., et al. (2012). Regulated recombinant protein production in the Antarctic bacterium *Pseudoalteromonas haloplanktis* TAC125. *Methods in Molecular Biology*, *824*, 203–218.

Ritala, A., Häkkinen, S. T., Toivari, M., & Wiebe, M. G. (2017). Single cell protein—state-of-the-art, industrial landscape and patents 2001–2016. *Frontiers in Microbiology*, *8*, 2009.

Rosano, G. L., & Ceccarelli, E. A. (2014). Recombinant protein expression in *Escherichia coli*: advances and challenges. *Frontiers in Microbiology*, *5*, 172.

Saqib, S., Akram, A., Halim, S. A., & Tassaduq, R. (2017). Sources of β-galactosidase and its applications in food industry. *3 Biotech*, *7*, 79.

Sasikala, C., & Ramana, C. V. (1995). Biotechnological potentials of anoxygenic phototrophic bacteria. I. Production of single-cell protein, vitamins, ubiquinone's, hormones, and enzymes and use in waste treatment. *Advances in Applied Microbiology*, *41*, 173–226.

Scales, B. S., Dickson, R. P., LiPuma, J. J., & Huffnagle, G. B. (2014). Microbiology, genomics, and clinical significance of the *Pseudomonas fluorescens* species complex, an unappreciated colonizer of humans. *Clinical Microbiology Reviews*, *27*, 927–948.

Sharma, A., & Shouche, Y. (2014). Microbial Culture Collection (MCC) and International Depositary Authority (IDA) at National Center for Cell Science, Pune. *Indian Journal of Microbiology*, *54*, 129–133.

Shivlata, L., & Satyanarayana, T. (2015). Thermophilic and alkaliphilic *Actinobacteria*: biology and potential applications. *Frontiers in Microbiology*, *6*, 1014.

Simon, B., Nomellini, J., Chiou, P., et al. (2001). Recombinant vaccines against infectious hematopoietic necrosis virus: production by the *Caulobacter crescentus* S-layer protein secretion system and evaluation in laboratory trials. *Diseases of Aquatic Organisms*, *44*, 17–27.

Singh, R., Kumar, M., Mittal, A., & Mehta, P. K. (2016). Microbial enzymes: industrial progress in 21st century. *Biotech*, *6*, 174.

Singh, V., Haque, S., Singh, H., Verma, J., Vibha, K., Singh, R., Jawed, A., & Tripathi, C. K. (2016). Isolation, screening, and identification of novel isolates of *Actinomycetes* from India for antimicrobial applications. *Frontiers in Microbiology*, *7*, 1921.

Swiecki, M., & Colonna, M. (2011). Type I interferons: Diversity of sources, production pathways and effects on immune responses. *Current Opinion in Virology*, *1*, 463–475.

Thompson, R. C., Moore, C. J., vom Saal, F. S., & Swan, S. H. (2009). Plastics, the environment and human health: current consensus and future trends. *Philosophical Transactions of the Royal Society B: Biological Sciences*, *364*, 2153–2166.

Toyokawa, Y., Takahara, H., Reungsang, A., et al. (2010). Purification and characterization of a halotolerant serine proteinase from thermotolerant *Bacillus licheniformis* RKK-04 isolated from Thai fish sauce. *Applied Microbiology and Biotechnology*, *86*, 1867–1875.

Tripathi, N. K., & Shrivastava, A. (2019). Recent developments in bioprocessing of recombinant proteins: expression hosts and process development. *Frontiers in Bioengineering and Biotechnology*, *7*, 420.

Vigentini, I., Merico, A., Tutino, M. L., Compagno, C., & Marino, G. (2006). Optimization of recombinant human nerve growth factor production in the psychrophilic *Pseudoalteromonas haloplanktis*. *Journal of Biotechnology*, *127*, 141–150.

Vitorino, L. C., & Bessa, L. A. (2017). Technological microbiology: development and applications. *Frontiers in Microbiology*, *8*, 827.

Vroman, I., & Tighzert, L. (2009). Biodegradable polymers. *Materials (Basel)*, *2*, 307–344.

Wingfield, P. T. (2015). Overview of the purification of recombinant proteins. *Current Protocols in Protein Science*, *80*, 6.1.1–6.1.35.

Wu, G. (2009). Amino acids: metabolism, functions, and nutrition. *Amino Acids*, *37*, 1–17.

Zamani, A., Khajavi, M., Nazarpak, M. H., & Gisbert, E. (2020). Evaluation of a bacterial single-cell protein in compound diets for rainbow trout (*Oncorhynchus mykiss*) fry as an alternative protein source. *Animals (Basel)*, *10*, 1676.

Zhao, L. L., Liu, M., Ge, J. W., Qiao, X. Y., Li, Y. J., & Liu, D. Q. (2012). Expression of infectious pancreatic necrosis virus (IPNV) VP2-VP3 fusion protein in *Lactobacillus casei* and immunogenicity in rainbow trout. *Vaccine*, *30*, 1823–1829.

CHAPTER 12

# Bacterial Nanocellulose: Evolution in Engineering, Enhanced Mass Production, and Wide-Ranging Application Rephrase

BABLI KUMARI,[1] OM PRAKASH,[1] SAURABH SINGH RATHORE,[1] ABHISHEK KUMAR,[2] AKHILESH KUMAR SINGH,[1,*] and BRIJESH PANDEY[1,*]

[1]*Department of Biotechnology, School of Life Sciences, Mahatma Gandhi Central University, Motihari, Bihar, India*

[2]*Parul Institute of Management and Research, Parul University, Vadodara, Gujarat, India*

*Corresponding author

## ABSTRACT

Bacterial nanocellulose (BNC) is gaining recognition as a highly versatile biomaterial due to its exceptional physicochemical and biological properties. However, its large-scale commercialization remains limited by high production costs, significant capital investment, and scalability challenges. To address these barriers, researchers are developing advanced production strategies, including bioreactor-based systems, static intermittent methods, and semi-continuous fed-batch processes. Efforts are also directed toward optimizing substrate formulations and utilizing cost-effective feedstocks to enhance industrial-scale BNC yields. This chapter highlights the pivotal role of genetic modification in improving BNC production, offering promising solutions to overcome key limitations and support commercial feasibility. It provides an overview of various production approaches, the

Industrial Biotechnology: Current Progress and Novel Technologies.
Prakash Kumar Sarangi, Akhilesh Kumar Singh, Rajesh Kumar Srivastava, and Brijesh Pandey (Eds.)


DOI: 10.1201/9781779642233-12

unique characteristics of BNC, and its expanding applications in food, personal care, biomedical devices, electronics, and advanced materials. By outlining recent advances and future opportunities, the chapter aims to support the continued development of BNC-based technologies. As innovations progress, BNC is expected to become a cornerstone biomaterial, driving sustainable industrial growth and enabling next-generation solutions across multiple sectors.

## 12.1 INTRODUCTION

Bacterial nanocellulose (BNC) stands out as a remarkable natural biopolymer, intricately synthesized by certain bacterial strains as an exopolysaccharide primarily composed of β-D glucopyranose. Despite its remarkable composition, consisting of 99% water, BNC showcases exceptional mechanical prowess (Gama et al., 2012; Numata et al., 2015). What makes BNC even more intriguing is its water retention capacity coupled with a nanostructured morphology akin to collagen, a protein found in the extracellular matrix (ECM), rendering BNC highly conducive for cellular adhesion and immobilization (El-Hoseny et al., 2015). In the realm of bioprocessing, researchers harness the capabilities of metabolically engineered microorganisms, such as *Escherichia coli* or *Saccharomyces cerevisiae*, to transform biomass into a spectrum of value-added biomaterials, spanning from biofuels to extracellular polymeric substances (Sharma et al., 2012, 2013). The versatility of bioprocessing techniques extends to utilizing a diverse array of biomasses, catering to myriad environmental applications. However, in light of the limitations posed by both synthetic and natural materials, the scientific community is gravitating towards the development of novel, more dynamic materials capable of addressing multifaceted challenges across various domains. Enter BNC, a potential game-changer in the realm of biopolymers, synthesized as an extracellular macromolecule of β-D-glucopyranose by select bacterial strains. Despite its predominantly aqueous composition, BNC boasts formidable mechanical properties (Sharma et al., 2015). The distinct attributes of BNC, delineated underscore its suitability for cellular adhesion and immobilization, owing to its nanostructured architecture reminiscent of collagen. Furthermore, being classified under the GRAS materials category, BNC emerges as a frontrunner for a plethora of applications. Primarily, BNC finds its niche in biocomposites, where it lends its prowess to domains such as wound healing, drug delivery, and tissue regeneration, with exemplary examples like Bofill leading the way (Numata et al., 2015). However, the widespread adoption of BNC in the biomedical arena hinges upon mitigating the high production costs through the application of sophisticated multifunctional culture mediums and the transition to high-efficiency bioreactors. Projections from global forecast analyses paint a promising picture, anticipating a threefold expansion in the BNC market over the next five years. To realize this potential, optimizing substrate selection, refining biosynthesis mechanisms, tackling genetic modifications, addressing instability challenges, and enhancing production feasibility stand as pivotal objectives. The biosynthetic route is gaining traction for its inherent ability to orchestrate the self-assembly of secreted fibrils endowed with unique physiochemical properties. Leveraging biosynthetic methods not only ensures unparalleled purity by circumventing the presence of pectin, lignin, and hemicellulose but also obviates the need for cumbersome purification processes. Moreover, delving into biosynthetic pathways facilitates the identification of potential microorganisms instrumental in BNC production (El-Hoseny et al., 2015). However, striking a delicate balance in biosynthetic pathway enzyme expression becomes imperative to prevent undue metabolic burden induced by overexpression or inadequate supply of critical precursors for downstream biosynthesis. In the quest for cost-effective BNC production, attention is increasingly shifting towards unconventional yet abundant feedstocks such as sugar-rich biowaste sourced from fruits, vegetables, sugar cane bagasse, and wood processing residues. Harnessing these resources not only optimizes production costs but also aligns with sustainability imperatives. Nevertheless, realizing the full commercial potential of BNC mandates targeted research endeavors aimed at refining production techniques and scaling up operations. Scaling up BNC production presents a myriad of challenges, ranging from the inherent nature of target metabolites to prolonged biosynthesis durations and modest yields. Enhancing fermentation technology emerges as a promising avenue for augmenting BNC yields. However, the obligate aerobic nature of microbial BNC producers necessitates thoughtful deliberation on culture management, be it static or dynamic. Pioneering efforts by Kralisch et al. (2010) exemplify the fusion of static and agitated cultivation methods to devise a semi-continuous culture strategy, leveraging horizontal lift reactors to harvest BNC biofilms. This innovative approach not only streamlines production processes but also significantly slashes costs. The characteristics of BNC render it amenable to diverse applications across biomedical, food packaging, cosmetics, and electronics domains. This chapter delves into various facets of BNC biosynthesis, effective substrate utilization strategies, current status, challenges, and future prospects, with a keen emphasis on devising cost-effective strategies to unlock its full potential.

## 12.2 STRUCTURAL MORPHOLOGY OF BNC FOR FUNCTIONAL NANOHYBRID DEVELOPMENT

BNC has garnered substantial attention owing to its unique characteristics, including purity, distinctive surface chemistry, fibrous and porous structure, and a host of other physico-mechanical and biological properties. Its standout features encompass high-water absorption and retention capabilities, sustained and prolonged release profiles, notable porosity, semi-crystalline nature, mechanical and thermal robustness, elevated crystallinity, as well as a fine fibrous network that lends itself to optical transparency and 3D structuring (Öz et al., 2023; Su et al., 2022; Ullah et al., 2022). Moreover, BNC exhibits biocompatibility, biodegradability, non-toxicity, non-immunogenicity, and hemocompatibility, rendering it a versatile and sought-after material across diverse research domains. The intricate fibril network of BNC manifests as meticulously organized 3D nanofibers, endowing BNC sheets with expansive surface area, enhanced porosity, and favorable aspect ratios. This structural arrangement not only facilitates efficient matrix formation but also positions BNC as an ideal candidate for reinforcement in composite materials. BNC seamlessly integrates with biocompatible polymers, conducting agents, nanomaterials, antimicrobial compounds, clays, and more, thereby conferring additional functionalities to the resultant composites. Consequently, BNC emerges as a frontrunner for a myriad of applications spanning various fields, encapsulating its versatility and potential impact (Revin et al., 2022).

### *12.2.1 SURFACE CHEMISTRY*

BNC represents a chain of glucose units, characterized by an abundance of free hydroxyl (OH) groups, averaging three OH groups per glucose moiety. Its elongated and slender fibrils contribute to a substantial surface area and aspect ratio. Notably, the cellulose chain displays an asymmetry, featuring a reducing aldehyde (CHO) group at one end, termed the reducing end, while the opposite end lacks this group, hence termed the non-reducing end (Habibi et al., 2014; Shahzad et al., 2023). The accessible OH groups render BNC amenable to chemical modifications (Eyley et al., 2014; Orlando et al., 2020), fostering interactions with diverse functional groups and facilitating the formation of composites with various materials. Surface modification of BNC not only introduces additional functionalities but also addresses inherent limitations. For instance, treatments such as TEMPO (2,2,6,6-tetramethyl-1-piperidinyloxy) oxidation or the incorporation of anionic sulfate groups onto its surface mitigate cellulose fibril aggregation by inducing repulsion among them (Khatta et al., 2021).

### 12.2.2 ULTRAFINE THIN FIBROUS STRUCTURE OF BNC

BNC is a highly specialized material characterized by an ultrafine and delicate fibrous structure, which imparts exceptional properties suitable for a wide range of applications. Notably, BNC fibers exhibit a substantial reduction in diameter, approximately two orders of magnitude smaller than plant-derived fibers, predominantly existing within the nanoscale range. When observed from the top surface, the cellulose fibers of BNC appear randomly distributed, a phenomenon attributed to the dynamic motility of bacterial cells. However, cross-sectional analysis via scanning electron microscopy reveals a stratified organization, conferring a distinct layered architecture to BNC. This reticulated configuration provides BNC with a robust and resilient appearance. Furthermore, the random arrangement of cellulose fibers forms an intricate web-like matrix, significantly contributing to its exceptional mechanical strength, thermal stability, and elevated crystalline characteristics. Consequently, the unique structural attributes of BNC not only differentiate it from conventional cellulose materials but also emphasize its potential for diverse applications across various industries (Ul-Islam et al., 2015).

### 12.2.3 POROSITY AND ADSORPTION POTENTIAL

BNC exhibits a significant degree of porosity, a characteristic influenced by several factors including synthesis methodologies, microbial strains employed, growth medium composition, and post-synthesis treatments. Its open fiber arrangement generates a multitude of pores, resulting in a highly porous matrix with a substantial surface area (Shah et al., 2013). This attribute is particularly important in applications where efficient absorption of bioactive substances is essential, such as in wound dressing materials, facilitating the absorption of wound exudates. The porosity of BNC is critical in determining its capacity to accommodate various absorption materials, ranging from solid particles such as nanoparticles to liquids such as solutions and polymers, as well as soluble molecules such as antibiotics (Lamboni et al., 2016). However, while the porosity of BNC can extend to the nanoscale level, this may impede the penetration of larger particles. Conversely, the small pore size of pristine BNC facilitates the infiltration of mammalian cells. Pyrogens, including sugars, salts, or other particles, are incorporated into its matrix to tailor the porosity of BNC for specific applications. These pyrogens function as space holders within the BNC structure, subsequently removed to generate well-defined pores (Khan et al., 2018; Vitta et al., 2012). Conversely, larger pores within BNC can be advantageous in certain scenarios, facilitating the rapid release of small molecules such as drugs or growth factors. However, achieving optimal porosity necessitates careful control over the size and shape of pores, ensuring compatibility with the intended application while preserving the fibrous morphology of BNC. Therefore, meticulous management of BNC's porosity is crucial for maximizing its utility across various fields (Torgbo et al., 2019).

### 12.2.4 MACROSTRUCTURE AND ORIENTATION

BNC exhibits remarkable versatility in both wet (hydrogel) and dry (paper, aerogel, powder, membrane) forms, with each variant offering distinct properties tailored to its specific physical state. The physical structure of BNC can be intricately controlled at macro-, micro-, and nano-scales during production by manipulating growth conditions or incorporating additives into the production medium (Gromovykh et al., 2020). This flexibility allows for the generation of diverse BNC forms such as sheets, pellets, and granules, achieved through static, shaking, and agitation cultivation methods, respectively (Shi et al., 2018). Naturally, BNC fibers display anisotropic characteristics, influenced by the movement of bacterial cells. Nonetheless, researchers have successfully engineered BNC with unique structural arrangements such as honeycomb, aligned, and patterned fibers by subjecting them to external stimuli like electric or magnetic fields (Uraki et al., 2007). Additionally, introducing templated structures into the culture medium during production, such as honeycomb-patterned microgrooves or poly-di-methyl-siloxane (PDMS) and microfluidic channels, has yielded patterned BNC variants (Putra et al., 2008). This suggests the feasibility of producing BNC with tailored structural patterns. Despite its anisotropic behavior, the overall structure of BNC remains compact and robust, rendering it highly suitable for a wide array of biomedical and non-medical applications. Whether in the form of hydrogels for wound dressings or membranes for filtration, BNC's adaptable physical properties make it an attractive material for various industrial and scientific endeavors (Wang et al., 2008).

### 12.2.5 SELF-ASSEMBLY AND CRYSTALLIZATION OF GLUCAN CHAINS

The predominant producer of BNC, *Komagataeibacter xylinum,* synthesizes two primary cellulose polymorphs: ribbon-like cellulose I and amorphous cellulose II. While cellulose I demonstrates a parallel alignment of uniaxially arranged glucan chains, cellulose II exhibits a more random arrangement. The distinctive reticulate structure and fibrous morphology of BNC are attributed to the dynamic movement and assembly of these glucan chains. Initiation of the process occurs through transmembrane cellulose synthase complexes (TCs) situated on the cell membrane. These complexes are responsible for the extrusion of cellulose fibrils. As a result, fibrils are formed, transitioning into protofibrils with a diameter typically ranging from 2 to 4 nm. These protofibrils then coalesce into bundles, eventually aggregating into ribbons measuring approximately 80 × 4 nm in size. An estimated 50 to 80 TCs are distributed along the cell axis, acting as the sites where cellulose fibril aggregation initiates. The spatial arrangement of TCs plays a crucial role in determining the orientation and organization of glucan chains within the BNC structure. Moreover, the assembly and crystallization processes of these glucan chains are meticulously regulated by genetic information encoded within the bcsABCS operon. This regulatory mechanism ensures precise control over BNC formation, facilitating the development of its complex and robust material properties (Mehta et al., 2015).

### 12.2.6 BIOCOMPATIBILITY

Biocompatibility, at its core, denotes a material's ability to interact with living cells or tissues directly, devoid of any adverse effects (Morais et al., 2010). While lacking adhesive sites for cell adhesion, BNC earns its biocompatible status primarily due to its non-toxic nature (Klemm et al., 2001). Notably, BNC exhibits moderate biocompatibility across various cell types, with no discernible foreign body reactions. Despite its inherent biocompatibility, BNC falls short of meeting the stringent requirements for many tissues engineering applications, necessitating enhancements such as the development of hybrids with other biocompatible polymers. Beyond its non-toxicity, BNC's biocompatibility is closely linked to its porous, fibrous, and three-dimensional structure, along with its remarkable liquid absorption and retention capacities, particularly in biomedical contexts. For instance, porous BNC serves as an excellent substrate for cell adhesion, while its three-dimensional architecture facilitates deep cellular infiltration into the matrix (Schumann et al., 2009). Moreover, the fibrous structure of BNC bears resemblance to natural collagen, rendering it valuable for tissue engineering endeavors. Additionally, BNC's high liquid absorption capability proves advantageous for wound care by effectively absorbing exudates at the wound site, while its superior water holding capacity maintains an optimal moist environment conducive to wound healing (Helenius et al., 2006).

### 12.2.7 BIODEGRADABILITY

The biodegradation of biomaterials presents both an intriguing prospect and a formidable challenge, particularly for materials with high crystallinity and density like BNC. The absence of cellulase enzymes in mammalian cells or tissues hinders the *in vivo* degradation of BNC in humans, necessitating alternative approaches to address this limitation. One such strategy involves periodate oxidation, which has been devised to facilitate the *in vivo* degradation of BNC. For instance, Li et al. demonstrated significant improvements in the biodegradation of BNC through periodate oxidation, resulting in enhanced degradation across various media without compromising the original fibrous network. This method yields 2,3-dialdehyde cellulose (DAC), a biodegradable cellulose derivative at physiological pH, generating safe degradation products (Li et al., 2009). However, specific applications of BNC, such as in bone tissue engineering, may require additional pre-treatment and chemical modifications like oxidation. Moreover, careful selection of reinforcement materials alongside BNC is paramount to ensure the biological safety of the resultant degradation products. It's noteworthy that the architecture of biological scaffolds may undergo changes during degradation, emphasizing the importance of considering such dynamics in the design and implementation of biomaterials. Overall, biodegradability stands as a crucial attribute for biomaterials in various biomedical applications, underscoring the need for innovative approaches to enhance degradation while maintaining biological safety and structural integrity (Li et al., 2009).

### 12.2.8 NON-IMMUNOGENICITY

Immunogenicity, defined as the ability of an antigen or foreign substance to trigger an immune response within the body, is a critical consideration in biomedical applications. While BNC is generally regarded as non-immunogenic, there remains a limited understanding of its interactions with immune cells. Consequently, the assessment of immunogenicity becomes imperative, particularly in the context of utilizing BNC-based scaffolds for tissue engineering, especially in *in vivo* scenarios where direct contact with cells, tissues, and blood occurs (Leitao et al., 2013). The extent of immunogenicity and ensuing response may vary based on several factors, including the composition of BNC-based scaffolds and their fabrication methods, the size and morphology of cellulose fibers, the potential for agglomeration and contamination, as well as interactions between cells and the scaffold, and between the scaffold and blood. Hence, a comprehensive comprehension of BNC's immunogenicity is essential to advance the development of safe and efficacious scaffolds for biomedical applications. Exploring the immunogenic properties of BNC entails evaluating its potential to provoke immune responses and understanding the mechanisms underlying such interactions with immune cells. By delving deeper into these aspects, researchers can refine scaffold design and fabrication techniques to mitigate any adverse immunological reactions, ultimately fostering the creation of BNC-based scaffolds that are both biocompatible and immunologically inert. This holistic approach is crucial for the continued advancement of BNC as a promising biomaterial for a diverse range of biomedical applications (Roman et al., 2019).

### 12.2.9 HEMOCOMPATIBILITY

Hemocompatibility, a critical characteristic of biomaterials, refers to their ability to interact with blood without inducing toxicity. In the realm of biomedical engineering, this property holds particular significance for BNC-based artificial organs such as heart valves and blood vessels (Scherner et al., 2014), which have been the focus of research by various investigators. Ensuring the hemocompatibility of BNC-based scaffolds is paramount to prevent adverse effects such as immune responses, inflammation, or infection upon implantation into the body. Numerous studies have indicated that BNC-based scaffolds generally exhibit hemocompatible properties, facilitating proper osteoconduction, integration, and induction within the host tissue (Andrade et al., 2011; Pang et al., 2020; Seyednejad et al., 2012). This favorable outcome is attributed to BNC's ability to deter platelet adhesion and activation, minimize Factor XII activation, and mitigate acute inflammatory responses. Moreover, these scaffolds must also facilitate the formation of new blood vessels and enable the exchange of nutrients and gases within newly formed tissues. While existing research underscores the inherent hemocompatibility of BNC-based scaffolds, further advancements are imperative to enhance their compatibility and ensure successful implantation in human recipients. Continued research and development efforts are essential to refine BNC-based devices, optimize their hemocompatible properties, and advance their safety and efficacy for clinical applications. By addressing these challenges, BNC-based artificial organs can fulfill their potential as safe and effective solutions in the field of regenerative medicine (Mirtalebi et al., 2019; Torgbo et al., 2018; Zheng et al., 2020).

## 12.3 BIOSYNTHESIS OF BACTERIAL NANOCELLULOSE (BNC)

BNC stands as an extracellular biopolymer renowned for its formation of a three-dimensional network at the interface of air and liquid culture mediums. The discovery of BNC traces back to A. J. Brown in 1886, who observed *Acetobacter xylinum* cells synthesizing cellulose using glucose and oxygen. Notably, *Acetobacter* has since been reclassified as *Komagataeibacter*, representing one of the premier rod-shaped Gram-negative acetic bacterial species. Recent research underscores the significance of focusing on bacterial strains within this species, given their propensity to serve as model organisms for molecular, biochemical, and genetic investigations, owing to their intriguing phenotypes and high cellulose production capabilities (Castro et al., 2015). In addition to *Komagataeibacter*, several other noteworthy organisms contribute to BNC production, including *Dickeya dadantii*, *Rhizobium leguminosarum*, *Agrobacterium tumefaciens*, *Salmonella enterica*, *Escherichia coli*, and *Pseudomonas putida* (Römling et al., 2015). One particularly compelling avenue for enhancing BNC production efficiency while simultaneously reducing costs lies in the development of GM strains capable of producing BNC. This innovative approach holds significant promise for advancing the field of BNC production (Moradi et al., 2021).

### 12.3.1 MOLECULAR MECHANISMS INVOLVED IN BIOSYNTHESIS

The synthesis of BNC is a meticulously orchestrated and tightly regulated process, encompassing multiple stages and involving a myriad of genes encoding specific enzymes and regulatory proteins organized into catalytic complexes. This intricate multistep process involves the coordinated action of various enzymes and regulatory proteins, all meticulously regulated to ensure precise control over BNC production. Central to BNC synthesis is the cellulose synthase, which plays a pivotal role in catalyzing the production of cellulose. Working in concert with enzymes such as endo β-1,4-glucanase, the complementing factor, and β-glucosidase, the cellulose synthase is responsible for orchestrating the polymerization of glucose units into cellulose chains. These genes are often located in the flanking regions of operons, highlighting their coordinated regulation. The biosynthetic pathways involved in BNC production are intertwined with various metabolic processes, including the phosphoglycerate pathway, the Embden Meyerhof Parnas route, gluconeogenesis, and the Krebs cycle (Gromet et al., 1957). These pathways play critical roles in providing the necessary precursors and energy for cellulose synthesis (Figure 12.1). BNC biosynthesis can be broken down into four main enzymatic stages: (i) conversion of glucose into glucose-6-phosphate through phosphorylation by glucokinase; (ii) production of glucose-1-phosphate from glucose-6-phosphate by phosphoglucomutase; (iii) synthesis of uridine diphosphate glucose (UDP-Glc) from glucose-1-phosphate using UDP-glucose pyrophosphorylase; and (iv) cellulose production through the polymerization of UDP-glucose via β-1,4 glucan linkages in the presence of cellulose synthase (Bcs) (Ross et al., 1991). The cellulose synthase complex (Bcs) comprises four distinct protein subunits: BcsA, BcsB, BcsC, and BcsD, all controlled by a single promoter within the BC synthase operon (bcs). BcsA serves as the catalytic subunit responsible for cellulose synthesis, forming transmembrane pores through the inner membrane (Ross et al., 1987). BcsB interacts with BcsA, facilitating the movement of the polymer through the periplasm to the outer membrane. BcsC, located in the outer membrane, is involved in complex assembly and facilitates the exit of cellulose from the cell (Morgan et al., 2013). The exact function of BcsD remains unclear, but it is speculated to play a role in cellulose sub-fiber extrusion or crystallization. Overall, the intricate molecular mechanisms underlying BNC synthesis highlight the complexity of this process and underscore the need for further research to fully elucidate the intricacies of cellulose biosynthesis in bacteria (Saxena et al., 1994).

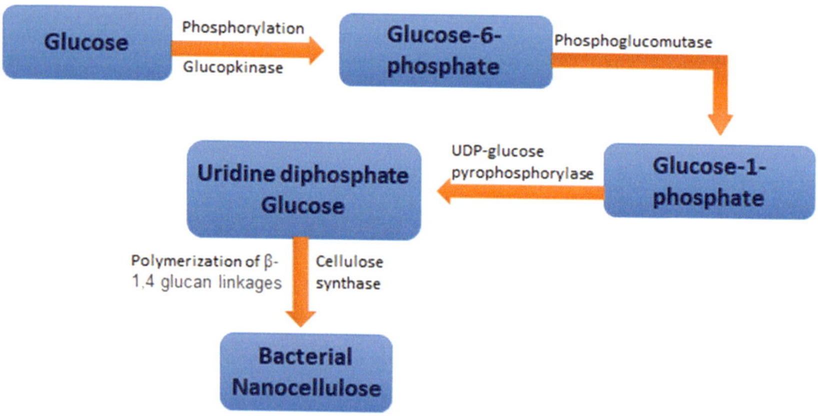


**FIGURE 12.1** Schematic representation of biosynthesis pathways of bacterial nanocellulose production.

### 12.3.2 GENETIC MODIFICATION POSSIBILITIES

The production of BNC from *Komagataeibacter* strains presents challenges due to low productivity and variability in nutritional requirements among strains. To address these challenges, extensive genetic manipulation is required to optimize BNC production. Genetic engineering techniques have been employed to enhance BNC synthesis efficiency and introduce structural modifications to the BNC network. Various strategies have been explored, including the expression of foreign genes or disruption of specific genes involved in BNC synthesis (Edwards et al., 1999). Techniques such as homologous recombination, heterologous gene expression, and CRISPR have been utilized to modify the genomes of BNC-producing bacteria. Gene sequencing has provided insights into the molecular mechanisms underlying BNC synthesis, guiding genetic engineering efforts. Electroporation, a common method for genetic manipulation, induces transient pores in cell membranes, facilitating the entry of macromolecules into cells. Target genes, such as those encoding phosphogluconate dehydrogenase and glucose 6-phosphate isomerase, have been identified for overexpression to enhance BNC synthesis. Additionally, conjugation with *Escherichia coli* cells and transposon mutagenesis have been employed to introduce genetic modifications in *Komagataeibacter* strains (Chen et al., 2019; Yadav et al., 2010). Despite progress in genetic engineering, further research and development are needed to overcome existing challenges and fully harness the potential of GM *Komagataeibacter* strains for BNC production (Moradi et al., 2021). Continued efforts to optimize genetic manipulation techniques and understand the molecular basis of BNC synthesis are essential for realizing the widespread utilization of BNC-based materials in various industries. In summary, genetic engineering offers promising avenues for enhancing BNC production efficiency and tailoring its properties to meet specific application requirements (Singhania et al., 2021). By leveraging advanced genetic manipulation techniques, researchers can address the challenges associated with BNC production and unlock its full potential for diverse industrial applications (Battad-Bernardo et al., 2004).

#### 12.3.3.1 INHIBITION OF GENE EXPRESSION

In 1990, groundbreaking research initiated the application of gene disruption techniques to understand the molecular mechanisms underlying BNC synthesis by targeting the bcsD gene using the plasmid pACYC184 (Kuo et al., 2015). Researchers observed a significant reduction, approximately 40%, in cellulose synthesis efficiency, underscoring the pivotal role of the bcsD gene in optimizing BNC production. Subsequent investigations by Saxena et al. unveiled that the disrupted bcsD mutant yielded both cellulose I and cellulose II, indicating the involvement of bcsD genes in cellulose crystallization. Further insights were gleaned by Mehta et al., who delineated the function of BcsD in aligning the linear terminal complex along the cell's longitudinal axis, a critical step in the final phase of cellulose hierarchical assembly (Mehta et al., 2015). Expanding on this understanding, Bae et al. employed genetic engineering to disrupt the dgc1 gene, implicated in stimulating BNC biosynthesis. Interestingly, while the disruption of dgc1 had minimal impact on BNC synthesis, it significantly altered the structural integrity of the resulting membranes, yielding scattered fibers. Moreover, disruption of the aceP gene, responsible for acetan production, led to the production of acetan with altered structural characteristics but maintained yield (Bae et al., 2004). Ishida et al. delved into the disruption of the aceA gene, involved in the acetan biosynthetic pathway, which surprisingly resulted in increased BNC production despite the anticipated suppression of acetan synthesis (Edwards et al., 1999). Conversely, disruption of the ghd gene, encoding glucose dehydrogenase (GDH), revealed intriguing findings (Shigematsu et al., 2005). This genetic manipulation led to heightened cellulose synthesis efficiency without the formation of gluconic acid, a common byproduct. The mutant strain exhibited enhanced BNC production, attributed to improved mass transfer of oxygen and nutrients in shaking culture conditions. Overall, these pioneering studies underscore the intricate interplay between gene expression and BNC synthesis (Ishida et al., 2002), laying the groundwork for targeted genetic modifications to optimize BNC production efficiency and tailor its properties for diverse applications (Kuo et al., 2015).

#### *12.3.3.2 GENE OVEREXPRESSION*

In a groundbreaking study, Mangayil et al. explored the potential of enhancing BNC production by overexpressing key genes involved in cellulose synthesis. By overexpressing the bcsA genes, bcsAB, and the entire cellulose synthase operon (bcsABCD) in *K. xylinus* DSM, the researchers observed a remarkable increase in BNC production efficiency. Mutants engineered with these genetic modifications exhibited two to four times higher BNC yield compared to wild-type strains, with the bcsABCD overexpression mutant demonstrating the highest efficiency (Mangayil et al., 2017). Similarly, Kawano et al. investigated the influence of the CMCax gene on BNC biosynthesis in *K. hansenii* ATCC 23769. They found that overexpression of the CMCax gene led to improved BNC output, and supplementation of the culture medium with CMCax protein further enhanced cellulose formation. This highlights the potential of leveraging CMCax gene expression to regulate BNC synthesis (Kawano et al., 2002). Subsequent research by Nakai et al. examined the impact of CMCax on BNC production using the BPR 2001 mutant of *K. xylinus*. Interestingly, disruption of the cmcax gene resulted in reduced BNC production compared to the wild-type strain, with the mutant exclusively producing cellulose II, suggesting a role of CMCax in influencing cellulose crystallinity (Nakai et al., 2013). Further insights into the structural influence of CMCax on cellulose fibers were provided by Kawano et al., who utilized electron microscopy to demonstrate that CMCax can modulate the structure of cellulose fibers. Cells of *K. hansenii* ATCC 23769 overexpressing the cmcax gene exhibited cellulose fibers with a more intact structure compared to wild-type strains, indicating the potential of CMCax to influence BNC morphology. Overall, these studies highlight the significance of genetic engineering approaches in optimizing BNC production and elucidating the molecular mechanisms underlying cellulose synthesis. Leveraging gene overexpression and disruption techniques offers promising avenues for enhancing BNC yield and tailoring its properties for various applications (Kawano et al., 2002).

### 12.3.3 GENETIC INSTABILITY CHALLENGES

The considerable diversity in dietary requirements and productivity among different *Komagataeibacter* strains poses a significant challenge to the widespread adoption of BNC biosynthesis in industry. One of the major obstacles is the genetic instability observed in some BNC-producing strains, which tend to spontaneously generate cellulose-negative mutants when subjected to agitation during fermentation. This phenomenon was first documented by Hestrin and Schramm in 1954, highlighting the need for a deeper understanding of the underlying mechanisms (Schramm et al., 1954). The emergence of cellulose-negative mutants in agitated liquid cultures, where aeration is homogeneous, presents a persistent challenge. Despite extensive research efforts, the precise chemical basis for the development of these mutants remains elusive. Strategies aimed at minimizing the formation of cellulose-negative mutants have been explored, including the substitution of glucose with fructose, supplementation of glucose medium with ethanol, and optimization of agitation speed (Krystynowicz et al., 2002). Additionally, the role of plasmids in BNC biosynthesis has been a subject of investigation, given that many BNC-producing strains harbor plasmids of varying sizes. However, it has been observed that some BNC-synthesizing strains do not possess plasmids, indicating a more complex relationship between plasmids and BNC production (Valla et al., 1983). Moreover, the presence of IS1031 insertion elements within the genomes of certain *Komagataeibacter* strains has been associated with the cellulose-negative morphotype. These insertion elements disrupt the coding sequences of essential enzymes involved in the cellulose biosynthesis pathway, such as phosphoglucomutase and glucose-1-phosphate uridylyl transferase. Understanding the interplay between genetic factors, culture conditions, and cellulose biosynthesis pathways is essential for overcoming these challenges and maximizing BNC production efficiency in industrial settings. Further research into the mechanisms underlying cellulose-negative mutant formation and the role of genetic elements will be crucial for the development of robust BNC production processes (Siguier et al., 2014).

## 12.4 DIFFERENT PRODUCTION TECHNIQUES FOR BACTERIAL NANOCELLULOSE BIOSYNTHESIS

BNC biosynthesis follows a well-regulated process consisting of two main stages: the formation of 1,4-glucan linkages and subsequent assembly and crystallization of cellulose. Initially, carbon sources like glucose or fructose are transported into the cell, where they are converted into the cellulose precursor UDPG. The cellulose synthase enzyme (Bcs) then polymerizes glucose from UDPG into 1,4-glucan strands. Finally, cellulose chains are secreted as sub-fibrils through pores in the cell membrane and assembled into ribbons within a 3D nanofiber network supported by hydrogen bonds. The production of BNC occurs through an oxidative fermentation process, typically involving the oxidation of sugars and organic acids in synthetic or non-synthetic media rich in sugars and nitrogen, at temperatures between 25 to 30°C and pH levels ranging from 4.5 to 7.5 (Jozala et al., 2016).

BNC produced under various culture conditions exhibits diverse structural properties, influencing its physicochemical characteristics and morphologies, rendering it suitable for a wide array of biomedical and industrial applications (Siguier et al., 2009). Various factors affect the biosynthetic production of BNC, as depicted in Figure 12.2. Currently, three main methods—static, agitated, and bioreactor-based bacterial culturing—are employed for cellulose production. Each method yields cellulose with distinct physicochemical features due to differences in cellulose assembly into nano- and micro-structures. Therefore, the choice of production technique is dictated by the desired properties of the BNC for specific applications. The culture environment, encompassing factors like bacterial strain, nutrients, oxygen availability, and pH, significantly influences BNC characteristics (Koizumi et al., 2008). Compared to cellulose produced via static culture, cellulose from agitated culture exhibits lower mechanical strength and reduced yields, with a higher risk of microbial mutations potentially impacting BNC production. However, static culture requires more cultivation area and time (Wang et al., 2019). When considering the characteristics necessary for BNC production, the composition of the culture medium is crucial for ensuring the effectiveness of the biotechnological process. The culture medium's composition directly affects various aspects of cellulose synthesis, including yield, morphology, structure, and physical properties, regardless of the production method employed. Therefore, careful consideration of the culture medium components is essential for optimizing BNC production (Mohammadkazemi et al., 2015).

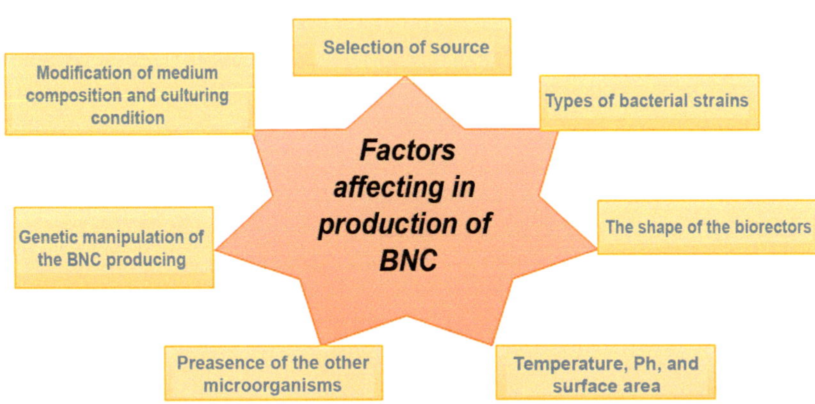


**FIGURE 12.2** Different factors affecting biosynthesis of bacterial nanocellulose.

### 12.4.1 STATIC FERMENTATION METHOD

Various methodologies have been employed in the creation of BNC, ranging from batch and fed-batch cultivation to continuous methods utilizing bioreactors. The choice of production process significantly impacts the supramolecular structure, mechanical, and physical properties of BNC, thus tailored to the intended application. Static cultivation, a standard method, yields highly uniform BNC structures ideal for applications like wound dressings due to its lamellar structure and minimal branching. The static culture method, widely employed in laboratory settings, involves placing a culture medium with a pH of 4.5 to 6.5 into containers of various shapes and sizes for incubation. This process yields BNC conforming to the shape of the container, consistently producing homogeneous structures. It is considered the gold standard for manufacturing flat BNC with excellent reproducibility for commercial use (Huang et al., 2016; Jozala et al., 2016). Dessert nata de coco stands as a prime example, produced via static cultivation, wherein BNC sheets are skimmed from the culture medium (Barja et al., 2021). Innovative approaches, such as semi-continuous planar BNC production, have been developed by Kralisch et al., utilizing a horizontal lift reactor. This technique combines continuous processing with static cultivation, yielding BNC with a uniform 3D structure akin to statically produced BNC. The process ensures smooth extraction of appropriately sized BNC sheets without damaging the medium (Kralisch et al., 2010). The composition of the culture medium plays a crucial role in BNC production. The medium described by Hestrin and Schramm in 1954 includes glucose, yeast extract, peptone, anhydrous $Na_2HPO_4$, and $C_6H_8O_7.H_2O$. However, due to its high cost, alternative mediums have been explored. Fruit juices, agricultural, and industrial waste have shown promise as cost-effective carbon and nutrient sources for BNC production (Hestrin and Schramm, 1954). To address cost concerns, researchers have explored alternative carbon sources such as corn steep liquor, molasses, and candied jujube wastewater. Researchers implemented static intermittent fed-batch technology using sweet lime pulp waste to enhance BNC synthesis. Similarly, other researchers also utilized lipid fermentation effluent as a substrate, demonstrating the potential to increase BNC production while minimizing costs (Dubey et al., 2017; Huang et al., 2016). Experimentation with different carbon sources has yielded promising results in increasing BNC yields while reducing manufacturing expenses. However, environmental parameters such as pH, temperature, and dissolved oxygen concentration must be carefully controlled to optimize cellulose synthesis. These advancements underscore the ongoing efforts to enhance BNC production efficiency and sustainability (Revin et al., 2018).

### 12.4.2 AGITATED FERMENTATION METHOD

In static culture systems, overcoming the challenges of high costs and limited production rates has been a focal point. Introducing an agitated or shaking culture presents a potential solution to these issues. Oxygen distribution stands out as a critical concern in static culture, directly impacting BNC formation. Interestingly, excessive oxygen supply has been found to hinder BNC formation, prompting the development of agitated culture methods aimed at optimizing oxygen delivery during bacterial culture. Factors such as culture duration, spinning speed, and additives in the culture medium all influence the size and shape of the resulting BNC structures (Hu et al., 2010). The continuous shear force exerted during agitated culture plays a significant role in generating spherical BNC structures, with rotationally agitated cultivation being a primary driver (Hu et al., 2013). Additionally, bacterial concentration affects the quantity and size of sphere-like BNC, with higher concentrations resulting in increased production (Hu et al., 2010). However, agitated culture presents its own set of challenges, including bacterial strain instability, non-newtonian behavior during BNC mixing, and significant shear forces. BNC produced through agitated culture exhibits microstructural and property alterations, including reduced polymerization degree, crystallinity index, and mechanical properties (Kouda et al., 1996). Comparing static and agitated cultures, the formation of BNC membranes differs: static culture forms membranes at the air-liquid interface, while agitated culture synthesizes BNC from the particle center, expanding outward (Hu et al., 2010). Despite its challenges, some studies propose agitated culture as a viable strategy for large-scale, cost-effective production (Hu et al., 2010). Researchers have explored various parameters in agitated culture, including rotation speed, to optimize the production of sphere-like BNC. Lower rotation speeds result in irregularly shaped BNC, while higher speeds facilitate the formation of sphere-like structures (Hu et al., 2010). Efforts to enhance

BNC production have led to the investigation of efficient bioreactors. Bioreactor cultures, particularly those employing continuous cultivation with spinning discs or airlift mechanisms for oxygen delivery, have demonstrated higher BNC production rates. However, BNC produced in bioreactors may exhibit lower crystallinity, elasticity, and polymerization degree compared to static or agitated culture methods (Wang et al., 2019). Various bioreactor types, including membrane, rotating disc, horizontal lift, and modified airlift reactors, have been explored for BNC production (Lin et al., 2014; Onodera et al., 2002; Wu et al., 2015). The use of bioreactors presents opportunities for increased BNC production, albeit on a limited scale. Fundamental research into BNC biosynthesis remains crucial, alongside the development of innovative biotechnological techniques to scale up production efficiently. Moreover, advancements in cell-free extract technology offer promising avenues for large-scale BNC production, with a focus on optimizing cellulose synthase complexes to enhance manufacturing processes (Ávila et al., 2015; Ludwicka et al., 2020). Despite significant progress in optimizing BNC production methods, challenges persist in scaling up cultivation for commercialization. Economic barriers, including high capital and operating costs, coupled with poor productivity, hinder widespread adoption. Nonetheless, the versatility of BNC in various industries, including food, personal care, biomedical, and electronics, highlights its potential for diverse applications (Jozala et al., 2016). Ongoing research endeavors aim to overcome these challenges and unlock the full commercial potential of BNC. Some major techniques for BNC are shown in Table 12.1.

## 12.5 BIOTECHNOLOGICAL APPLICATIONS OF BNC

### *12.5.1 BIOMEDICAL APPLICATIONS*

BNC is a desirable material for biomedical applications because of its special qualities, which include high purity, biocompatibility, and mechanical strength. BNC has been researched extensively as a wound dressing, both alone and in hybrid form, because it can maintain a moist environment that encourages tissue regeneration and lowers the risk of infection. Furthermore, BNC-based scaffolds have been created for use in tissue engineering processes involving the regeneration of vascular, cartilage, and bone tissue. It has also been investigated to employ BNC

**TABLE 12.1** Major Production Techniques for Bacterial Nanocellulose Production

| Production Method | Description | Advantage | Disadvantage | References |
|---|---|---|---|---|
| Bioreactor assisted production (Rotary disc and Air lift reactors) | A novel approach to the Rotating Biological Contactor (RBC) has been developed, involving the immersion of organisms in a nutrient-rich medium followed by exposure to air via rotating discs. | The revamped Rotating Biological Contactor (RBC) demonstrates heightened productivity, streamlined work-up processes, and is conducive to efficient scaling-up. | Optimal productivity hinges on meticulous maintenance of culture media and conditions, underscoring the criticality of stringent protocols in ensuring high yields. | Mahmood et al. (2015) |
| Static intermittent fed batch technique | The utilization of specific fresh media plays a pivotal role in fostering rapid pellicle growth, often exhibiting irregular time intervals of accelerated proliferation. | rate in irregular time intervals. Simple process; Highly improved production; Large scale productivity | Insufficient oversight of fermentation conditions may lead to cellulose separation occurring as either a pellicle or, at times, a reticulated slurry. | Sharma et al. (2021) |
| Agitated fermentation | Reciprocal agitation maintained at 90–100 rpm; stirring promotes accelerated cell growth. | Suitable for large-scale industrial production; Overcoming diffusion is straightforward; User-friendly for operators. | BNC takes the form of irregular spheres rather than a pellicle; agitation at high rpm poses potential for culture mutations; yields are low; instability issues plague the culture. | Zhou et al. (2018) |
| Static fermentation | At the outset, assorted media components are introduced; BNC production occurs within the vessel at the interface between air and liquid. | Simple technique; No need of sophisticated instruments. | The process is time-consuming; monitoring fermentation conditions proves challenging; BNC yield is influenced by two cellulose forms: pellicle or reticulated slurry. | Meereboer et al. (2020) |
| Cell-free extract technique | Cell lysis releases the majority of enzymes required for BNC synthesis directly into the medium. | Simple procedure; Suitable for large-scale implementation; Improved yield due to shortened culture processing time. | No proper control on fermentation parameter. | Patel et al. (2016); Ranjan et al. (2018) |

and its hybrids as carriers of medications or growth factors in drug delivery systems. All things considered, BNC's biomedical uses show off its promise as a flexible biomaterial for regenerative medicine (Sharma et al., 2019). Some of the promising biomedical applications of BNC have been summarized below:

#### *12.5.1.1 WOUND HEALING*

In biomedical research, BNC is a fundamental component, especially when it comes to the field of wound healing in human organs. Its complex structure of fibers and pores serves as a three-dimensional scaffold that promotes migration, proliferation, and adhesion of cells while simultaneously serving as a barrier against the infiltration of pathogens. Moreover, BNC is able to effectively absorb exudates from wounded tissues, enable gas exchange, and demonstrate exceptional moisture retention properties. Its remarkable purity adds even more allure; it is non-toxic, non-allergenic, and biocompatible, which attests to its effectiveness and safety (Picheth et al., 2017; Portela et al., 2019). The Food and Drug Administration (FDA) has approved BNC as a wound dressing, highlighting its importance in clinical practice and the wide range of commercially accessible choices. Notably, the innovative Biofill skin substitute has transformed wound care and shown promise in the management of dermabrasions, skin cancer, severe burns, and persistent ulcers. Its rapid detachment after re-epithelization and tight attachment to wound beds provide instant pain relief, which is essential for patient comfort. Moreover, a considerable proportion of patients suffer from chronic varicose ulcers, for which BNC is useful as a dry membrane. Products such as XCell, a BNC wound dressing that never dries, are excellent for preserving wound moisture, speeding up tissue granulation, and assisting with autolytic debridement. Furthermore, a number of trustworthy solutions for managing burns and ulcers, reducing infections, and reducing pain have surfaced, including Bioprocess, Bionext, Dermafill, and Membracel BC membranes. These developments have contributed to improving the wound healing process. In summary, BNC is a highly important resource for wound healing applications. A wide variety of commercial solutions have been shown to effectively treat burns, chronic ulcers, and other skin problems. It has a clear revolutionary effect on wound care, and current research in cutting-edge biomedical fields is exploring its potential, which attests to its persistent relevance and promise in changing healthcare paradigms (Pavel et al., 2020; Zhong et al., 2020).

#### 12.5.1.2 CARDIOVASCULAR DEVICES

Though it is still in its early phases, the study of BNC in cardiac tissue regeneration is a rapidly expanding subject. Thus far, minimal studies have been undertaken with the aim of revealing the potential of BNC in the creation of cardiovascular devices. In order to protect the cardiac muscles from harmful effects and pathological remodeling in ischemic heart disease, skeletal myoblasts and mesenchymal stem cells (MSC) were delivered via BNC (Simeoni et al., 2021). This method shows how BNC can act as a protective matrix to promote the regeneration and repair of heart tissue. Additionally, the creation of a scaffold made of BNC and polyurethane (BNC/PU) that demonstrated improved mechanical strength and favorable conditions for the survival and operation of natively anisotropic cardiac cells was pioneered. This novel scaffold has potential for supporting physiological function and offering structural support in heart tissue engineering. Furthermore, studies on cellulose acetate and decreased cellulose-based scaffolds have demonstrated their ability to improve electrical and gap junction performance, which will help cardiomyocytes grow *in vitro*. These developments highlight how BNC-based materials can be easily tailored to specific requirements in cardiac tissue engineering by changing the scaffold's characteristics (Chiono et al., 2014). While the application of BNC in cardiac tissue regeneration is still in its early stages, these research encouraging results highlight the material's potential as a useful instrument in this field. The potential uses of BNC in the creation of cardiovascular devices are quite promising in terms of enhancing cardiac patient treatment options. Significant advancements in the field of cardiac tissue engineering and regeneration are expected from ongoing research and development in this subject, opening up new possibilities for patient care and therapeutic intervention (Entcheva et al., 2004).

#### 12.5.1.3 NEURAL TISSUES

Biocompatible neural interfaces have great promise for improving cognitive and motor function, as well as treating neurological conditions. However, the stiff construction and dense inorganic materials of existing neural interfaces sometimes pose issues since they might cause tissue injury. BNC is a superior substitute for neural implants because of its remarkable flexibility, biocompatibility, and suitability for subcutaneous implantation over the long term. Research has demonstrated that functionalizing BNC with recombinant proteins improves the adherence and survival of MSC, which causes neurotrophins to be upregulated and neuronal regeneration to occur (Pertile et al., 2012). Furthermore, in conditions similar to the brain, BNC/graphene oxide (GO) hybrids have been shown to support neural cells, and oxidized BNC-based scaffolds have excellent biocompatibility and hemocompatibility with neurons of the peripheral nervous system. Furthermore, BNC membranes have demonstrated efficacy in impeding epidural fibrosis and peridural adhesions. Furthermore, BNC that has been loaded with growth factors has demonstrated encouraging results in the treatment of spinal cord injuries (Hou et al., 2018; Kim et al., 2017;). In conclusion, BNC-based neural implants offer a compelling solution with their flexibility, biocompatibility, and support for neuronal regeneration. Consequently, the application of BNC-based neural interfaces holds significant promise for future advancements in neuroscience and tissue engineering (Stumpf et al., 2020).

#### *12.5.1.4 BONE AND CARTILAGE*

Hydroxyapatite (HAp) has been added to BNC matrices as a result of research efforts to replicate the natural bone environment. This has shown encouraging results in the creation of biomimetic environments (Duan et al., 2010). Furthermore, the incorporation of growth factors is essential for the maturation of bone stem cells. This has led to research into the combination of growth factors, nanofillers, and natural and synthetic polymers with BNC scaffolds to more closely mimic the natural environment needed for bone regeneration (Favi et al., 2013). According to recent research, MSCs that receive structural support from bone grafting scaffolds differentiate quickly into osteocytes and chondrocytes. BNC scaffolds coated with calcium phosphate have shown to enhance MSC differentiation towards an osteoblastic phenotype, while loading osteogenic growth factors like osteogenic growth peptide (OGP) further amplifies bone cell osteogenic potential (Bab et al., 1992; Sundberg et al., 2015). Specifically, OGP regulates the osteogenesis structure of osteoprogenitor cells, with

CHOeK1 cells seeded on OGP-BNC membranes exhibiting significantly enhanced osteoblastic phenotype characteristics (Saska et al., 2012). Moreover, BNC scaffolds loaded with BMP-2 exhibit robust osteogenic potential, with BMP-2-coated BNC scaffolds leading to greater bone formation and higher calcium levels in rat subcutaneous models (Shi et al., 2012). Another study demonstrated that a 3D BNC scaffold loaded with BMP-2 promotes osteodifferentiation of murine MSCs. Additionally, BNC has shown promise in aiding the regeneration of damaged cartilage by facilitating chondrocyte attachment, migration, and proliferation, resulting in the formation of ECM. Metabolically engineered bacterial cellulose (MBC) produced under N-acetyl glucosamine (GlcNAc) conditions has been shown to effectively facilitate the attachment, proliferation, and differentiation of human MSCs. Nonetheless, optimal cell growth and penetration necessitate scaffolds with a highly interconnected network structure and appropriate pore size, which the inherent pore size of BNC does not provide for cartilage cell growth and penetration. Various studies have thus focused on enhancing the porosity of BNC scaffolds to address this issue, such as designing BNC scaffolds with altered porosity using agarose particles as templates and developing a 3D-composite scaffold composed of micro-fibrillated BNC and poly(3-hydroxybutyrate) (P(3HB)) to enhance cell attachment, proliferation, and migration (Dubey et al., 2020).

#### *12.5.1.5 DRUG DELIVERY*

In recent years, both natural and synthetic polymers have been extensively studied for their potential in drug delivery applications (Dasari et al., 2022). Notably, researchers have delved into exploring the capabilities of BNC-based hydrogel scaffolds for drug delivery, leveraging their fine network structure, high reactive surface, and significant porosity (Eslahi et al., 2020). Through various techniques such as blending, nanoparticle impregnation, and surface modifications, it is possible to achieve exact medication release profiles by customizing BNC. As an illustration, a study created a glutaraldehyde crosslinked hydrogel with BNC and gelatin that showed excellent thermal stability, controlled release properties, and chemical and mechanical resistance for a model medication. Likewise, BNC and chitosan-based pH-sensitive semi-interpenetrating hydrogels demonstrated superior quetiapine fumarate release characteristics. Furthermore, using a non-Fiskian diffusion mechanism, researchers developed a BNC and GO nanohybrid loaded with ibuprofen to demonstrate its effectiveness in controlled-release drug delivery systems. Additionally, a biocompatible BNC-acrylamide hydrogel was created as a pH-sensitive smart carrier for theophylline oral drug delivery. At pH 7.4, the drug releases more *in vivo* while still being hemocompatible and non-cytotoxic at higher doses, guaranteeing its safety for use in oral drug delivery applications. Promising results have been achieved with BNC-based hydrogel scaffolds for drug delivery, which take advantage of BNC's special qualities to meet certain drug release needs. In the future, BNC-based hydrogel scaffolds have a great chance to become a top drug delivery platform with additional improvement and investigation of modification methods (Pandey et al., 2014).

#### *12.5.1.6 DIAGNOSTICS AND BIOSENSING*

Biosensors are becoming increasingly important in tissue engineering and regenerative medicine, where they are used in early disease identification in clinical settings. These biosensors often track biological signals *in vivo* in real time, such as reactions to tissue injury, inflammatory processes, and different medical disorders, using biosensing components including antibodies, receptors, and enzymes (Marques et al., 2008). BNC-Silver (Ag) nanocomposites were prepared and employed for bioanalysis as surface-enhanced Raman scattering (SERS) lamellas, facilitating the analysis of amino acids such as L-glutamine, L-phenylalanine, and L-histidine. Another study focused on glucose oxidase reactions using BNC as an external lamella in a glucose biosensor, where BNC nanofibers containing Au nanoparticles (BC-A) were utilized for glucose determination in human blood samples (Eisele et al., 1994). This biosensor demonstrated high sensitivity, detecting glucose levels as low as 2.3 μM with a linear range of 10–400 μM (Wang et al., 2010). Furthermore, BNC Nano paper was utilized for the first time as a substrate for the development of high-performance artificial tongues. Hydrophobic walls were constructed on the BNC nano paper substrates using laser printing technology, and the photoluminescence properties of an immobilized radiometric probe (carbon dot-Rhodamine B nanohybrids) on the nano paper platform were employed to improve visual discrimination analysis (Abbasi-Moayed et al., 2018). These nano paper-based artificial tongues offer a modern approach to designing optical sensor arrays for advanced biochemical analysis (Lv et al., 2018). Another cutting-edge biosensor creates a highly adaptable, self-powered glucose detector by combining BNC with the deposition of gold nanoparticles. One of the earliest biosensors in this category to be described was glucose oxidase, which is crucial for glucose monitoring in the management of diabetes. Furthermore, direct electron transfer between glucose and glucose oxidase is made possible by a sensor created by immobilizing the enzyme on BNC-filtered carbon nanotube composites (Kim et al., 2013). Recently, affinity ligands, enzymes, and cells were immobilized using magnetically modified BNC, which was generated by *Komagataeibacter sucrofermentans*, and perchloric acid-stabilized magnetic fluid. This modified BNC demonstrates the adaptability and potential of BNC-based biosensors in healthcare applications and shows promise as a useful tool in medical diagnostics (Baldikova et al., 2017).

## 12.6 NON-BIOMEDICAL APPLICATIONS OF BNC-BASED NANOHYBRIDS

### *12.6.1 BIOSENSING*

Bacterial cellulose (BC) is a very promising material for the development of flexible sensors because of its large surface area, high surface hydroxyl (OH) group content, and remarkable water absorption and retention characteristics. In a noteworthy study, scientists used potassium hydroxide (KOH) and BNC nanofibers to create a flexible humidity sensor. By varying the BNC networks, the sensor's performance was improved. The BNC/KOH sensor demonstrated exceptional properties such as flexibility, tensile strength, folding endurance, and a notably strong reaction to humidity (Ma et al., 2022). In another innovative approach, BNC nanofibers were utilized to coat quartz crystal microbalance (QCM) for the development of a straightforward and cost-effective humidity sensor. Imidazolium perchlorate ($ImClO_4$) molecular ferroelectric was infused into the BNC matrix to create recyclable and ecologically benign flexible piezoelectric sensors. These sensors showed a wide operating range and remarkable sensitivity (Lu et al., 2014). Furthermore, researchers developed bi-enzymatic glucose biosensors by synthesizing Au nanoparticles using a BNC suspension, forming BC/Au nanocomposites. These composites' surfaces were then combined with myoglobin (Mb), hemoglobin (Hb), and horseradish peroxidase to create electrocatalytic activity. This produced biocatalytic properties for $H_2O_2$ biosensing that were very sensitive and had a low detection limit. Recently, carboxylate multi-walled carbon nanotubes (MW-CNTs) were used to modify BNC, and then poly(ethyleneimine) (PEI) was used to modify the surface. High density and directed phage immobilization, electrical conductivity, antibacterial activity, and exceptionally selective and specific bacterial detection in both pure and mixed cultures were among the features displayed by this hybrid surface. Furthermore, it had a high degree of accuracy in differentiating between live and dead bacterial cells. Because of its large surface area and surface roughness, BNC has great promise for the design of humidity, piezoelectric, and biosensors, among other applications, owing to its substantial surface area and the presence of surface OH groups. The future outlook for BNC-based sensor development appears promising, and further research holds the potential to unlock even more advanced and efficient sensor designs (Song et al., 2009).

### 12.6.2 COSMETICS

In the world of cosmetics, BNC is a useful resource since it is a versatile substance that can blend in seamlessly with a variety of compounds, such as essential oils and plant extracts (Hasan et al., 2012). Its surface is covered in hydroxyl (OH) groups, which help the active chemicals in the BNC matrix connect and ensure regulated release when applied to the skin. This is a desirable property for face mask compositions (Campano et al., 2016). Because of their remarkable moisturizing qualities and low toxicity, BNC-based face masks have shown efficacy in treating dry skin diseases (Lin et al., 2015). A recent study found that BNC loaded with propolis extract using both *in situ* and *ex situ* methods produced skincare products with encouraging outcomes. The BNC hybrids showed an amazing ability to retain water at 98.01 ± 0.17% and a notable 15.16% suppression of oxidant activity (Amorim et al., 2022). Furthermore, BNC fragments used to cosmetics (0.05% to 1.0% by weight) show significant improvements in skin exfoliation and moisturizing properties (Ougiya et al., 1998). developed a face scrub recipe that uses powdered BC that is enhanced with glutinous rice, aloe vera, vitamin C, and olive oil. The goal of the recipe is to improve skincare Hasan et al. (2012). Personal cleaning formulas represent another intriguing application for BNC. Traditional surfactants, which may inadvertently harm skin constituents and result in allergic reactions and skin irritation, are frequently used in such formulations. It has been found that BNC loaded with silver nanoparticles has an extraordinary ability to stabilize oil/water emulsions. The BNC's fine fibrils obstruct the coalescence of oil droplets by functioning as a mechanical barrier and scaffold. This emulsion's ability to withstand temperature and pH variations is another feature that highlights its potential for use in cleaning product compositions. When taken as a whole, these studies highlight the several advantages that BNC offers the cosmetics sector. Because of its low toxicity profile, ability to combine with active substances, controlled release during application, and moisturizing power, it is a great option for face masks and personal cleansing formulations. In essence, the findings underscore the versatility and immense potential of BNC in elevating cosmetic product formulations (Amnuaikit et al., 2011).

### 12.6.3 FOOD

BNC has emerged as a promising material in the food industry for several reasons (Liu et al., 2023). First of all, the FDA has approved it as safe, citing its excellent purity and moldability as reasons for its suitability for many uses. Its adaptability in food production is further enhanced by its capacity to undergo *in situ* modifications. Additionally, BNC has the ability to aid in digestion and has been connected to the prevention of chronic illnesses including diabetes and cardiovascular disease (Zhai al., 2018). Its use in producing low-calorie foods like surimi (Lin et al., 2011) underscores its potential for healthier food options. Studies have also demonstrated the cholesterol reduction and fat substitution benefits of BNC, as evidenced by experiments with hamsters and mayonnaise (Dourado et al., 2017). Additionally, research has shown positive effects on health markers such as triglycerides, total serum cholesterol, and liver cholesterol (Akoglu et al., 2018; Chau et al., 2008), adding to the evidence for its ability to improve cardiovascular health. BNC has shown to be a very successful food packaging material in terms of improving food safety and prolonging shelf life. Active BNC-based packaging materials can be customized to fulfill individual requirements by adding different additives, such as taint removers, moisture controllers, ethylene and oxygen scavengers, and antibacterial agents. By adding materials like succinic acid (SA), researchers have successfully created biodegradable, antibacterial BNC-based monolayer and multilayer composites, such as BNC-SA (Jipa et al., 2012) films. These films demonstrate the flexibility in their design with water sensitivity and SA release rates based on BNC and SA concentrations. Similarly, to generate antimicrobial films for food packaging, BNC fibers have been mixed with SA and a poly (vinyl alcohol) (PVA) matrix (Dobre et al., 2012). Edible antimicrobial BNC membranes have also been developed, utilizing substances like lactoferrin (Padrao et al., 2016). Moreover, fruit packaging has been investigated using multifunctional BNC-based hybrids that incorporate zein protein nanoparticles (ZNs) or other additives such carboxymethylcellulose (CMC), glycerol, yeast, silver nanoparticles, olive, and ginger oils (Gao et al., 2020). These composites have a number of advantages, including improved water solubility, high tensile strength, non-toxicity, antibacterial and antifungal activity, and sensory qualities like color and odor (Atta et al., 2022). With its nutritional fiber qualities that help with both digestion and the prevention of chronic illnesses, BNC is a safe substitute that shows a lot of promise for a variety of uses in the food sector. Its adaptability to different food products' packaging adds even more allure, providing increased safety and longer shelf lives (Atta et al., 2022).

### *12.6.4 ADDITIVE MANUFACTURING*

When it comes to scaffold and biomedical device manufacturing, the materials that are used need to have qualities that are scalable, which is typically accomplished by using composites or blends. Through 3D printing or additive manufacturing, these materials are meticulously created to fulfill precise specifications for biological uses. The process of additive manufacturing involves layer-by-layer construction, and BNC is a material of note that is utilized in the creation of 3D scaffolds. The incorporation of BNC into different composite materials for 3D printing has been the subject of numerous investigations. For instance, in order to create 3D printed scaffolds, researchers have investigated a mixture of BNC, alginate, and laponite nano clay. The release of proteins such as bovine serum albumin (BSA) and the degradability of the scaffold were impacted by changes in the concentration of laponite nano clay. On the other hand, too much laponite nano clay might prevent cells from proliferating (Wei et al., 2020). A different work (Gutierrez et al., 2019) presented a BNC/alginate hydrogel composite with copper nanostructures, which enhanced the antibacterial capabilities of the 3D printed material. They created a creative hydrogel ink that combines BNC with gelatin, glycerol, and silk fibroin. Excellent printability was demonstrated by this composite, which produced scaffolds with strengthened mechanical qualities. The scaffolds' capacity for self-repair and tensile strength was significantly improved with the addition of BNC. Another study investigated a composite of polyvinyl alcohol (PVA), hexagonal boron nitride, and BNC to create bone tissue scaffolds using 3D printing (Huang et al., 2019). Human osteoblast cell viability on the printed scaffolds was much increased by the ideal composite material; however, the inclusion of BNC somewhat decreased the scaffold's tensile strength. In conclusion, it has been shown that 3D-printed BNC mixes or composites have better mechanical qualities and increased cell survivability. To get the best results, however, great thought must be given to the kind and quantity of composite material. All things considered, there is great potential for improving material science for biomedical applications through the continued investigation and improvement of composite materials and 3D printing techniques (Aki et al., 2020).

### 12.6.5 ENVIRONMENTAL

Water treatment, pollution monitoring, and air filtration are just a few of the environmental applications where BNC membranes offer a viable and sustainable alternative to traditional synthetic polymer-based membranes (Habibi et al., 2014; Shahzad et al., 2023). Because nanotechnology has made it possible to integrate polymers and nanoparticles, it has aided in the development of nanocomposite materials (Seshadri et al., 2020). BNC has attracted a lot of interest as a possible pollution sensor in environmental sensing applications. For example, designed nanocomposites that detect hydrogen sulfide ($H_2S$) by coating BNC nanocrystals (BCNCs) with silver nanoparticles (AgNPs). Even at low concentrations, these hybrid films showed remarkable sensitivity to H2S (Sukhavattanakul et al., 2020).

Similarly, BNC and polyethyleneimine (PEI) double-layer nanofilms were devised for formaldehyde gas detection, showcasing optimal sensing performance. Moreover, BNC membranes have been enhanced with metal oxides like zinc oxide (ZnO) or titanium oxide ($TiO_2$) to bolster their sensing capabilities. The incorporation of ZnO semiconductor onto BNC surfaces showed outstanding reactivity to a variety of contaminants, including ethanol, nitrogen dioxide, and acetone, with a notable sensitivity to nitrogen dioxide at room temperature (Wang et al., 2020). BNC-based composites have demonstrated efficacy not only in sensing applications but also in photocatalytic destruction of organic contaminants. They created a BNC/$TiO_2$ composite to degrade contaminants such as bisphenol-A, phenol, and methyl orange. Moreover, BNC has been used in the creation of air filters, either by itself or in conjunction with other substances like silver nanowires (AgNW) or soy protein isolate (SPI), reaching excellent removal effectiveness for hazardous compounds and particulate matter (PM) (Liu et al., 2020). BNC membranes offer an eco-friendly and versatile solution for addressing environmental challenges, demonstrating remarkable sensitivity towards pollutants and exceptional efficiency in air filtration. Continued research and development in this field hold promise for advancing sustainable environmental technologies (Rocha Santana et al., 2023).

### *12.6.6 ENERGY*

Highly valued for its remarkable mechanical characteristics and thermal stability, BNC is a potential candidate for energy storage applications that extend beyond supercapacitors and include dielectric materials. Novel approaches to BNC-based conductive composites have opened the door to a wide range of energy applications (Prilepskii et al., 2023). Because of BNC's exceptional catalytic ability, palladium (Pd) precipitates, producing high surface area BNC/Pd hybrids that are perfect for energy storage applications. Additionally, BNC is used in fuel cells and polyelectrolyte membranes. Examples of this include BNC/Pt composites that demonstrate strong electrocatalytic activity and BNC films doped with protonic acid that demonstrate significant proton conductivity for fuel cell membranes. Novel techniques that highlight BNC's adaptability include pyrolyzing BNC into interwoven carbon nanofibers and creating electrically conducting BNC/polyaniline (BC/PANI) composites (Evans et al., 2003). These techniques produce 3D conducting networks with remarkable electrical conductivity that are structurally strong and crucial for materials used in energy storage. BNC has advantages for supercapacitor development as well. The potential of BNC in this field is demonstrated by $MnO_2$-coated BNC supercapacitors and all-biomaterial supercapacitors that use activated pyrolyzed BNC electrodes and exhibit exceptional energy density, cycling stability, and specific capacitance (Yang et al., 2009). Essentially, BNC shows itself to be a flexible material suitable for various energy storage uses. Its conductivity, mechanical strength, and catalytic potential make it a good fit for next-generation energy storage technologies. Further developments in BNC-based conductive composites could lead to increased energy density, stability, and efficiency—a major step toward sustainable energy sources (Truong et al., 2021).

## 12.7 CHALLENGES AND FUTURE PERSPECTIVES

The debate over whether BNC can replace or rival traditional cellulose sources remains contentious, with a definitive answer pending advancements in scaling up BNC production and fermentation bioprocesses. Despite extensive research efforts dedicated to BNC production, achieving economically feasible production at a commercial scale has proven elusive. illustrates the challenges hindering successful BNC production and utilization. These challenges can be categorized into four main areas: (i) Production-based hurdles; (ii) Substrate-based limitations; (iii) Strain-related obstacles; and (iv) Clinical progress and marketing of BNC-based therapeutics. Thus far, the primary obstacle to scaling up BNC production lies in its high production costs, primarily attributed to the expensive culture media and slow production processes. The substantial capital investment and operational expenses pose significant barriers to the commercialization of BNC at a competitive cost. Further research is warranted, particularly in exploring alternative, cost-effective substrates for bacterial growth in BNC production. Scientists are increasingly exploring novel feedstock options to address the demand for more economical BNC production processes (Gama et al., 2016).

### 12.7.1 PRODUCTION-BASED CHALLENGES

There is a noticeable scarcity of bioreactor-based studies in BNC production, with the majority focusing on static or agitated methods. This underscores the urgent need to explore bioreactor-based cultivation techniques to achieve revolutionary advancements in BNC production. Bioreactors offer the potential for meticulous control over all crucial parameters, laying the foundation for groundbreaking progress. Presently, bioreactors utilized in BNC production feature rudimentary designs (Zahan et al., 2010). To unlock the full potential of BNC production, it is imperative to employ more intricate and sophisticated bioreactor designs. Enhancements could include the integration of advanced features such as optimized pH probes and water jackets, enabling precise regulation of pH and temperature within the bioreactor environment (Keshk et al., 2017). Maintaining pH, oxygen levels, and temperature at optimal values throughout the fermentation process is crucial. Achieving this could lead to a substantial increase in microbial cellulose production. Moreover, leveraging modified production methods like the static intermittent fed-batch strategy and cell-free extract system holds promise for enhancing BNC production efficiency. Exploration of various combinations of agro/industrial wastes and strains, alongside innovative production techniques, is essential. This approach aims to identify the most suitable combination of cultivation technique, substrate, and strain to significantly boost BNC production. By harnessing the potential of bioreactor-based cultivation and implementing advanced design improvements, the path towards groundbreaking BNC production can be paved (Zahan et al., 2010).

### 12.7.2 SUBSTRATE-BASED CHALLENGES

The culture media employed in BNC production accounts for a significant portion of the total production costs, underscoring the critical need to identify new cost-effective substrates to enhance BNC yields efficiently and rapidly. Currently, there is a growing focus on utilizing agro/industrial wastes as economical substrates for BNC production, which not only addresses cost concerns but also offers environmental benefits by repurposing waste materials. However, to maximize the potential of these substrates, studies need to be conducted under controlled conditions in advanced bioreactors. This approach ensures optimal BNC productivity and quality, paving the way for sustainable and scalable production. Moreover, exploring co-cultures of different bacterial strains, particularly with cost-effective substrates, holds promise for enhancing BNC production. Efforts to isolate and characterize microorganisms with superior BNC production capabilities should be intensified, focusing on both individual strains and symbiotic associations (Florea et al., 2016). Additionally, investigating microbial populations involved in fermentative processes like those found in kombucha and nata de coco could unveil novel pathways for BNC synthesis. Furthermore, understanding the molecular basis of BNC synthesis, including the complex interplay of catalytic and regulatory protein complexes, is crucial for optimizing production efficiency. Genetic engineering offers a promising avenue for strain improvement, with recent advancements showcasing the potential to enhance BNC yields while reducing production costs. For instance, the isolation of strains like *Komagataeibacter rheticus* iGEM, which exhibit high BNC yields under nitrogen stress, highlights the potential of genetic manipulation to optimize production conditions and decrease costs. However, regulatory considerations must be addressed, particularly in industries like medicine and food. In summary, addressing the challenges associated with BNC production requires a multidisciplinary approach encompassing genetic engineering, metabolic modeling, and advanced bioreactor design. By harnessing the potential of these technologies, we can unlock the full capabilities of BNC for various applications while ensuring sustainability and cost-effectiveness (de Oliveira et al., 2016).

### 12.7.3 CLINICAL STUDIES AND MARKETING RELATED CHALLENGES

The translation of *in vitro* and animal study results into clinical applications for BNC-based products poses significant challenges, hindering their introduction to the market. Despite the availability of numerous BNC-based therapeutics, only a few have been approved for patient use. This limited approval stems from various factors, including challenges in scaling up manufacturing, high development costs, concerns regarding sterility, and issues related to patents. Moreover, regulatory barriers further impede the approval process, requiring stringent quality assurance for consistent manufacturing, comprehensive quality control, and comparability evaluations for component and process changes (Achi et al., 2005). Establishing appropriate shipping and storage conditions and determining shelf life also present regulatory hurdles. One approach to address these challenges is to develop cost-effective BNC-based biodevices, which could help streamline manufacturing processes and reduce development costs. Additionally, further research efforts are needed to explore BNC's potential in specific biomedical areas such as neurological disorders, diabetes, cancer, and vaccines. Innovative research is already underway to explore future trends in BNC applications, particularly in nanotechnology, including the development of nanoparticles for drug delivery systems and BNC-based biodevices for treating challenging disorders like Alzheimer's, cancer, and diabetes. However, it is essential for BNC to demonstrate clear therapeutic advantages over existing treatment options *in vivo*, ensuring its efficacy and safety compared to conventional biodevices and drugs on the market. Through continued research and development, BNC has the potential to revolutionize various biomedical fields and offer novel solutions to complex medical challenges (Oliveira et al., 2015).

## 12.8 CONCLUSION

BNC is a material of enormous industrial concern and known to have applicability in versatile fields; therefore, additional impetus is obligatory to make this greener material a competitive product while being economically viable. BNC has wide usage in different technological applications, including biomedical areas like wound healing, drug delivery, tissue engineering, biosensing device fabrication, and medical implants. Efforts to enhance BNC production have focused on reducing manufacturing costs, increasing yields, and improving overall performance through tailored physico-chemical and biological characteristics. Metabolic engineering of microbes, innovative strategies using bioreactors in both agitated and static modes, and replacing traditional cultural strains with cost-effective agricultural feedstocks are three main approaches for increasing BNC production. However, BNC faces challenges such as low antibacterial activity, poor processing solubility, and limited porosity. To address these drawbacks, bio-agents such as medicinal plant extracts can be incorporated to impart antimicrobial properties to BNC. Moreover, features like cell adhesion, pore size, and porosity can be modified by blending BNC with various biopolymers. With these enhancements, BNC could find applications in biomedical scaffolds and personal care items, provided it can be produced in large quantities at an affordable cost.

## KEYWORDS


- **bacterial nanocellulose**
- **biomedical applications**
- **industrial scalability**
- **nanohybrid synthesis**
- **substrate optimization**
- **surface chemistry**


## REFERENCES


Abbasi-Moayed, S., Golmohammadi, H., & Hormozi-Nezhad, M. R. (2018). A nanopaper-based artificial tongue: A ratio metric fluorescent sensor array on bacterial nanocellulose for chemical discrimination applications. *Nanoscale*, *10*(5), 2492–2502.

Achi, O. K. (2005). The potential for upgrading traditional fermented foods through biotechnology. *African Journal of Biotechnology*, *4*(5), 375–380.

Akaraonye, E., Filip, J., Safarikova, M., Salih, V., Keshavarz, T., Knowles, J. C., & Roy, I. (2016). Composite scaffolds for cartilage tissue engineering based on natural polymers of bacterial origin, thermoplastic poly (3-hydroxybutyrate) and micro-fibrillated bacterial cellulose. *Polymer International*, *65*(7), 780–791.

Aki, D., Ulag, S., Unal, S., Sengor, M., Ekren, N., Lin, C. C., & Gunduz, O. (2020). 3D printing of PVA/hexagonal boron nitride/bacterial cellulose composite scaffolds for bone tissue engineering. *Materials & Design*, *196*, 109094.

Akoglu, A., Cakır, I., Karahan, A. G., & Çakmakçı, M. L. (2018). Effects of bacterial cellulose as a fat replacer on some properties of fat-reduced mayonnaise. *Romanian Biotechnological Letters*, *23*(3).

Amnuaikit, T., Chusuit, T., Raknam, P., & Boonme, P. (2011). Effects of a cellulose mask synthesized by a bacterium on facial skin characteristics and user satisfaction. *Medical Devices: Evidence and Research*, *4*, 77–81.

Amorim, J. D., Nascimento, H. A., Silva Junior, C. J. G., Medeiros, A. D., Silva, I. D. L., Costa, A. F. S., & Sarubbo, L. A. (2022). Obtainment of bacterial cellulose with added propolis extract for cosmetic applications. *Polymer Engineering & Science*, *62*(2), 565–575.

Andrade, F. K., Silva, J. P., Carvalho, M., Castanheira, E. M., Soares, R., & Gama, M. (2011). Studies on the hemocompatibility of bacterial cellulose. *Journal of Biomedical Materials Research Part A*, *98*(4), 554–566.

Atta, O. M., Manan, S., Ul-Islam, M., Ahmed, A. A. Q., Ullah, M. W., & Yang, G. (2022). Development and characterization of plant oil-incorporated carboxymethyl cellulose/bacterial cellulose/glycerol-based antimicrobial edible films for food packaging applications. *Advanced Composites and Hybrid Materials*, *5*, 1–18.

Ávila, M., Feldmann, H., & Pleumeekers, E. M. (2015). Novel bilayer bacterial nanocellulose scaffold supports neocartilage formation *in vitro* and *in vivo*. *Biomaterials*, *44*, 1–44.

Bab, I., Gazit, D., Chorev, M., Muhlrad, A., Shteyer, A., Greenberg, Z., & Kahn, A. (1992). Histone H4-related osteogenic growth peptide (OGP): a novel circulating stimulator of osteoblastic activity. *The EMBO Journal*, *11*(5), 1867–1873.

Bae, S. O., Sugano, Y., & Ohi, K. (2004). Features of bacterial cellulose synthesis in a mutant generated by disruption of the diguanylate cyclase 1 gene of *Acetobacter xylinum* BPR 2001. *Applied Microbiology and Biotechnology*, *65*, 315–322.

Baldikova, E., Pospiskova, K., Ladakis, D., Kookos, I. K., Koutinas, A. A., Safarikova, M., & Safarik, I. (2017). Magnetically modified bacterial cellulose: a promising carrier for immobilization of affinity ligands, enzymes, and cells. *Materials Science and Engineering: C*, *71*, 214–221.

Barja, F. (2021). Bacterial nanocellulose production and biomedical applications. *Journal of Biomedical Research*, *35*(4), 310.

Battad-Bernardo, E., McCrindle, S. L., Couperwhite, I., & Neilan, B. A. (2004). Insertion of an *E. coli lacZ* gene in *Acetobacter xylinus* for the production of cellulose in whey. *FEMS Microbiology Letters*, *231*(2), 253–260.

Campano, C., Balea, A., Blanco, A., & Negro, C. (2016). Enhancement of the fermentation process and properties of bacterial cellulose: a review. *Cellulose*, *23*, 57–91.

Castro, C., Cordeiro, N., Faria, M., Zuluaga, R., Putaux, J. L., Filpponen, I., & Gañán, P. (2015). *In-situ* glocalization during biosynthesis of bacterial cellulose. *Carbohydrate Polymers*, *126*, 32–39.

Chandana, A., Mallick, S. P., Dikshit, P. K., Singh, B. N., & Sahi, A. K. (2022). Recent developments in bacterial nanocellulose production and its biomedical applications. *Journal of Polymers and the Environment*, *30*(10), 4040–4067.

Chen, G., Chen, L., Wang, W., Chen, S., Wang, H., Wei, Y., & Hong, F. F. (2019). Improved bacterial nanocellulose production from glucose without the loss of quality by evaluating thirteen agitator configurations at low speed. *Microbial Biotechnology*, *12*(6), 1387–1402.

Chiono, V., Mozetic, P., Boffito, M., Sartori, S., Gioffredi, E., Silvestri, A., Rainer, A., Giannitelli, S. M., Trombetta, M., Nurzynska, D., Di Meglio, F., Castaldo, C., Miraglia, R., Montagnani, S., & Ciardelli, G. (2014). Polyurethane-based scaffolds for myocardial tissue engineering. *Interface Focus*, *4*(1), 20130045. https://doi.org/10.1098/rsfs.2013.0045 (accessed on 5th November 2025).

Dasari, S., Njiki, S., Mbemi, A., Yedjou, C. G., & Tchounwou, P. B. (2022). Pharmacological effects of cisplatin combination with natural products in cancer chemotherapy. *International Journal of Molecular Sciences*, *23*(3), 1532.

de Oliveira Barud, H. G., Da Silva, R. R., da Silva Barud, H., Tercjak, A., Gutierrez, J., Lustri, W. R., & Ribeiro, S. J. (2016). A multipurpose natural and renewable polymer in medical applications: Bacterial cellulose. *Carbohydrate Polymers*, *153*, 406–420.

Dobre, L. M., Stoica-Guzun, A., Stroescu, M., Jipa, I. M., Dobre, T., Ferdeş, M., & Ciumpiliac, Ş. (2012). Modeling of sorbic acid diffusion through bacterial cellulose-based antimicrobial films. *Chemical Papers*, *66*, 144–151.

Dourado, F., Gama, M., & Rodrigues, A. C. (2017). A review on the toxicology and dietetic role of bacterial cellulose. *Toxicology Reports*, *4*, 543–553.

Duan, B., Wang, M., Zhou, W. Y., Cheung, W. L., Li, Z. Y., & Lu, W. W. (2010). Three-dimensional nanocomposite scaffolds fabricated via selective laser sintering for bone tissue engineering. *Acta Biomaterial*, *6*(12), 4495–4505.

Dubey, S., & Singh, J., & Singh, R. P. (2018). Biotransformation of sweet lime pulp waste into high-quality nanocellulose with an excellent productivity using *Komagataeibacter europaeus* SGP37 under static intermittent fed-batch cultivation. *Bioresource Technology*, *247*, 73–80.

Dubey, S., Mishra, R., Roy, P., & Singh, R. P. (2021). 3-D macro/microporous-nanofibrous bacterial cellulose scaffolds seeded with BMP-2 preconditioned mesenchymal stem cells exhibit remarkable potential for bone tissue engineering. *International Journal of Biological Macromolecules*, *167*, 934–946.

Edwards, K. J., Jay, A. J., Colquhoun, I. J., Morris, V. J., Gasson, M. J., & Griffin, A. M. (1999). Generation of a novel polysaccharide by inactivation of the aceP gene from the acetan biosynthetic pathway in *Acetobacter xylinum*. *Microbiology*, *145*(6), 1499–1506.

Eisele, S., Ammon, H. P. T., Kindervater, R., Gröbe, A., & Göpel, W. (1994). Optimized biosensor for whole blood measurements using a new cellulose-based membrane. *Biosensors and Bioelectronics*, *9*(2), 119–124.

El-Hoseny, S. M., Basmaji, P., de Olyveira, G. M., Costa, L. M. M., Alwahedi, A. M., da Costa Oliveira, J. D., & Francozo, G. B. (2015). Natural ECM-bacterial cellulose wound healing—Dubai study. *Journal of Biomaterials and Nanobiotechnology*, *6*(4), 237–246.

Entcheva, E., Bien, H., Yin, L., Chung, C. Y., Farrell, M., & Kostov, Y. (2004). Functional cardiac cell constructs on cellulose-based scaffolding. *Biomaterials*, *25*(26), 5753–5762.

Eslahi, N., Mahmoodi, A., Mahmoudi, N., Zandi, N., & Simchi, A. (2020). Processing and properties of nanofibrous bacterial cellulose-containing polymer composites: a review of recent advances for biomedical applications. *Polymer Reviews*, *60*(1), 144–170.

Evans, B. R., O'Neill, H. M., Malyvanh, V. P., Lee, I., & Woodward, J. (2003). Palladium-bacterial cellulose membranes for fuel cells. *Biosensors and Bioelectronics*, *18*(7), 917–923.

Eyley, S., & Thielemans, W. (2014). Surface modification of cellulose nanocrystals. *Nanoscale*, *6*(14), 7764–7779.

Favi, P. M., Benson, R. S., Neilsen, N. R., Hammonds, R. L., Bates, C. C., Stephens, C. P., & Dhar, M. S. (2013). Cell proliferation, viability, and *in vitro* differentiation of equine mesenchymal stem cells seeded on bacterial cellulose hydrogel scaffolds. *Materials Science and Engineering: C*, *33*(4), 1935–1944.

Florea, M., Hagemann, H., Santosa, G., Abbott, J., Micklem, C. N., Spencer-Milnes, X., & Ellis, T. (2016). Engineering control of bacterial cellulose production using a genetic toolkit and a new cellulose-producing strain. *Proceedings of the National Academy of Sciences*, *113*(24), E3431–E3440.

Gama, M., Dourado, F., & Bielecki, S. (2016). *Bacterial Nanocellulose: From Biotechnology to Bio-Economy*. Elsevier.

Gama, M., Gatenholm, P., & Klemm, D. (2012). *Bacterial Nanocellulose: A Sophisticated Multifunctional Material*. CRC Press.

Gromet, Z., Schramm, M., & Hestrin, S. (1957). Synthesis of cellulose by *Acetobacter xylinum*. 4. Enzyme systems present in a crude extract of glucose-grown cells. *Biochemical Journal*, *67*(4), 679.

Gromovykh, T. I., Pigaleva, M. A., Gallyamov, M. O., Ivanenko, I. P., Ozerova, K. E., Kharitonova, E. P., & Kiselyova, O. I. (2020). Structural organization of bacterial cellulose: The origin of anisotropy and layered structures. *Carbohydrate Polymers*, *237*, 116140.

Gutierrez, E., Burdiles, P. A., Quero, F., Palma, P., Olate-Moya, F., & Palza, H. (2019). 3D printing of antimicrobial alginate/bacterial-cellulose composite hydrogels by incorporating copper nanostructures. *ACS Biomaterials Science & Engineering*, *5*(11), 6290–6299.

Habibi, Y. (2014). Key advances in the chemical modification of nanocelluloses. *Chemical Society Reviews*, *43*(5), 1519–1542.

Hasan, N., Biak, D. R. A., & Kamarudin, S. (2012). Application of bacterial cellulose (BC) in natural facial scrub. *International Journal on Advanced Science Engineering and Information Technology*, *2*(4), 1–4.

Helenius, G., Bäckdahl, H., Bodin, A., Nannmark, U., Gatenholm, P., & Risberg, B. (2006). *In vivo* biocompatibility of bacterial cellulose. *Journal of Biomedical Materials Research Part A*, *76*(2), 431–438. https://doi.org/10.1002/jbm.a.30570 (accessed on 5th November 2025).

Hou, Y., Wang, X., Yang, J., Zhu, R., Zhang, Z., & Li, Y. (2018). Development and biocompatibility evaluation of biodegradable bacterial cellulose as a novel peripheral nerve scaffold. *Journal of Biomedical Materials Research Part A*, *106*(5), 1288–1298.

Hu, Y., & Catchmark, J. M. (2010). Formation and characterization of sphere-like bacterial cellulose particles produced by *Acetobacter xylinum* JCM 9730 strain. *Biomacromolecules*, *11*(7), 1727–1734.

Hu, Y., Catchmark, J. M., & Vogler, E. A. (2013). Factors impacting the formation of sphere-like bacterial cellulose particles and their biocompatibility for human osteoblast growth. *Biomacromolecules*, *14*, 3444–3452.

Huang, C., Guo, H. J., & Xiong, L. (2016). Using wastewater after lipid fermentation as substrate for bacterial cellulose production by *Gluconacetobacter xylinus*. *Carbohydrate Polymers*, *136*, 198–202.

Huang, L., Du, X., Fan, S., Yang, G., Shao, H., Li, D., & Zhang, Y. (2019). Bacterial cellulose nanofibers promote stress and fidelity of 3D-printed silk-based hydrogel scaffold with hierarchical pores. *Carbohydrate Polymers*, *221*, 146–156.

Ishida, T., Sugano, Y., & Nakai, T. (2002). Effects of acetan on production of bacterial cellulose by *Acetobacter xylinum*. *Bioscience, Biotechnology, and Biochemistry*, *66*, 1677–1681.

Jipa, I. M., Stoica-Guzun, A., & Stroescu, M. (2012). Controlled release of sorbic acid from bacterial cellulose-based mono and multilayer antimicrobial films. *LWT*, *47*(2), 400–406.

Jozala, A. F., de Lencastre-Novaes, L. C., & Lopes, A. M. (2016). Bacterial nanocellulose production and application: A 10-year overview. *Applied Microbiology and Biotechnology*, *100*, 2063–2072.

Kawano, S., Tajima, K., Kono, H., Erata, T., Munekata, M., & Takai, M. (2002). Effects of endogenous endo-β-1,4-glucanase on cellulose biosynthesis in *Acetobacter xylinum* ATCC23769. *Journal of Bioscience and Bioengineering*, *94*(3), 275–281.

Keshk, S. M., & El-Kott, A. F. (2017). Natural bacterial biodegradable medical polymers: Bacterial cellulose. In *Science and Principles of Biodegradable and Bioresorbable Medical Polymers* (pp. 295–319). Woodhead Publishing.

Khan, S., Ul-Islam, M., Ikram, M., Islam, S. U., Ullah, M. W., Israr, M., & Park, J. K. (2018). Preparation and structural characterization of surface-modified microporous bacterial cellulose scaffolds: A potential material for skin regeneration applications *in vitro* and *in vivo*. *International Journal of Biological Macromolecules*, *117*, 1200–1210.

Khattak, S., Qin, X. T., Wahid, F., Huang, L. H., Xie, Y. Y., Jia, S. R., & Zhong, C. (2021). Permeation of silver sulfadiazine into TEMPO-oxidized bacterial cellulose as an antibacterial agent. *Frontiers in Bioengineering and Biotechnology*, *8*, 616467.

Kim, D., Park, S., Jo, I., Kim, S. M., Kang, D. H., Cho, S. P., & Yoon, M. H. (2017). Multiscale modulation of nanocrystalline cellulose hydrogel via nanocarbon hybridization for 3D neuronal bilayer formation. *Small*, *13*(26), 1700331.

Kim, Y. H., Park, S., Won, K., Kim, H. J., & Lee, S. H. (2013). Bacterial cellulose–carbon nanotube composite as a biocompatible electrode for the direct electron transfer of glucose oxidase. *Journal of Chemical Technology & Biotechnology*, *88*(6), 1067–1070.

Klemm, D., Schumann, D., Udhardt, U., & Marsch, S. (2001). Bacterial synthesized cellulose—artificial blood vessels for microsurgery. *Progress in Polymer Science*, *26*(9), 1561–1603.

Koizumi, S., Yue, Z., & Tomita, Y. (2008). Bacterium organizes hierarchical amorphous structure in microbial cellulose. *European Physical Journal E*, *26*, 137–142.

Kouda, T., Yano, H., & Yoshinaga, F. (1996). Characterization of non-Newtonian behavior during mixing of bacterial cellulose in a bioreactor. *Journal of Fermentation and Bioengineering*, *82*, 382–386.

Kralisch, D., Hessler, N., Klemm, D., Erdmann, R., & Schmidt, W. (2010). White biotechnology for cellulose manufacturing—The HoLiR concept. *Biotechnology and Bioengineering*, *105*(4), 740–747.

Krystynowicz, A., Czaja, W., Wiktorowska-Jezierska, A., Gonçalves-Miśkiewicz, M., Turkiewicz, M., & Bielecki, S. (2002). Factors affecting the yield and properties of bacterial cellulose. *Journal of Industrial Microbiology and Biotechnology*, *29*(4), 189–195.

Kuo, C. H., Teng, H. Y., & Lee, C. K. (2015). Knock-out of glucose dehydrogenase gene in *Gluconacetobacter xylinus* for bacterial cellulose production enhancement. *Biotechnology and Bioprocess Engineering*, *20*, 18–25.

Lamboni, L., Li, Y., Liu, J., & Yang, G. (2016). Silk sericin-functionalized bacterial cellulose as a potential wound-healing biomaterial. *Biomacromolecules*, *17*(9), 3076–3084.

Leitao, A. F., Gupta, S., Silva, J. P., Reviakine, I., & Gama, M. (2013). Hemocompatibility study of a bacterial cellulose/polyvinyl alcohol nanocomposite. *Colloids and Surfaces B: Bio Interfaces*, *111*, 493–502.

Li, J., Wan, Y., Li, L., Liang, H., & Wang, J. (2009). Preparation and characterization of 2,3-dialdehyde bacterial cellulose for potential biodegradable tissue engineering scaffolds. *Materials Science and Engineering: C*, *29*(5), 1635–1642.

Lin, S. B., Chen, L. C., & Chen, H. H. (2011). Physical characteristics of surimi and bacterial cellulose composite gel. *Journal of Food Process Engineering*, *34*(4), 1363–1379.

Lin, S. P., Hsieh, S. C., Chen, K. I., Demirci, A., & Cheng, K. C. (2014). Semi-continuous bacterial cellulose production in a rotating disk bioreactor and its materials properties analysis. *Cellulose*, *21*, 835–844.

Lin, Y. C., Wey, Y. C., Lee, M. L., & Lin, P. C. (2015). U.S. Patent Application No. 14/614,855.

Liu, L., Ode Boni, B. O., Ullah, M. W., Qi, F., Li, X., Shi, Z., & Yang, G. (2023). Cellulose: A promising and versatile Pickering emulsifier for healthy foods. *Food Reviews International*, *39*(9), 7081–7111.

Lu, H., & Jiang, X. (2014). Structure and properties of bacterial cellulose produced using a trickling bed reactor. *Applied Biochemistry and Biotechnology*, *172*, 3844–3861.

Ludwicka, K., Kaczmarek, M., & Białkowska, A. (2020). Bacterial nanocellulose—a biobased polymer for active and intelligent food packaging applications: recent advances and developments. *Polymers (Basel)*, *12*, 1–23.

Lv, P., Zhou, H., Mensah, A., Feng, Q., Wang, D., Hu, X., & Wei, Q. (2018). A highly flexible self-powered biosensor for glucose detection by epitaxial deposition of gold nanoparticles on conductive bacterial cellulose. *Chemical Engineering Journal*, *351*, 177–188.

Ma, H., Li, X., Lou, J., Gu, Y., Zhang, Y., Jiang, Y., & Han, W. (2022). Strong bacterial cellulose-based films with natural laminar alignment for highly sensitive humidity sensors. *ACS Applied Materials & Interfaces*, *14*(2), 3165–3175.

Mahmood, K. A., Wilkinson, S. J., & Zimmerman, W. B. (2015). Airlift bioreactor for biological applications with microbubble mediated transport processes. *Chemical Engineering Science*, *137*, 243–253.

Mangayil, R., Rajala, S., & Pammo, A. (2017). Engineering and characterization of bacterial nanocellulose films as low-cost and flexible sensor material. *ACS Applied Materials & Interfaces*, *9*, 19048–19056.

Marques, P. A., Nogueira, H. I., Pinto, R. J., Neto, C. P., & Trindade, T. (2008). Silver-bacterial cellulosic sponges as active SERS substrates. *Journal of Raman Spectroscopy*, *39*(4), 439–443.

Meereboer, K. W., Misra, M., & Mohanty, A. K. (2020). Review of recent advances in the biodegradability of polyhydroxyalkanoate (PHA) bioplastics and their composites. *Green Chemistry*, *22*, 2–40.

Mehta, K., Pfeffer, S., & Brown, R. M. (2015). Characterization of an acsD disruption mutant provides additional evidence for the hierarchical cell-directed self-assembly of cellulose in *Gluconacetobacter xylinus*. *Cellulose*, *22*, 119–137.

Mirtalebi, S. S., Almasi, H., & Khaledabad, M. A. (2019). Physical, morphological, antimicrobial and release properties of novel MgO-bacterial cellulose nanohybrids prepared by *in-situ* and *ex-situ* methods. *International Journal of Biological Macromolecules*, *128*, 848–857.

Mohammadkazemi, F., Doosthoseini, K., Ganjian, E., & Azin, M. (2015). Manufacturing of bacterial nano-cellulose reinforced fiber–cement composites. *Construction and Building Materials*, *101*, 958–964.

Moradi, M., Jacek, P., Farhangfar, A., Guimaraes, J. T., & Forough, M. (2021). The role of genetic manipulation and *in situ* modifications on production of bacterial nanocellulose: A review. *International Journal of Biological Macromolecules*, *183*, 635–650.

Morais, J. M., Papadimitrakopoulos, F., & Burgess, D. J. (2010). Biomaterials/tissue interactions: Possible solutions to overcome foreign body response. *The AAPS Journal*, *12*, 188–196.

Morgan, J. L., Strumillo, J., & Zimmer, J. (2013). Crystallographic snapshot of cellulose synthesis and membrane translocation. *Nature*, *493*(7431), 181–186.

Nakai, T., Sugano, Y., Shoda, M., Sakakibara, H., Oiwa, K., Tuzi, S., & Mineyuki, Y. (2013). Formation of highly twisted ribbons in a carboxymethylcellulase gene-disrupted strain of a cellulose-producing bacterium. *Journal of Bacteriology*, *195*(5), 958–964.

Numata, Y., Sakata, T., Furukawa, H., & Tajima, K. (2015). Bacterial cellulose gels with high mechanical strength. *Materials Science and Engineering: C*, *47*, 57–62.

Oliveira, C., Carvalho, V., Domingues, L., & Gama, F. M. (2015). Recombinant CBM-fusion technology—Applications overview. *Biotechnology Advances*, *33*(3, 4), 358–369.

Onodera, M., Harashima, I., & Toda, K. (2002). Silicone rubber membrane bioreactors for bacterial cellulose production. *Biotechnology and Bioprocess Engineering*, *7*(5), 289–294.

Orlando, I., Basnett, P., Nigmatullin, R., Wang, W., Knowles, J. C., & Roy, I. (2020). Chemical modification of bacterial cellulose for the development of an antibacterial wound dressing. *Frontiers in Bioengineering and Biotechnology*, *8*, 557885.

Ougiya, H., Hioki, N., Watanabe, K., Morinaga, Y., Yoshinaga, F., & Samejima, M. (1998). Relationship between the physical properties and surface area of cellulose derived from adsorbates of various molecular sizes. *Bioscience, Biotechnology, and Biochemistry*, *62*(10), 1880–1884.

Öz, Y. E., & Kalender, M. (2023). A novel static cultivation of bacterial cellulose production from sugar beet molasses: Series static culture (SSC) system. *International Journal of Biological Macromolecules*, *225*, 1306–1314.

Padrão, J., Gonçalves, S., Silva, J. P., Sencadas, V., Lanceros-Méndez, S., Pinheiro, A. C., & Dourado, F. (2016). Bacterial cellulose–lactoferrin as an antimicrobial edible packaging. *Food Hydrocolloids*, *58*, 126–140.

Pandey, M., Mohamad, N., & Amin, M. C. I. M. (2014). Bacterial cellulose/acrylamide pH-sensitive smart hydrogel: Development, characterization, and toxicity studies in ICR mice model. *Molecular Pharmaceutics*, *11*(10), 3596–3608.

Pang, M., Huang, Y., Meng, F., Zhuang, Y., Liu, H., Du, M., & Cai, Y. (2020). Application of bacterial cellulose in skin and bone tissue engineering. *European Polymer Journal*, *122*, 109365.

Patel, S. N., Sharma, M., & Lata, K. (2016). Improved operational stability of D-psicose 3-epimerase by a novel protein engineering strategy, and D-psicose production from fruit and vegetable residues. *Bioresource Technology*, *216*, 121–127.

Pavel, T. I., Chircov, C., Rădulescu, M., & Grumezescu, A. M. (2020). Regenerative wound dressings for skin cancer. *Cancers*, *12*(10), 2954.

Pertile, R., Moreira, S., Andrade, F., Domingues, L., & Gama, M. (2012). Bacterial cellulose modified using recombinant proteins to improve neuronal and mesenchymal cell adhesion. *Biotechnology Progress*, *28*(2), 526–532.

Picheth, G. F., Pirich, C. L., Sierakowski, M. R., Woehl, M. A., Sakakibara, C. N., de Souza, C. F., & de Freitas, R. A. (2017). Bacterial cellulose in biomedical applications: A review. *International Journal of Biological Macromolecules*, *104*, 97–106.

Portela, R., Leal, C. R., Almeida, P. L., & Sobral, R. G. (2019). Bacterial cellulose: a versatile biopolymer for wound dressing applications. *Microbial Biotechnology*, *12*(4), 586–610.

Pourramezan, G. Z., Roayaei, A. M., & Qezelbash, Q. R. (2009). Optimization of culture conditions for bacterial cellulose production by *Acetobacter* sp. 4B-2. *Biotechnology*, *8*, 150–154.

Prilepskii, A., Nikolaev, V., & Klaving, A. (2023). Conductive bacterial cellulose: From drug delivery to flexible electronics. *Carbohydrate Polymers*, 120850.

Putra, A., Kakugo, A., Furukawa, H., Gong, J. P., Osada, Y., Uemura, T., & Yamamoto, M. (2008). Production of bacterial cellulose with well-oriented fibril on PDMS substrate. *Polymer Journal*, *40*(2), 137–142.

Ranjan, B., Pillai, S., Permaul, K., & Singh, S. (2018). A novel strategy for the efficient removal of toxic cyanate by the combinatorial use of recombinant enzymes immobilized on amino silane-modified magnetic nanoparticles. *Bioresource Technology*, *253*, 105–111.

Revin, V. V., Liyaskina, E. V., Parchaykina, M. V., Kuzmenko, T. P., Kurgaeva, I. V., Revin, V. D., & Ullah, M. W. (2022). Bacterial cellulose-based polymer nanocomposites: A review. *Polymers*, *14*(21), 4670.

Revin, V., Liyaskina, E., & Nazarkina, M. (2018). Cost-effective production of bacterial cellulose using acidic food industry by-products. *Brazilian Journal of Microbiology*, *49*, 151–159.

Rocha Santana, R. M., Napoleão, D. C., Rodriguez-Diaz, J. M., de Mendonça Gomes, R. K., Silva, M. G., de Lima, V. M. E., & Duarte, M. M. M. B. (2023). Efficient microbial cellulose/Fe3O4 nanocomposite for photocatalytic degradation by advanced oxidation process of textile dyes. *Chemosphere*, *326*, 138453.

Roman, M., Haring, A. P., & Bertucio, T. J. (2019). The growing merits and dwindling limitations of bacterial cellulose-based tissue engineering scaffolds. *Current Opinion in Chemical Engineering*, *24*, 98–106.

Römling, U., & Galperin, M. Y. (2015). Bacterial cellulose biosynthesis: Diversity of operons, subunits, products, and functions. *Trends in Microbiology*, *23*(9), 545–557.

Ross, P., Mayer, R., & Benziman, M. (1991). Cellulose biosynthesis and function in bacteria. *Microbiological Reviews*, *55*, 35–58.

Ross, P., Weinhouse, H., & Aloni, Y. (1987). Regulation of cellulose synthesis in *Acetobacter xylinum* by cyclic dianalytic acid. *Nature*, *325*, 279–281.

Saska, S., Scarel-Caminaga, R. M., Teixeira, L. N., Franchi, L. P., Dos Santos, R. A., Gaspar, A. M. M., & Marchetto, R. (2012). Characterization and *in vitro* evaluation of bacterial cellulose membranes functionalized with osteogenic growth peptide for bone tissue engineering. *Journal of Materials Science: Materials in Medicine*, *23*, 2253–2266.

Saxena, I. M., Kudlicka, K., Okuda, K., & Brown, R. M. Jr. (1994). Characterization of genes in the cellulose-synthesizing operon (acs operon) of *Acetobacter xylinum*: Implications for cellulose crystallization. *Journal of Bacteriology*, *176*(18), 5735–5752.

Scherner, M., Reutter, S., Klemm, D., Sterner-Kock, A., Guschlbauer, M., Richter, T., & Wippermann, J. (2014). *In vivo* application of tissue-engineered blood vessels of bacterial cellulose as small arterial substitutes: Proof of concept? *Journal of Surgical Research*, *189*(2), 340–347.

Schramm, M., & Hestrin, S. (1954). Factors affecting production of cellulose at the air/liquid interface of a culture of *Acetobacter xylinum*. *Microbiology*, *11*(1), 123–129.

Schumann, D. A., Wippermann, J., Klemm, D. O., Kramer, F., Koth, D., Kosmehl, H., & Salehi-Gelani, S. (2009). Artificial vascular implants from bacterial cellulose: Preliminary results of small arterial substitutes. *Cellulose*, *16*, 877–885.

Seshadri, A., Vedula, G., & Naguib, H. E. (2020). Scalable sensing of hydrocarbon pollutants using soluble Chemi resistive polymer composites. *Materials Chemistry and Physics*, *239*, 122119.

Seyednejad, H., Gawlitta, D., Kuiper, R. V., de Bruin, A., van Nostrum, C. F., Vermonden, T., & Hennink, W. E. (2012). *In vivo* biocompatibility and biodegradation of 3D-printed porous scaffolds based on a hydroxyl-functionalized poly (ε-caprolactone). *Biomaterials*, *33*(17), 4309–4318.

Shah, N., Ul-Islam, M., Khattak, W. A., & Park, J. K. (2013). Overview of bacterial cellulose composites: A multipurpose advanced material. *Carbohydrate Polymers*, *98*(2), 1585–1598.

Shahzad, A., Ullah, M. W., Ali, J., Aziz, K., Javed, M. A., Shi, Z., & Yang, G. (2023). The versatility of nanocellulose, modification strategies, and its current progress in wastewater treatment and environmental remediation. *Science of The Total Environment*, *858*, 159937.

Sharma, C., & Bhardwaj, N. K. (2019). Bacterial nanocellulose: Present status, biomedical applications and future perspectives. *Materials Science and Engineering: C*, *104*, 109963.

Sharma, C., Bhardwaj, N. K., & Pathak, P. (2021). Static intermittent fed-batch production of bacterial nanocellulose from black tea and its modification using chitosan to develop antibacterial green packaging material. *Journal of Cleaner Production*, *279*, 123608.

Sharma, C., Dinda, A. K., & Mishra, N. C. (2012). Synthesis and characterization of glycine modified chitosan–gelatin–alginate composite scaffold for tissue engineering applications. *Journal of Biomaterials and Tissue Engineering*, *2*(2), 133–142.

Sharma, C., Dinda, A. K., & Mishra, N. C. (2013). Fabrication and characterization of natural origin chitosan-gelatin-alginate composite scaffold by foaming method without using surfactant. *Journal of Applied Polymer Science*, *127*(4), 3228–3241.

Sharma, C., Dinda, A. K., Potdar, P. D., & Mishra, N. C. (2015). Fabrication of quaternary composite scaffold from silk fibroin, chitosan, gelatin, and alginate for skin regeneration. *Journal of Applied Polymer Science*, *132*(44).

Shi, Q., Li, Y., Sun, J., Zhang, H., Chen, L., Chen, B., & Wang, Z. (2012). The osteogenesis of bacterial cellulose scaffold loaded with bone morphogenetic protein-2. *Biomaterials*, *33*(28), 6644–6649.

Shi, Z., Shi, X., Ullah, M. W., Li, S., Revin, V. V., & Yang, G. (2018). Fabrication of nanocomposites and hybrid materials using microbial bio templates. *Advanced Composites and Hybrid Materials*, *1*, 79–93.

Shigematsu, T., Takamine, K., Kitazato, M., et al. (2005). Cellulose production from glucose using a glucose dehydrogenase gene (gdh)-deficient mutant of *Gluconacetobacter xylinus* and its use for bioconversion of sweet potato pulp. *Journal of Bioscience and Bioengineering*, *99*, 415–422.

Siguier, P., Gourbeyre, E., & Chandler, M. (2014). Bacterial insertion sequences: Their genomic impact and diversity. *FEMS Microbiology Reviews*, *38*, 865–891.

Simeoni, R. B., Mogharbel, B. F., Francisco, J. C., Miyague, N. I., Irioda, A. C., Souza, C. M., & Carvalho, K. A. (2021). Beneficial roles of cellulose patch-mediated cell therapy in myocardial infarction: A preclinical study. *Cells*, *10*(2), 424.

Singhania, R. R., Patel, A. K., Tsai, M. L., Chen, C. W., & Di Dong, C. (2021). Genetic modification for enhancing bacterial cellulose production and its applications. *Bioengineered*, *12*(1), 6793–6807.

Song, H. J., Li, H., Seo, J. H., Kim, M. J., & Kim, S. J. (2009). Pilot-scale production of bacterial cellulose by a spherical type bubble column bioreactor using saccharified food wastes. *Korean Journal of Chemical Engineering*, *26*, 141–146.

Stumpf, T. R., Sandarage, R. V., Galuta, A., Fournier, P., Li, T., Kirkwood, K., & Cao, X. (2020). Design and evaluation of a biosynthesized cellulose drug releasing duraplasty. *Materials Science and Engineering: C*, *110*, 110677.

Su, T., Liu, N., Lei, D., Wang, L., Ren, Z., Zhang, Q., & Gao, Y. (2022). Flexible MXene/bacterial cellulose film sound detector based on piezoresistive sensing mechanism. *ACS Nano*, *16*(5), 8461–8471.

Sukhavattanakul, P., & Manuspiya, H. (2020). Fabrication of hybrid thin film based on bacterial cellulose nanocrystals and metal nanoparticles with hydrogen sulfide gas sensor ability. *Carbohydrate Polymers*, *230*, 115566.

Sun, L., Vella, P., Schnell, R., Polyakova, A., Bourenkov, G., Li, F., & Römling, U. (2018). Structural and functional characterization of the BcsG subunit of the cellulose synthase in *Salmonella typhimurium*. *Journal of Molecular Biology*, *430*(18), 3170–3189.

Sundberg, J., Götherström, C., & Gatenholm, P. (2015). Biosynthesis and *in vitro* evaluation of macroporous mineralized bacterial nanocellulose scaffolds for bone tissue engineering. *Bio-Medical Materials and Engineering*, *25*(1), 39–52.

Torgbo, S., & Sukyai, P. (2018). Bacterial cellulose-based scaffold materials for bone tissue engineering. *Applied Materials Today*, *11*, 34–49.

Torgbo, S., & Sukyai, P. (2019). Fabrication of microporous bacterial cellulose embedded with magnetite and hydroxyapatite nanocomposite scaffold for bone tissue engineering. *Materials Chemistry and Physics*, *237*, 121868.

Truong, D. H., Dam, M. S., Bujna, E., Rezessy-Szabo, J., Farkas, C., Vi, V. N. H., & Nguyen, Q. D. (2021). *In situ* fabrication of electrically conducting bacterial cellulose-polyaniline-titanium-dioxide composites with the immobilization of *Shewanella xiamenensis* and its application as bioanode in microbial fuel cell. *Fuel*, *285*, 119259.

Ul-Islam, M., Khan, S., Ullah, M. W., & Park, J. K. (2015). Bacterial cellulose composites: Synthetic strategies and multiple applications in biomedical and electro-conductive fields. *Biotechnology Journal*, *10*(12), 1847–1861.

Ullah, M. W., Ul-Islam, M., Wahid, F., & Yang, G. (2022). Nanocellulose: A multipurpose advanced functional material, Volume II. *Frontiers in Bioengineering and Biotechnology*, *10*, 931256.

Uraki, Y., Nemoto, J., Otsuka, H., Tamai, Y., Sugiyama, J., Kishimoto, T., & Shimomura, M. (2007). Honeycomb-like architecture produced by living bacteria, *Gluconacetobacter xylinus*. *Carbohydrate Polymers*, *69*(1), 1–6.

Valla, S., Coucheron, D. H., & Kjosbakken, J. (1983). *Acetobacter xylinum* contains several plasmids: Evidence for their involvement in cellulose formation. *Archives of Microbiology*, *134*, 9–11.

Vitta, S., & Thiruvengadam, V. J. C. S. (2012). Multifunctional bacterial cellulose and nanoparticle-embedded composites. *Current Science*, 1398–1405.

Wang, G., Chen, X. F., Shi, X. D., Yu, L. J., Liu, B. F., & Yang, G. (2008). Bio-fabrication of patterned cellulose nano-fibers. *Advanced Materials Research*, *47*, 1359–1362.

Wang, J., Tavakoli, J., & Tang, Y. (2019). Bacterial cellulose production, properties and applications with different culture methods–a review. *Carbohydrate Polymers*, *219*, 63–76.

Wang, W., Li, H. Y., Zhang, D. W., Jiang, J., Cui, Y. R., Qiu, S., & Zhang, X. X. (2010). Fabrication of bienzymatic glucose biosensor based on novel gold nanoparticles-bacteria cellulose nanofibers nanocomposite. *Electroanalysis*, *22*(21), 2543–2550.

Wei, J., Wang, B., Li, Z., Wu, Z., Zhang, M., Sheng, N., & Chen, S. (2020). A 3D-printable TEMPO-oxidized bacterial cellulose/alginate hydrogel with enhanced stability via nano clay incorporation. *Carbohydrate Polymers*, *238*, 116207.

Wu, S. C., & Li, M. H. (2015). Production of bacterial cellulose membranes in a modified airlift bioreactor by *Gluconacetobacter xylinus*. *Journal of Bioscience and Bioengineering*, *120*, 444–449.

Yadav, V., Panilaitis, B. J., Shi, H., Lee, K., Cebe, P., & Kaplan, D. L. (2010). Novel *in vivo*-degradable cellulose-chitin copolymer from metabolically engineered *Gluconacetobacter xylinus*. *Applied and Environmental Microbiology*, *76*(18), 6257–6265.

Yadav, V., Sun, L., Panilaitis, B., & Kaplan, D. L. (2015). *In vitro* chondrogenesis with lysozyme susceptible bacterial cellulose as a scaffold. *Journal of Tissue Engineering and Regenerative Medicine*. https://doi.org/10.1002/term.1644 (accessed on 5th November 2025).

Yang, J., Sun, D., Li, J., Yang, X., Yu, J., Hao, Q., & Gu, J. (2009). *In situ* deposition of platinum nanoparticles on bacterial cellulose membranes and evaluation of PEM fuel cell performance. *Electrochimica Acta*, *54*(26), 6300–6305.

Yin, N., Stilwell, M. D., Santos, T. M., Wang, H., & Weibel, D. B. (2015). Agarose particle-templated porous bacterial cellulose and its application in cartilage growth *in vitro*. *Acta Biomaterial*, *12*, 129–138.

Zahan, K., Fadhrullah, M., Pa'e, N., Ng, C., & Muhamad, I. (2010). Designing economical production of microbial cellulose from waste using modified bioreactor. In *Proceedings of the ICPE*.

Zhai, X., Lin, D., Zhao, Y., Li, W., & Yang, X. (2018). Enhanced anti-obesity effects of bacterial cellulose combined with konjac glucomannan in high-fat diet-fed C57BL/6J mice. *Food & Function*, *9*(10), 5260–5272.

Zheng, L., Li, S., Luo, J., & Wang, X. (2020). Latest advances on bacterial cellulose-based antibacterial materials as wound dressings. *Frontiers in Bioengineering and*

*Biotechnology, 8*, 593768. https://doi.org/10.3389/fbioe.2020.593768 (accessed on 5th November 2025).

Zhong, C. (2020). Industrial-scale production and applications of bacterial cellulose. *Frontiers in Bioengineering and Biotechnology, 8*, 605374. https://doi.org/10.3389/fbioe.2020.605374 (accessed on 5th November 2025).

Zhou, Y., Han, L. R., He, H. W., Sang, B., Yu, D. L., Feng, J. T., & Zhang, X. (2018). Effects of agitation, aeration and temperature on production of a novel glycoprotein GP-1 by *Streptomyces kanasenisi* ZX01 and scale-up based on volumetric oxygen transfer coefficient. *Molecules, 23*(1), 125. https://doi.org/10.3390/molecules23010125 (accessed on 5th November 2025).

# CHAPTER 13

# Bioreactors: Unlocking the Full Potential of Microorganisms for Industrial Metabolite Production

SUJEET PRATAP SINGH,[1,*] RAJESH KUMAR SRIVASTAVA,[2] and RAVI DESHWAL[3]

[1]*Amity Institute of Biotechnology, Amity University Uttar Pradesh, Lucknow Campus, Lucknow, Uttar Pradesh, India*

[2]*Department of Biotechnology, School of Core Engineering, GITAM (Deemed to be University), Visakhapatnam, Andhra Pradesh, India*

[3]*Institute of Bioscience and Technology, Sri Ramswaroop Memorial University, Lucknow, Uttar Pradesh, India*

*Corresponding author

## ABSTRACT

Microorganisms possess a vast potential for industrial production of valuable compounds, but large-scale utilization often requires optimized growth conditions. Bioreactors serve as controlled environments that cater to the specific needs of these microscopic workhorses. This abstract explores the role of bioreactors in unlocking the full potential of microorganisms for industrial applications. It discusses how bioreactors provide precise control over factors like temperature, pH, nutrients, and oxygen availability, creating ideal conditions for efficient production of enzymes, biofuels, pharmaceuticals, and other valuable products. The abstract also highlights the ongoing advancements in bioreactor design and monitoring

Industrial Biotechnology: Current Progress and Novel Technologies.
Prakash Kumar Sarangi, Akhilesh Kumar Singh, Rajesh Kumar Srivastava, and Brijesh Pandey (Eds.)


DOI: 10.1201/9781779642233-13

systems, paving the way for even more efficient and sustainable biomanufacturing processes.

## 13.1 INTRODUCTION

Bioreactor application has nowadays become mandatory for metabolite production from various microbial fermentations. This reactor helps to control various parameters like temperature, pH, aeration, and mixing of media components and microbial cells. Further, metabolites from microbial cell systems need optimum cultivation conditions that can help in the reduction of byproduct formation with enhanced desired products. Normally, bioreactor application can be done from laboratory to pilot and then industrial scale. This can help with metabolite production at large quantities with batch, fed-batch, and continuous modes of fermentation. Bioreactors are designed at different configurations with facilities to promote different types of microbial cell competency and better cultivation conditions that can help in flux analysis. Imagine a controlled environment teeming with microscopic life, diligently producing the goods we rely on. This is not science fiction; it's the world of bioreactors, the unsung heroes of modern industrial production. These vessels act as miniature ecosystems, fostering the growth of cells or organisms for a vast array of applications. At their core, bioreactors are essentially advanced containers designed to provide optimal conditions for living organisms. They function by precisely regulating factors like temperature, pH, nutrients, and oxygen levels. This controlled environment allows for the efficient production of various products, from life-saving drugs to sustainable biofuels (Nikita et al., 2023). The advent of recombinant DNA technology in the 1970s opened new avenues for bioreactor applications, particularly in the production of recombinant proteins and pharmaceuticals. Bioreactors became integral to the manufacturing processes of biopharmaceuticals such as insulin, GHs, and vaccines, driving further advancements in bioreactor design and scale-up methodologies (Vandermies and Fickers, 2019). In recent decades, the emergence of bioreactor systems capable of supporting a wide range of microorganisms and biochemical processes has expanded the scope of bioreactor applications. From microbial fermentation to cell culture and tissue engineering, bioreactors now play a central role in diverse fields such as biotechnology, agriculture, environmental remediation, and regenerative medicine (Nikita et al., 2023; Vandermies and Fickers, 2019). This chapter provides an overview of bioreactor designs and applications that can help in microbial product formation. Bioreactor design and methods have also become mandatory for various metabolite production.

## 13.2 BIOREACTORS

Bioreactor utility can be done for different types of fermentation processes that can help in high quantity of metabolites.

### *13.2.1 UNDERSTANDING THE ROLE OF BIOREACTORS IN INDUSTRIAL PRODUCTION*

Here's how bioreactors play a crucial role in different industries:

- **Pharmaceuticals:** Bioreactors are instrumental in the production of vaccines, antibiotics, and other vital medications. They enable the large-scale cultivation of microorganisms that produce these drugs, ensuring consistent quality and meeting the high demands of healthcare.
- **Food and Beverage:** Fermentation, a process heavily reliant on bioreactors, is the backbone of numerous food and beverage products. From the familiar fizz of your favorite beer to the tang of yogurt, bioreactors create ideal environments for yeast and bacteria to perform their magic. Additionally, bioreactors can produce enzymes used in food processing, enhancing texture, flavor, and shelf life (Desobgo, 2018).
- **Biofuels:** As the world seeks sustainable energy solutions, bioreactors are at the forefront of biofuel production. They cultivate organisms like algae that can be converted into biodiesel, offering a cleaner alternative to fossil fuels.
- **Waste Management:** Bioreactors can be eco-warriors too! They play a vital role in wastewater treatment by harnessing the power of microbes to break down pollutants. This bioremediation process helps purify wastewater before it rejoins the environment.

- **Emerging Fields:** The potential of bioreactors extends beyond traditional industries. Researchers are exploring their use in bioprinting tissues for transplants and creating lab-grown meat, a potential solution to the environmental impact of conventional meat production (Chen et al., 2022).

The benefits of bioreactors are undeniable. They offer:

- **Efficiency:** Bioreactors optimize production processes, leading to higher yields and consistent product quality.
- **Scalability:** The size of bioreactors can be adjusted to meet production needs, allowing for large-scale manufacturing.
- **Control:** The controlled environment minimizes contamination and ensures optimal conditions for the desired output.

However, bioreactor technology also faces challenges. Maintaining sterile environments and ensuring the viability of living organisms are complex tasks. Additionally, research and development to optimize bioprocesses for new products requires ongoing investment.

Despite these challenges, bioreactors are revolutionizing industrial production. As technology advances and research delves deeper, these versatile tools hold the potential to unlock a future filled with sustainable, efficient, and innovative products that improve our lives (Baudequin et al., 2021).

### *13.2.2 HISTORICAL OVERVIEW AND EVOLUTION OF BIOREACTOR TECHNOLOGY*

The historical overview and evolution of bioreactor technology trace a fascinating journey marked by significant milestones, breakthroughs, and innovations that have shaped its present-day applications and capabilities.

The roots of bioreactor technology can be traced back to ancient civilizations, where fermentation processes were utilized for food and beverage production. Early civilizations, such as the Mesopotamians and Egyptians, employed fermentation to produce bread, beer, and wine, albeit in rudimentary vessels such as clay pots and wooden barrels.

However, it was not until the 20th century that bioreactor technology began to emerge as a distinct field of study and engineering. The pioneering work of scientists such as Louis Pasteur and Eduard Buchner laid the foundation for understanding the microbial processes underlying fermentation.

Pasteur's discoveries on microbial fermentation and the role of microorganisms in food spoilage revolutionized the field of microbiology and paved the way for controlled fermentation processes (Szkodny and Lee, 2022).

The advent of industrial microbiology in the late 19th and early 20th centuries further propelled the development of bioreactor technology. With the rise of the pharmaceutical, chemical, and food industries, there was a growing demand for large-scale production of microbial products such as antibiotics, enzymes, and organic acids. This demand spurred the development of specialized vessels capable of supporting microbial growth and metabolism under controlled conditions.

The early bioreactors were simple vessels equipped with basic instrumentation for monitoring and controlling key parameters such as temperature, pH, and agitation. Glass and stainless steel were commonly used materials for construction, providing durability and ease of sterilization. These early bioreactors laid the groundwork for subsequent advancements in bioreactor design and engineering.

The latter half of the 20th century witnessed rapid progress in bioreactor technology driven by advancements in microbiology, biochemistry, and engineering. The introduction of stirred-tank bioreactors revolutionized the field by enabling better mixing and aeration of culture media, leading to improved microbial growth and product formation. Concurrently, developments in sensor technology, automation, and control systems enhanced the precision and efficiency of bioreactor operations.

Looking ahead, the evolution of bioreactor technology is poised to continue, fueled by ongoing research and innovation in areas such as synthetic biology, metabolic engineering, and process optimization. As industries seek sustainable and cost-effective solutions for producing high-value products, bioreactors are likely to play an increasingly prominent role in shaping the future of industrial production (Table 13.1).

### *13.2.3 IMPORTANCE OF MICROORGANISMS IN INDUSTRIAL PROCESSES*

Microorganisms, including bacteria, fungi, yeast, and algae, play a pivotal role in numerous industrial processes, contributing to the production of a wide range of valuable products. Their importance stems from their remarkable ability to catalyze biochemical reactions, produce enzymes, and synthesize various compounds of industrial significance. Understanding the

**TABLE 13.1** Historical Development of Bioreactor Technology

| Era | Bioreactor Technology | Applications |
|---|---|---|
| Ancient Origins (10,000 BC Onwards) | Primitive containers like clay pots and animal skins | Unintentional fermentation leading to foods like yogurt and beverages like wine and beer |
| Rise of Deliberate Fermentation (3,000 BC Onwards) | More controlled fermentation processes | Bread making, pickling vegetables |
| Scientific Revolution (18th and 19th Centuries) | Simple glass containers with basic controls | Laboratory-scale fermentation experiments |
| 20th Century: The Age of Industrial Bioreactors | Development of first commercial fermenters | Large-scale production of antibiotics and other fermented products |
| Mid-20th Century Onwards: Rise of Cell Culture | Specialized bioreactors for adherent and suspension cultures | Vaccine production and other applications requiring mammalian cell growth |
| Late 20th Century Onwards: Bioreactors Beyond Fermentation | More sophisticated bioreactors with advanced materials and engineering | Bioremediation, biofuel production, bioprinting tissues in addition to fermentation and cell culture |

multifaceted roles of microorganisms in industrial processes is essential for optimizing production efficiency, improving product quality, and developing sustainable manufacturing strategies (Behera et al., 2019).

- **Microbial Fermentation:** One of the most prominent roles of microorganisms in industrial processes is in fermentation. Microbes are adept at metabolizing diverse substrates, such as sugars, starches, and organic acids, to produce a plethora of products including ethanol, acetone, butanol, lactic acid, and citric acid. Fermentation processes are widely used in industries such as food and beverage, pharmaceuticals, biofuels, and chemicals.
- **Enzyme Production:** Microorganisms are prolific producers of enzymes, which serve as biocatalysts in numerous industrial applications. Enzymes such as amylases, proteases, lipases, and cellulases find widespread use in food processing, detergent manufacturing, the textile industry, pulp and paper production, and biofuel synthesis. Microbial fermentation processes are often employed for large-scale enzyme production.
- **Biopharmaceutical Manufacturing:** Microorganisms are harnessed for the production of a variety of biopharmaceuticals, including therapeutic proteins, antibodies, vaccines, and antibiotics. Recombinant DNA technology allows for the genetic engineering of microorganisms to produce specific proteins of interest, which are then synthesized in bioreactors using microbial fermentation processes.
- **Bioremediation:** Microorganisms play a crucial role in environmental remediation by metabolizing and degrading pollutants in soil, water, and air. Certain bacteria and fungi possess the ability to break down harmful contaminants such as hydrocarbons, heavy metals, pesticides, and industrial chemicals, thereby facilitating the cleanup of contaminated sites and reducing environmental pollution.
- **Agricultural Applications:** Microorganisms contribute to agricultural productivity through processes such as nitrogen fixation, phosphate solubilization, and plant growth promotion. Certain strains of bacteria, such as rhizobia and mycorrhizae, form symbiotic relationships with plants, enhancing nutrient uptake and

improving crop yields. Additionally, microbial biofertilizers and biopesticides offer sustainable alternatives to chemical inputs in agriculture.

- **Biomineralization and Biocementation:** Microorganisms possess the remarkable ability to induce mineral precipitation and cementation, a process known as biomineralization or biocementation. This phenomenon has applications in construction, geotechnical engineering, and environmental remediation, where microbial activities are harnessed to strengthen soil, stabilize slopes, and mitigate erosion.

## 13.3 DESIGN AND OPERATION OF BIOREACTORS

### *13.3.1 PRINCIPLES OF BIOREACTOR DESIGN*

The principles of bioreactor design encompass a range of considerations aimed at creating an optimal environment for microbial growth and product formation. These principles are essential for maximizing the efficiency, productivity, and scalability of bioprocesses in various industrial applications (Yu et al., 2020) (Figure 13.1).

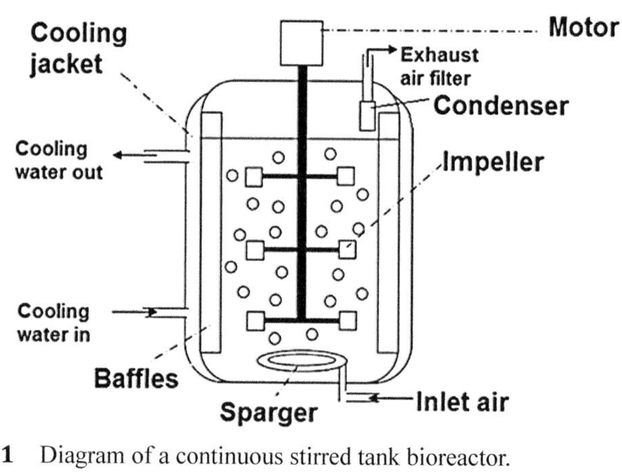


**FIGURE 13.1** Diagram of a continuous stirred tank bioreactor.

- **Bioreactor Geometry:** The geometry of a bioreactor influences the distribution of nutrients, gases, and heat within the culture medium. Common geometries include stirred-tank reactors, airlift reactors, and packed bed reactors, each offering advantages depending on the specific requirements of the bioprocess.

- **Mass Transfer:** Efficient mass transfer of oxygen, nutrients, and waste products is crucial for supporting microbial growth and metabolic activity. Design parameters such as agitation rate, aeration strategy, and reactor configuration are optimized to enhance mass transfer rates and prevent substrate limitations.
- **Heat Transfer:** Proper control of temperature is essential for maintaining optimal microbial growth and protein stability. Bioreactor design incorporates mechanisms for heat removal, such as cooling jackets or internal heat exchangers, to regulate temperature and prevent thermal stress on the microorganisms.
- **Sterilization:** Maintaining a sterile environment is critical for preventing contamination and ensuring the purity of the final product. Bioreactor design includes features such as autoclavable components, steam-in-place systems, and sterile filters to achieve and maintain sterility throughout the fermentation process.
- **Mixing and Homogeneity:** Effective mixing of the culture medium promotes uniform distribution of nutrients and enhances microbial contact with substrates. Bioreactor design features such as impellers, baffles, and spargers are optimized to ensure thorough mixing and homogeneity of the culture.
- **Instrumentation and Control:** Bioreactor systems are equipped with sensors and control systems to monitor and regulate key process parameters such as pH, dissolved oxygen, and agitation speed. Advanced instrumentation enables real-time monitoring and automated control, allowing for precise adjustments to optimize bioprocess performance.
- **Scale-Up Considerations:** Scaling up bioprocesses from laboratory-scale to industrial-scale operations requires careful consideration of factors such as mixing dynamics, mass transfer limitations, and reactor geometry. Bioreactor design incorporates scale-up principles to ensure reproducibility and consistency across different production scales.

By adhering to these principles of bioreactor design, engineers can create robust and efficient bioprocesses capable of meeting the demands of industrial production while maximizing product yield, quality, and economic viability (Mandenius, 2016).

### 13.3.2 TYPES OF BIOREACTORS: BATCH, CONTINUOUS, AND FED-BATCH

Bioreactors are pivotal in industrial bioprocessing, providing controlled environments for the growth of microorganisms or cells to produce various valuable products. Among the primary types of bioreactors are batch, continuous, and fed-batch systems, each offering distinct advantages and applications (Shanmugam et al., 2022) (Figure 13.2).

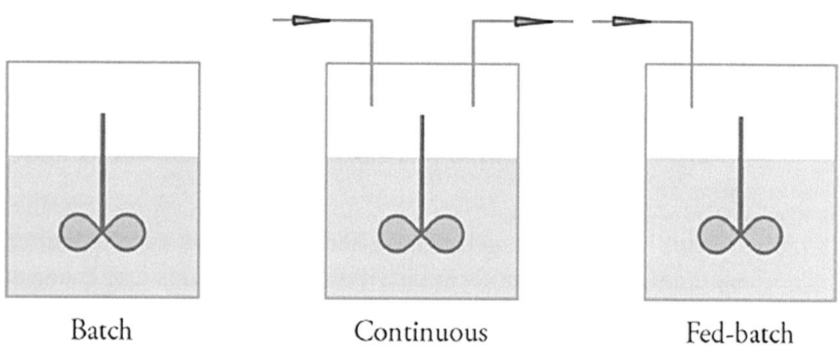


**FIGURE 13.2** Mode of operations.

#### 13.3.2.1 BATCH BIOREACTORS

Batch bioreactors are the simplest and most commonly used type of bioreactor. In a batch system, all ingredients, including nutrients and microorganisms, are added to the reactor vessel at the start of the process. The culture then grows and metabolizes under controlled conditions until the desired product is obtained or the process is complete.

##### 13.3.2.1.1 *Advantages*

- Simple setup and operation.
- Well-suited for small-scale production and research purposes.
- Easy to monitor and control key parameters.

##### *13.3.2.1.2 Limitations*

- Lower productivity compared to continuous systems.
- Downtime between batches for cleaning and sterilization.
- Inefficiencies due to start-up and shutdown procedures.

#### *13.3.2.2 CONTINUOUS BIOREACTORS*

Continuous bioreactors operate continuously, with fresh nutrients continuously or intermittently fed into the reactor while culture broth is withdrawn at a constant rate to maintain a steady-state condition. This allows for sustained microbial growth and product formation over extended periods.

##### *13.3.2.2.1 Advantages*

- Higher productivity and efficiency compared to batch systems.
- Reduced downtime and labor associated with batch-to-batch operations.
- Well-suited for large-scale production of high-value products.

##### *13.3.2.2.2 Limitations*

- More complex setup and operation compared to batch systems.
- Requires sophisticated control systems to maintain steady-state conditions.
- Higher operating and maintenance costs.

#### *13.3.2.3 FED-BATCH BIOREACTORS*

Fed-batch bioreactors combine elements of both batch and continuous systems. In a fed-batch process, nutrients are added to the reactor incrementally throughout the fermentation process to maintain optimal growth conditions while preventing substrate inhibition or overflow metabolism.

#### *13.3.2.3.1 Advantages*

- Higher cell densities and product yields compared to batch systems.
- Improved control over product quality and process parameters.
- Well-suited for applications requiring high product concentrations.

#### *13.3.2.3.2 Limitations*

- More complex setup and control compared to batch systems.
- Requires careful monitoring and adjustment of feeding rates.
- Higher operating costs compared to batch systems.

Now, let us compare these three types of bioreactors in a tabular format (Table 13.2).

**TABLE 13.2** Comparison Among Different Types of Bioreactor System

| Feature | Batch Culture | Continuous Culture | Fed-Batch Culture |
|---|---|---|---|
| Mode of operation | Discontinuous | Continuous | Semi-continuous |
| Nutrient addition | All added at the beginning | Continuous feeding of fresh medium | Initial addition, followed by feeding of limiting substrate |
| Product harvest | Entire culture broth harvested at the end | Continuous removal of culture broth | Entire culture broth harvested at the end |
| Cell density and product concentration | Variable throughout the process | Constant | Extends the high-production phase of batch cultures |
| Complexity | Simple | Complex | Moderately complex |
| Suitability | Studying cell growth kinetics, simple products | Consistent product quality, high cell density | Higher product yield than batch cultures, wider range of applications |

### *13.3.3 PARAMETERS INFLUENCING BIOREACTOR PERFORMANCE*

Bioreactors provide a controlled environment for cultivating biological organisms, but their success hinges on maintaining optimal conditions for the desired process. Several key parameters significantly influence bioreactor performance, impacting cell growth, product yield, and overall efficiency (Ntwampe et al., 2010). Here is a look at some of the most critical factors:

- **Physical Environment:**
  - **Temperature:** Every organism has an optimal temperature range for growth and product formation. Deviation from this range can slow growth, reduce product yield, or even kill the cells. Bioreactors typically employ heating and cooling systems for precise temperature control.
  - **pH:** Cellular activity and enzyme functionality are highly dependent on the culture's pH level. Acids or bases can be added to the bioreactor to maintain the desired pH throughout the process.
  - **Dissolved Oxygen (DO):** Aerobic organisms require oxygen for respiration and growth. Bioreactors often utilize agitation and sparging with air or pure oxygen to ensure sufficient DO levels.
  - **Agitation and Mixing:** Proper mixing of the culture broth is crucial for maintaining a uniform environment within the bioreactor. Agitators like impellers provide this mixing, ensuring even distribution of nutrients, oxygen, and metabolites.
- **Chemical Environment:**
  - **Nutrients:** Cells require specific nutrients for growth and product formation. The type and concentration of these nutrients (sugars, amino acids, minerals) need to be carefully controlled to optimize cell activity and product yield.
  - **Substrates:** For product formation, specific substrates may be needed. In some cases, the concentration of these substrates can be adjusted during the process to influence product quality or quantity.
  - **Product Inhibition:** As the desired product accumulates in the culture broth, it can sometimes inhibit cell growth or product formation. Strategies like continuous product removal or manipulating growth phases can be employed to mitigate this effect.

- **Aseptic Conditions:** Maintaining a sterile environment within the bioreactor is paramount. Contamination by unwanted micro-organisms can disrupt the process, ruin the product, and even pose safety risks. Strict sterilization procedures and aseptic techniques are essential throughout the bioreactor operation.
- **Additional Factors:**
  - **Shear Stress:** Agitation can generate shear stress on the cells. While some mixing is necessary, excessive shear stress can damage or even lyse the cells. Bioreactor design and operating parameters need to be optimized to balance mixing efficiency with minimizing shear stress.
  - **Foam Formation:** Certain culture broths can foam excessively, hindering mixing and oxygen transfer. Antifoam agents can be added to control foam formation.

By carefully monitoring and controlling these critical parameters, bioreactor operators can create an optimal environment for their chosen organism, maximizing cell growth, product yield, and overall process efficiency (Vasumathi et al., 2012).

## 13.4 ENGINEERING BIOREACTOR SYSTEMS

### *13.4.1 SCALING UP FROM LAB TO INDUSTRIAL SCALE*

Scaling up a bioprocess from laboratory-scale to industrial-scale production is a complex and challenging endeavor that requires careful planning, optimization, and validation. While laboratory-scale experiments provide valuable insights into process kinetics, microbial behavior, and product formation, translating these findings to large-scale production environments involves addressing numerous technical, logistical, and economic considerations (Berenjian, 2020) (Figure 13.3).

- **Process Understanding and Optimization:** Before scaling up a bioprocess, it is essential to thoroughly understand the underlying biochemical and physiological principles governing microbial growth and product formation. This includes optimizing key process parameters such as nutrient composition, pH, temperature, and agitation to maximize productivity and product quality at the laboratory scale.

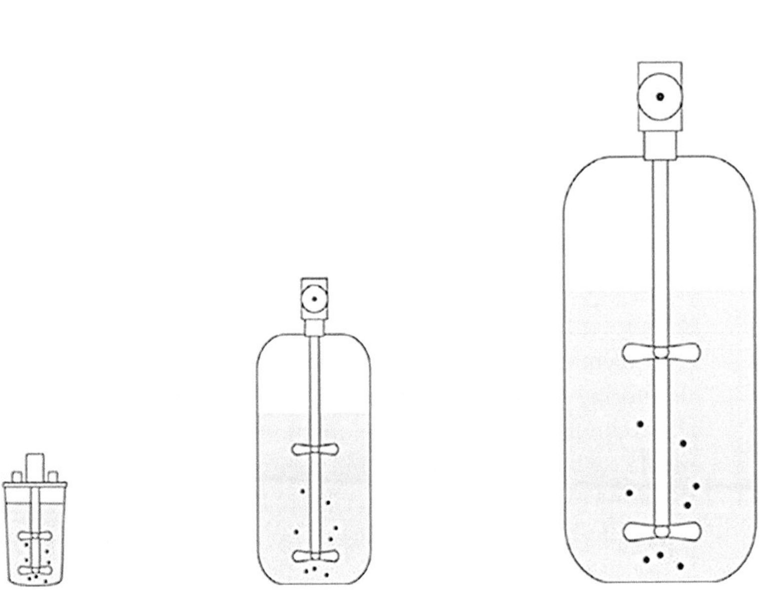

**FIGURE 13.3** Scaling up bioreactor.

- **Scale-Up Criteria:** Determining the appropriate criteria for scaling up a bioprocess is crucial for ensuring successful translation to industrial-scale production. Common scale-up criteria include maintaining similar mass transfer rates, mixing characteristics, and shear stresses across different scales to achieve comparable growth kinetics and product yields.
- **Bioreactor Design and Engineering:** Selecting the appropriate bioreactor design and engineering specifications is essential for successful scale-up. Factors such as reactor geometry, vessel size, agitation mechanisms, and aeration strategies must be carefully optimized to accommodate larger volumes while maintaining optimal growth conditions and process efficiency.
- **Mass Transfer and Mixing Dynamics:** Ensuring efficient mass transfer and mixing dynamics is critical for achieving uniform distribution of nutrients, gases, and cells within the bioreactor at industrial scale. Scaling up may require modifications to agitation systems, sparger designs, and reactor configurations to maintain optimal mixing and oxygen transfer rates.

- **Heat Transfer and Temperature Control:** Managing heat transfer and temperature control becomes increasingly challenging at larger scales due to greater heat generation and dissipation rates. Scaling up may necessitate the use of advanced cooling and heating systems, such as jacketed reactors, internal heat exchangers, or external cooling loops, to maintain the culture temperature within the optimal range.
- **Instrumentation and Process Control:** Implementing robust instrumentation and process control systems is essential for monitoring and regulating key process parameters at industrial scale. Advanced sensors, automation, and control algorithms enable real-time monitoring and adjustment of temperature, pH, dissolved oxygen, and agitation speed to maintain optimal growth conditions and maximize productivity.
- **Validation and Quality Assurance:** Validating the scaled-up bioprocess and ensuring product quality and consistency are critical steps in the scale-up process. This may involve conducting pilot-scale trials, process optimization studies, and comprehensive risk assessments to identify and mitigate potential challenges and uncertainties associated with scaling up.
- **Economic Considerations:** Assessing the economic feasibility and cost-effectiveness of scaling up a bioprocess is essential for decision-making and investment planning. Economic factors such as capital investment, operating costs, raw material availability, and market demand must be carefully evaluated to determine the viability and profitability of industrial-scale production.
- **Regulatory Compliance:** Ensuring regulatory compliance with applicable guidelines and standards is essential for scaling up bioprocesses in industries such as pharmaceuticals, biotechnology, and food manufacturing. This may involve obtaining regulatory approvals, conducting validation studies, and implementing quality assurance and quality control measures to ensure product safety, efficacy, and consistency (Lim et al., 2021).

In conclusion, scaling up a bioprocess from laboratory-scale to industrial-scale production requires a systematic and multidisciplinary approach encompassing process optimization, bioreactor design, engineering, validation, economic analysis, and regulatory compliance. By addressing these key considerations and challenges, bioprocess engineers can successfully transition from laboratory experimentation to commercial-scale production, unlocking the full potential of biotechnology for industrial applications.

### *13.4.2 BIOREACTOR INSTRUMENTATION AND CONTROL*

Bioreactors are the workhorses of the biotechnology industry, providing a controlled environment for cultivating cells and microorganisms responsible for producing a vast array of products, from life-saving drugs to biofuels. However, these vessels would not be nearly as effective without a sophisticated network of instruments and control systems that act as the silent conductors of the biological symphony within.

- **The Role of Instrumentation:** Bioreactor instrumentation plays a vital role in monitoring and measuring critical parameters that influence cell growth, product formation, and overall process efficiency (Robles et al., 2015). These parameters can be broadly categorized into two main groups:
    - **Physical Environment:** Temperature, pH, dissolved oxygen (DO), agitation speed, and pressure are some of the key physical parameters that directly impact cell health and activity. Sensors like thermocouples, pH probes, DO electrodes, and pressure transducers continuously monitor these factors.
    - **Chemical Environment:** Nutrient concentrations (sugars, amino acids), substrate levels, and product accumulation are crucial aspects of the chemical environment. While some analytes can be measured offline through sampling and analysis, advanced bioreactors utilize online sensors for real-time monitoring of these parameters. Examples include biosensors for specific nutrients or analytical instruments like chromatography for metabolite profiling.
- **Control Systems:** Maintaining the Symphony

  The collected data from the bioreactor's instrumentation feeds into the control system, the brain of the operation. This system compares the measured values to pre-defined setpoints and implements corrective actions to maintain optimal conditions. Here is a breakdown of some key control elements:

- **Controllers:** These electronic devices analyze the sensor data and determine if adjustments are necessary. Different types of controllers exist, ranging from simple on/off switches to sophisticated PID (proportional-integral-derivative) controllers that can implement complex control algorithms (Alimberti et al., 2021).
- **Actuators:** Based on the controller's output, actuators physically manipulate the bioreactor environment. Examples include:
- **Heating/Cooling Units:** Maintain the desired temperature.
- **Acid/Base Pumps:** Adjust the culture broth's pH.
- **Sparging Systems:** Control the flow of air or pure oxygen to maintain DO levels.
- **Feed Pumps:** Regulate the addition of fresh nutrients or substrates.
- **Agitator Motors:** Control the speed and intensity of mixing within the bioreactor.

- **Benefits of Effective Control:** A well-designed and implemented bioreactor control system offers numerous benefits:
- **Optimized Cell Growth and Product Yield:** By maintaining optimal conditions, the control system ensures efficient utilization of nutrients and substrates, leading to maximized cell growth and product formation.
- **Process Stability and Repeatability:** Precise control minimizes fluctuations in critical parameters, resulting in consistent and reproducible processes with minimal batch-to-batch variations.
- **Improved Process Safety:** The control system can be programmed with alarms and safety interlocks to prevent deviations from safe operating conditions, protecting both personnel and equipment.
- **Data Acquisition and Analysis:** Modern control systems often integrate data logging capabilities, allowing for real-time

monitoring and historical trend analysis. This data can be invaluable for process optimization and troubleshooting.

- **Advanced Control Strategies:** Bioreactor control systems are constantly evolving, incorporating sophisticated algorithms and advanced techniques like:
- **Model-Predictive Control (MPC):** This approach utilizes a mathematical model of the bioprocess to predict future behavior and adjust control actions proactively (Oh et al., 2022).
- **Adaptive Control:** These systems can learn and adapt to changing process dynamics, ensuring optimal control even under variable conditions.
- **Computer-Aided Process Optimization (CAPO):** Software tools can analyze bioreactor data and suggest optimal control strategies for maximizing process efficiency and product yield (Di Gravina et al., 2023).

Bioreactor instrumentation and control systems are the unsung heroes of bioprocessing. By meticulously monitoring critical parameters and implementing precise adjustments, they ensure a harmonious environment for the biological processes taking place within the bioreactor. This orchestration of life forms the foundation for the production of a wide range of valuable products, contributing significantly to advancements in healthcare, renewable energy, and other fields.

### *13.4.3 CHALLENGES AND SOLUTIONS IN BIOREACTOR ENGINEERING*

Bioreactors are powerful tools for cultivating cells and microorganisms, but their successful operation hinges on overcoming several engineering challenges. Here is a look at some key hurdles and innovative solutions driving advancements in bioreactor design and operation (Zhong, 2010).

#### *13.4.3.1 CHALLENGES*

- **Mimicking the *In Vivo* Environment:** Cells in their natural environment experience complex interactions with other cells, extracellular matrix (ECM), and gradients of nutrients and oxygen. Replicating these intricate conditions within a bioreactor remains a challenge.

- **Scalability:** Transitioning a bioprocess from lab-scale to industrial production requires significant adjustments. Issues like heat transfer, mixing efficiency, and nutrient delivery become more complex at larger scales.
- **Shear Stress:** Agitation, essential for mixing and oxygen transfer, can also generate shear stress on cells. Balancing efficient mixing with minimizing cell damage is a crucial consideration.
- **Aseptic Operation:** Maintaining sterility throughout the bioprocess is paramount to prevent contamination. However, large-scale operations and complex feeding strategies increase the risk of contamination events.
- **Process Monitoring and Control:** Precise monitoring and real-time control of critical parameters are essential for optimal cell growth and product yield. Developing robust and cost-effective sensor technologies remains an ongoing pursuit.

#### *13.4.3.2 SOLUTIONS*

- **Biomimetic Bioreactors:** Researchers are developing bioreactors that incorporate features mimicking the natural cellular environment, such as microfluidic devices that create gradients of nutrients and oxygen (Drapal et al., 2021).
- **Computational Modeling:** Advanced computer models can help predict bioreactor behavior at larger scales, facilitating smoother transitions from lab to industry.
- **Novel Mixing Strategies:** Innovative designs like oscillating bioreactors or microfluidic chips can achieve efficient mixing while minimizing shear stress on delicate cells.
- **Single-Use Bioreactors:** These disposable bioreactors eliminate the need for sterilization cycles, reducing contamination risks and simplifying operation in large-scale settings (Jossen et al., 2019).
- **Advanced Sensor Technologies:** Biosensors and online analytical tools are being developed to provide real-time, non-invasive monitoring of key parameters within the bioreactor.

- **Model-Predictive Control (MPC):** This advanced control strategy utilizes process models to predict future behavior and adjust control actions proactively, optimizing process performance (Oh et al., 2022).

#### *13.4.3.3 THE FUTURE OF BIOREACTOR ENGINEERING*

Bioreactor engineering is a constantly evolving field. By addressing these challenges through innovative design solutions, sensor development, and advanced control strategies, researchers are creating bioreactors that are more efficient, scalable, and capable of mimicking complex biological environments. These advancements will pave the way for the development of new and improved bioprocesses, leading to breakthroughs in medicine, biofuels, and other bio-based products.

## 13.5 APPLICATIONS OF BIOREACTORS IN INDUSTRIAL PRODUCTION

### *13.5.1 BIOPHARMACEUTICAL PRODUCTION*

Bioreactors have revolutionized the production of biopharmaceuticals; a rapidly growing class of drugs derived from living organisms or their biological processes. These drugs, including vaccines, therapeutic proteins, monoclonal antibodies, and gene therapies, offer highly targeted and often lifesaving treatments for various diseases. Bioreactors provide a controlled environment to cultivate the cells responsible for producing these complex biomolecules, ensuring consistent quality and large-scale production (Al-Zyoud et al., 2018).

Here is a closer look at how bioreactors are used in biopharmaceutical production:

- **Cell Culture:** Biopharmaceuticals are often produced by genetically engineered mammalian cells, such as Chinese Hamster Ovary (CHO) cells. Bioreactors provide a sterile and controlled environment for these cells to grow and proliferate. Nutrients, temperature, pH, and dissolved oxygen levels are meticulously maintained to optimize cell health and maximize product yield (O'Flaherty et al., 2020).

- **Upstream Processing:** This stage encompasses all steps before the actual product recovery. Bioreactors play a central role in this phase by:
  - **Seed Train Expansion:** Starting from a small vial of cells, bioreactors are used to gradually increase the cell population to a sufficient volume for large-scale production.
  - **Production Culture:** Once the desired cell density is achieved, bioreactors are used for large-scale production of the biopharmaceutical. Different bioreactor operation modes (batch, fed-batch, continuous) can be employed depending on the specific product and cell line.
  - **Product Secretion:** The desired biopharmaceutical is typically secreted by the cells into the culture broth. Bioreactors can be designed to facilitate product secretion, such as by utilizing perfusion techniques for continuous product removal.
  - **Downstream Processing:** After cultivation, the product needs to be purified and isolated from the culture broth. This downstream processing typically involves several steps like filtration, centrifugation, chromatography, and potentially viral inactivation steps to ensure product safety and purity.
- **Advantages of Bioreactors in Biopharmaceutical Production:**
  - **Scalability:** Bioreactors can be scaled up from research labs to large-scale industrial production, enabling the manufacture of biopharmaceuticals in sufficient quantities to meet patient needs.
  - **Controlled Environment:** Bioreactors provide a tightly controlled environment that minimizes contamination risks and ensures consistent product quality.
  - **Process Optimization:** Bioreactor design and operation can be optimized for specific cell lines and products, leading to higher yields and improved production efficiency.
- **Challenges and Future Directions:**
  - Despite their advantages, biopharmaceutical production using bioreactors faces challenges such as high production costs,

complex downstream processing, and the need for robust cell lines with high productivity.

- Future advancements in bioreactor design, single-use technologies, and process automation are expected to further streamline and improve biopharmaceutical production, making these life-saving drugs more accessible and affordable for patients worldwide.

### 13.5.2 BIOFUEL SYNTHESIS

Bioreactors are playing a key role in the development and production of biofuels, a promising alternative to traditional fossil fuels. Biofuels are derived from renewable biological sources like algae, microorganisms, or plant materials. Bioreactors provide a controlled environment to cultivate the organisms or process the feedstocks necessary for biofuel production (Chandra et al., 2020).

Here is a breakdown of how bioreactors are utilized in different biofuel production methods:

- **Biodiesel Production:** Biodiesel is a fatty acid methyl ester (FAME) fuel derived from vegetable oils or animal fats. Bioreactors can be used in two main ways for biodiesel production:
- **Microbial Transesterification:** Certain microorganisms can be used as biocatalysts to convert triglycerides (fats) in the feedstock into biodiesel through a process called transesterification. Bioreactors cultivate these microbes and facilitate the efficient conversion of feedstock into biodiesel.
- **Enzymatic Transesterification:** Enzymes isolated from specific organisms can also be used for transesterification. Bioreactors can be employed to produce these enzymes in large quantities for subsequent biodiesel production processes.
- **Bioethanol Production:** Bioethanol is an alcohol fuel derived from the fermentation of sugars by yeasts. Bioreactors play a crucial role in this process by:
  - **Biomass Pretreatment:** Lignocellulosic biomass, such as corn stover or switchgrass, needs pretreatment to break down

the tough cell walls and release fermentable sugars. Bioreactors can be used for enzymatic or microbial pretreatment processes.

  - **Microbial Fermentation:** Yeasts are cultivated in bioreactors to ferment the released sugars into bioethanol. Fermentation parameters like temperature, pH, and nutrient availability are precisely controlled to maximize ethanol yield.

- **Biohydrogen Production:** Biohydrogen, a clean-burning fuel, can be produced through various biological processes. Bioreactors are being explored for:

  - **Dark Fermentation:** Certain bacteria can produce hydrogen from organic matter through a fermentation process that does not require sunlight. Bioreactors provide the optimal environment for these bacteria to generate biohydrogen (Sarangi and Nanda, 2020).

  - **Biological Photolysis:** Algae or photosynthetic bacteria can be cultivated in bioreactors to produce hydrogen through a process involving sunlight and water. Research is ongoing to optimize bioreactor designs for efficient light utilization and hydrogen production.

- **Advantages of Bioreactors in Biofuel Synthesis**

  - **Controlled Environment:** Bioreactors ensure consistent and efficient conversion of feedstocks into biofuels by maintaining optimal conditions for the biological processes involved.

  - **Renewable Feedstocks:** Bioreactors enable the utilization of renewable biomass sources for fuel production, promoting sustainability and reducing dependence on fossil fuels.

  - **Process Optimization:** Bioreactor design and operation can be tailored to specific biofuel types and feedstocks, leading to higher yields and improved efficiency.

- **Challenges and Future Directions:**

  - Biofuel production using bioreactors faces challenges such as the need for cost-effective feedstocks, optimizing conversion efficiencies, and minimizing environmental impacts.

- Future advancements in bioreactor design, metabolic engineering of organisms, and integration with renewable energy sources like solar and wind power hold promise for making biofuel production even more sustainable and cost-competitive, paving the way for a cleaner energy future.

### *13.5.3 FOOD AND BEVERAGE PROCESSING*

Bioreactors are not just for high-tech pharmaceuticals and alternative fuels. They also play a surprisingly significant role in the food and beverage industry, contributing to the production of a variety of familiar products (Mitra and Murthy, 2021).
Here is a glimpse into how bioreactors are used to create some of our favorite foods and beverages:

- **Fermentation:** Fermentation is a metabolic process where microorganisms like bacteria or yeast convert sugars and other carbohydrates into various products. Bioreactors provide a controlled environment for these microbes to thrive, leading to efficient and consistent fermentation processes.
- **Bread and Bakery Products:** Baker's yeast, cultivated in bioreactors, ferments sugars in dough, leading to the characteristic rise and fluffy texture.
- **Alcoholic Beverages:** Beer, wine, and spirits all rely on fermentation by yeasts or bacteria for alcohol production. Bioreactors ensure consistent and high-quality fermentation for these beverages.
- **Dairy Products:** Yogurt, cheese, and other fermented dairy products involve the controlled fermentation of milk sugars by specific bacterial cultures. Bioreactors can be used to cultivate these cultures and ensure consistent product quality.
- **Enzyme Production:** Bioreactors are used to cultivate microorganisms that produce specific enzymes. These enzymes can then be used in various food and beverage applications:
    - **Cheesemaking:** Enzymes like rennet are used to curdle milk during cheese production. Bioreactors can produce these enzymes efficiently and at scale.

  - **Fruit Juice Clarification:** Pectinase enzymes help clarify fruit juices by breaking down pectin, a naturally occurring thickening agent. Bioreactors provide a reliable source of these enzymes for the juice industry.
  - **Sugar Production:** Enzymes are used to break down complex carbohydrates into simpler sugars during some stages of sugar production. Bioreactors can cultivate the microbes that produce these enzymes.
- **Bioconversions:** Bioreactors can be used for various bioconversion processes that create ingredients or additives for food and beverages:
  - **Vinegar Production:** Bacteria convert ethanol in alcoholic beverages into acetic acid, the key component of vinegar. Bioreactors can optimize this bioconversion process for efficient vinegar production.
  - **Organic Acid Production:** Citric acid, lactic acid, and other organic acids used as food additives can be produced through microbial fermentation in bioreactors.
  - **Food Colorings:** Some natural food colorings can be produced by cultivating specific microorganisms in bioreactors.
- **Advantages of Bioreactors in Food and Beverage Processing:**
  - **Controlled Quality:** Bioreactors provide consistent and controlled environments for fermentation and enzyme production, leading to consistent product quality and taste.
  - **Efficiency and Scalability:** Bioreactors enable efficient production of large quantities of enzymes, cultures, and fermented products.
  - **Improved Safety:** Bioreactor-based processes minimize contamination risks compared to traditional methods, leading to safer food and beverage products.

Bioreactors in food and beverage processing face challenges such as optimizing fermentation processes for specific products and ensuring cost-effectiveness.

### 13.5.4 ENVIRONMENTAL REMEDIATION

The damaging effects of pollution on our environment are a growing concern. Bioreactors are emerging as a powerful tool for environmental remediation, offering a natural and sustainable approach to cleaning up contaminated sites (Bosu et al., 2023). Here's how bioreactors are used to tackle various environmental challenges:

- **Wastewater Treatment:** Municipal and industrial wastewater often contains pollutants like organic matter, nutrients, and harmful chemicals. Bioreactors play a crucial role in wastewater treatment by:
    - **Activated Sludge Process:** This widely used method utilizes bioreactors filled with suspended flocs of microorganisms that break down organic matter in wastewater. Bioreactors provide optimal conditions for these microbes to thrive and efficiently treat the wastewater.
    - **Anaerobic Digestion:** Bioreactors can create oxygen-depleted environments suitable for anaerobic bacteria. These bacteria can degrade various pollutants, including organic matter and some toxic compounds, in wastewater.
- **Biodegradation of Pollutants:** Bioreactors can be used to treat soil and water contaminated with various pollutants:
    - **Hydrocarbon Remediation:** Certain microorganisms can break down petroleum-based hydrocarbons like oil spills. Bioreactors can cultivate these microbes and be used for *ex situ* (off-site) treatment of contaminated soil or *in situ* (on-site) bioremediation efforts.
    - **Heavy Metal Removal:** Bioreactors can be designed to harbor microbes that can accumulate or transform heavy metals like lead or mercury from contaminated water or soil.
- **Bioaugmentation and Biostimulation:** Bioaugmentation involves introducing specific microorganisms into a contaminated environment to enhance biodegradation. Bioreactors can be used to cultivate these microbes before their introduction to the contaminated site. Biostimulation, on the other hand, focuses

on providing nutrients and optimizing conditions to stimulate the growth of native microbial populations capable of degrading pollutants. Bioreactors can be used to develop and test suitable nutrient formulations for biostimulation strategies.

- **Advantages of Bioreactors in Environmental Remediation:**
  - **Sustainable Approach:** Bioreactors utilize natural biological processes for remediation, minimizing the need for harsh chemicals and promoting environmental sustainability.
  - **Targeted Treatment:** Bioreactors can be designed to target specific pollutants by selecting appropriate microbial communities or optimizing environmental conditions (Meena et al., 2021).
- **Efficiency and Control:** Bioreactors provide a controlled environment for biodegradation processes, leading to efficient and predictable pollutant removal.

Bioremediation using bioreactors faces challenges such as ensuring the survival and activity of microbes in contaminated environments and optimizing biodegradation rates for various pollutants.

## 13.6 ADVANCES IN BIOREACTOR TECHNOLOGY

### *13.6.1 INTEGRATION OF BIOREACTOR SYSTEMS WITH ANALYTICAL TOOLS*

The integration of bioreactor systems with analytical tools represents a significant advancement in bioreactor technology, enabling real-time monitoring, analysis, and control of key process parameters to enhance bioprocess performance, productivity, and product quality. This integration facilitates a deeper understanding of bioprocess dynamics, facilitates process optimization, and accelerates bioprocess development and scale-up (Gerzon et al., 2022).

Here is an exploration of the integration of bioreactor systems with analytical tools and its impact on bioprocessing:

- **Online Monitoring and Control:** Integration of bioreactor systems with online analytical tools allows for real-time monitoring and control of critical process parameters such as temperature, pH, dissolved oxygen (DO), biomass concentration, and metabolite concentrations. Online sensors and probes continuously measure these parameters within the bioreactor, providing instant feedback to control systems for automated adjustment of process conditions. This real-time monitoring and control enable rapid response to deviations from setpoints, optimization of process parameters, and prevention of process upsets, leading to improved process stability and productivity.

- **Sensors and Probes:** Online sensors and probes are essential components of integrated bioreactor systems, providing accurate and reliable measurements of key process parameters. These sensors include pH electrodes, temperature probes, DO sensors, biomass sensors, and online analyzers for measuring metabolites such as glucose, lactate, ethanol, and amino acids. Advances in sensor technology have led to the development of miniaturized, robust, and multiparameter sensors that can be integrated directly into bioreactor systems, enabling continuous monitoring of multiple parameters simultaneously.
- **Data Acquisition and Analysis:** Integration of bioreactor systems with data acquisition and analysis tools allows for the collection, storage, and analysis of large volumes of data generated during bioprocesses. Data acquisition systems capture real-time sensor data from bioreactor systems and store it in databases for further analysis. Data analysis tools, including statistical analysis software, machine learning algorithms, and process modeling software, analyze the collected data to identify trends, correlations, and patterns, providing insights into bioprocess behavior and performance. This data-driven approach enables informed decision-making, process optimization, and predictive modeling to improve bioprocess outcomes (Van Neste et al., 2023).
- **Process Understanding and Optimization:** Integration of bioreactor systems with analytical tools enhances process understanding and optimization by providing detailed insights into bioprocess kinetics, metabolic pathways, and cellular physiology. Online monitoring of biomass growth, substrate utilization, and product formation kinetics allows for the characterization of microbial

behavior and metabolic fluxes in real time. This information can be used to optimize process conditions, media formulations, and feeding strategies to maximize product yield, quality, and productivity. Additionally, advanced data analysis techniques such as multivariate analysis and metabolic flux analysis enable the identification of key process parameters and optimization targets for further process improvement.

- **Scale-Up and Tech Transfer:** Integrated bioreactor systems with analytical tools facilitate scale-up and technology transfer by providing consistent and reproducible process conditions across different scales. Real-time monitoring of critical process parameters ensures that process conditions remain within the optimal range during scale-up, minimizing variability and ensuring consistent product quality. Additionally, data-driven process optimization strategies developed at laboratory scale can be transferred to larger production scales with confidence, accelerating the scale-up process and reducing time-to-market for biopharmaceuticals and other bioproducts.
- **Quality Assurance and Regulatory Compliance:** Integration of bioreactor systems with analytical tools enhances quality assurance and regulatory compliance by enabling real-time monitoring and control of process parameters to ensure product quality and consistency. Online monitoring of critical quality attributes such as product purity, potency, and stability allows for early detection of deviations from specifications and timely intervention to prevent product failures or non-compliance. This proactive approach to quality assurance helps to ensure regulatory compliance and product safety, reducing the risk of batch failures, recalls, and regulatory sanctions.

### *13.6.2 BIOREACTOR AUTOMATION AND ROBOTICS*

Bioreactor automation and robotics represent significant advances in bioreactor technology, revolutionizing the way bioprocesses are conducted and managed. These advancements enable increased process control, efficiency, reproducibility, and scalability while reducing human intervention and error (Morschett et al., 2021).

Here is an overview of the key aspects of bioreactor automation and robotics:

- **Automated Process Control:** Bioreactor automation involves the integration of advanced control systems to automate the monitoring and regulation of key process parameters such as temperature, pH, dissolved oxygen, agitation speed, and nutrient feeding. Automated control systems utilize feedback from sensors and probes to continuously adjust process conditions in real-time, optimizing microbial growth, metabolism, and product formation. This automated approach enhances process stability, reproducibility, and productivity while minimizing the need for manual intervention.
- **Robotic Sampling and Analysis:** Robotic systems are employed to automate sampling and analysis tasks in bioreactor operations, reducing the time and labor required for manual sampling and analysis. Robotic samplers can collect samples at predefined time points or based on user-defined criteria, enabling frequent and consistent monitoring of bioprocess parameters. These samples can be analyzed using automated analytical instruments or online sensors, providing real-time insights into bioprocess performance, and facilitating process optimization.
- **Cell Culture Automation:** Automated cell culture systems utilize robotic platforms to automate cell culture maintenance tasks such as media exchange, cell passaging, and cell counting. These systems feature integrated robotics, liquid handling systems, and imaging technologies to automate routine cell culture operations, reducing hands-on time and minimizing variability between experiments. Automated cell culture systems enable high-throughput screening (HTS), process optimization, and scalability in bioprocess development and production.
- **High-Throughput Screening:** Robotics-enabled HTS platforms allow for the rapid screening of large numbers of microbial strains, cell lines, or culture conditions to identify optimal bioprocess conditions or high-producing cell clones. These systems feature robotic liquid handlers, microplate readers, and imaging systems to automate the screening process, enabling the evaluation of

thousands of samples in parallel. HTS platforms accelerate bioprocess development, strain engineering, and biopharmaceutical discovery by enabling rapid data generation and analysis (Zeng et al., 2020).

- **Integration with Data Management Systems:** Automated bioreactor systems are often integrated with data management and analysis software platforms to streamline data collection, storage, and analysis. These systems feature user-friendly interfaces, data visualization tools, and advanced analytics capabilities to facilitate real-time monitoring, process optimization, and decision-making. Integration with data management systems enables seamless data transfer between bioreactor systems, laboratory information management systems (LIMS), and process control systems, improving workflow efficiency and data integrity (Rodríguez-García et al., 2023).

### 13.6.3 EMERGING TRENDS IN BIOREACTOR DESIGN

Emerging trends in bioreactor design reflect innovative approaches aimed at addressing challenges, improving performance, and expanding the capabilities of bioprocessing systems. These trends leverage advancements in materials science, engineering principles, and biotechnology to enhance process control, scalability, and flexibility. Here is an overview of some key emerging trends in bioreactor design:

- **Single-Use Bioreactors:** Single-use bioreactors (SUBs) have gained popularity in recent years due to their flexibility, scalability, and cost-effectiveness. SUBs eliminate the need for cleaning and sterilization between batches, reducing downtime and contamination risks. These disposable bioreactors feature flexible plastic bags or liners that can be easily disposed of after use, making them ideal for small-scale and multiproduct manufacturing. Emerging trends in SUBs include the development of larger-scale systems, improved sensor integration, and advanced mixing technologies to enhance process performance and productivity (Jossen et al., 2019).
- **Modular Bioreactor Systems:** Modular bioreactor systems consist of interconnected bioreactor units that can be easily

assembled, disassembled, or reconfigured to accommodate different process requirements and production scales. These modular systems offer greater flexibility and scalability compared to traditional fixed-bed reactors or stirred-tank reactors. Emerging trends in modular bioreactor systems include the development of standardized modules, plug-and-play integration, and automation capabilities to streamline process development and scale-up (Schuerlein et al., 2016).

- **Microfluidic Bioreactors:** Microfluidic bioreactors utilize microscale channels and chambers to culture cells or microorganisms in controlled environments, offering precise control over fluid flow, mass transfer, and cellular interactions. These miniaturized bioreactors enable high-throughput experimentation, real-time imaging, and single-cell analysis, facilitating rapid prototyping and optimization of bioprocesses. Emerging trends in microfluidic bioreactors include the integration of advanced sensors, automation, and multiplexing capabilities to enhance throughput, sensitivity, and reproducibility (Blesken et al., 2016).
- **Bioreactor Integration with Artificial Intelligence (AI):** Integration of bioreactor systems with artificial intelligence (AI) and machine learning algorithms enables autonomous operation, predictive modeling, and adaptive control of bioprocesses. AI-powered bioreactors can analyze large volumes of data generated during bioprocessing operations to identify patterns, optimize process parameters, and predict outcomes in real time. Emerging trends in AI-enabled bioreactors include the development of predictive modeling tools, closed-loop control systems, and autonomous bioprocess optimization platforms to enhance productivity and efficiency (Kamali et al., 2021).
- **3D Bioprinter Bioreactors:** 3D bioprinting technology enables the fabrication of complex bioreactor structures with precise control over geometry, porosity, and material properties. 3D bioprinter bioreactors can mimic the physiological environment of cells or tissues, facilitating organ-on-a-chip models, tissue engineering, and regenerative medicine applications. Emerging trends in 3D bioprinter bioreactors include the incorporation of bioactive materials, cell-laden hydrogels, and vascular networks

to create functional tissue constructs for drug screening, disease modeling, and personalized medicine (Zhang et al., 2021).

By embracing these emerging trends, bioprocessing industries can accelerate bioprocess development, improve product quality, and meet the evolving demands of healthcare, biotechnology, and biomanufacturing sectors.

## 13.7 CHALLENGES AND FUTURE DIRECTIONS

### *13.7.1 BIOREACTOR LIMITATIONS AND BOTTLENECKS*

Despite the remarkable advancements in bioreactor technology, several limitations and bottlenecks continue to hinder the full potential of bioprocessing. Addressing these challenges is crucial for further optimizing bioprocesses and unlocking new frontiers in various fields. Here is a closer look at some key limitations:

- **Mimicking the *In Vivo* Environment:** Cells in their natural environment exist in a complex interplay with other cell types, ECM, and gradients of nutrients and oxygen. Replicating this intricate microenvironment within a bioreactor remains a challenge. Current designs often struggle to provide the necessary spatial organization, dynamic interactions, and controlled gradients that cells experience *in vivo*. This can limit cell growth, viability, and ultimately product yield (Mitchell et al., 2023).
- **Scalability Challenges:** Transitioning a bioprocess from successful lab-scale development to large-scale production can be fraught with difficulties. Factors like heat transfer, efficient mixing, and nutrient delivery become more complex at larger scales. Bioreactor design needs to adapt to ensure homogenous conditions and optimal cell health throughout the culture, even in large-scale production settings.
- **Shear Stress and Cell Damage:** Agitation is essential for mixing nutrients and oxygen within the bioreactor. However, excessive shear forces generated by agitation can damage delicate cells, impacting their viability and productivity. Balancing efficient

mixing with minimizing shear stress remains a critical consideration in bioreactor design and operation.

- **Aseptic Operation and Contamination Risks:** Maintaining sterility throughout the bioprocess is paramount to prevent contamination. However, large-scale operations with complex feeding strategies and frequent interventions increase the risk of contamination events. New strategies for sterile operation, along with robust and rapid contamination detection methods, are needed to minimize risks and ensure product safety.
- **Process Monitoring and Control Limitations:** Traditional bioreactor monitoring often relies on manual sampling and offline analysis, providing a limited snapshot of the culture state. Real-time monitoring of crucial parameters like cell viability, metabolite levels, and product formation remains a challenge. This limits the ability to make proactive adjustments and optimize the bioprocess in real-time (Lim et al., 2021).
- **Future Directions:** Overcoming these limitations requires innovation across various disciplines. Here are some promising future directions:
  - **Biomimetic Design Principles:** Bioreactors incorporating features like microfluidic channels, 3D scaffolds, and controlled flow patterns can provide a more natural environment for cells, leading to improved growth and productivity.
  - **Advanced Computational Modeling:** Simulations can help predict bioreactor behavior at larger scales, facilitating smoother transitions from lab to industry and optimizing design parameters before implementation.
  - **Novel Mixing Strategies:** Innovative approaches like oscillating bioreactors or microfluidic chips can achieve efficient mixing while minimizing shear stress on sensitive cells.
  - **Single-Use Bioreactors and Closed Systems:** Disposable bioreactors can simplify operation and reduce contamination risks. Additionally, closed systems with minimal human intervention can minimize contamination risks and improve sterility.

- **Advanced Sensor Technologies and Online Monitoring:** Development of robust and cost-effective biosensors and online analytical tools will enable real-time monitoring of critical parameters, facilitating proactive process control and optimization.

By addressing these limitations and embracing innovative solutions, researchers and engineers are paving the way for a future where bioreactors become even more efficient, scalable, and capable of fostering intricate biological processes. This progress will ultimately translate into advancements in various fields, from biopharmaceuticals and biofuels to regenerative medicine and environmental applications.

### *13.7.2 REGULATORY CONSIDERATIONS FOR BIOREACTOR-BASED PRODUCTION*

Regulatory considerations for bioreactor-based production are crucial aspects that influence the development, implementation, and commercialization of bioprocesses in various industries, including pharmaceuticals, biotechnology, and food production. Regulatory agencies such as the Food and Drug Administration (FDA), European Medicines Agency (EMA), and other national regulatory bodies establish guidelines and requirements to ensure the safety, efficacy, and quality of bioproducts manufactured using bioreactor technology (Valdiani et al., 2018).

Here are some key regulatory considerations for bioreactor-based production:

- **Good Manufacturing Practices (GMP):** Compliance with Good Manufacturing Practices (GMP) is essential for bioreactor-based production to ensure consistent quality, safety, and efficacy of biopharmaceuticals, vaccines, and other bioproducts. GMP regulations provide guidelines for facility design, equipment qualification, process validation, personnel training, and documentation practices to ensure that bioprocesses are conducted in a controlled and reproducible manner (Elseberg et al., 2014).
- **Quality Management Systems (QMS):** Implementing a robust Quality Management System (QMS) is essential for ensuring the quality and compliance of bioreactor-based production processes.

QMS encompasses quality control, quality assurance, and quality risk management activities to identify, assess, and mitigate potential risks and deviations throughout the bioproduction lifecycle. QMS principles such as batch recordkeeping, deviation management, change control, and CAPA (Corrective and Preventive Actions) are critical for maintaining product quality and regulatory compliance.

- **Process Validation and Qualification:** Process validation and qualification are essential components of regulatory compliance for bioreactor-based production. Process validation involves demonstrating that bioprocesses consistently produce products that meet predefined quality attributes and specifications. Qualification of bioreactor systems, equipment, and software ensures that they are suitable for their intended use and meet regulatory requirements. Validation studies include process characterization, equipment qualification, and validation of analytical methods to ensure the reliability and reproducibility of bioproduction processes.
- **Product Characterization and Testing:** Product characterization and testing are critical aspects of regulatory compliance for bioreactor-based production. Regulatory agencies require comprehensive characterization of bioproducts to assess their identity, purity, potency, and safety. Analytical methods such as chromatography, mass spectrometry, and immunoassays are used to evaluate product quality attributes, including protein structure, post-translational modifications, and impurity profiles. Stability testing is also required to assess the shelf-life and storage conditions of bioproducts.
- **Risk Assessment and Mitigation:** Conducting risk assessments and implementing risk mitigation strategies are essential for regulatory compliance in bioreactor-based production. Risk assessment involves identifying potential hazards, vulnerabilities, and failure modes associated with bioproduction processes and implementing measures to mitigate these risks. Risk mitigation strategies may include process design improvements, equipment redundancy, personnel training, and contingency planning to minimize the likelihood and impact of adverse events on product quality and patient safety.

By adhering to regulatory guidelines and requirements, bioprocessing companies can ensure the integrity and reliability of bioproduction processes and maintain public trust in the safety and efficacy of bioproducts.

## 13.8 CONCLUSION

Bioreactors have emerged as powerful tools that are revolutionizing industrial production across diverse sectors. From pharmaceuticals and biofuels to food and beverages and even environmental remediation, these versatile vessels are enabling the creation of sustainable and innovative products. As bioreactor technology continues to evolve with advancements in automation, design, and monitoring, we can expect even greater efficiency, scalability, and control over biological processes. This will undoubtedly lead to breakthroughs in various fields, fostering a future powered by bioreactors and the marvels they create.

In the years to come, the continued evolution and integration of bioreactor technology with cutting-edge innovations in biotechnology, materials science, and process engineering will further enhance the capabilities and impact of bioreactors in industrial production, paving the way for a more sustainable and prosperous future.

## KEYWORDS

- **bioreactor**
- **byproducts**
- **fermentation**
- **metabolites**
- **microbes**
- **substrates**

## REFERENCES

Alimberti, R., Chauhan, V., & Jaiswal, D. (2021). Bioreactor temperature control system using PID controller. https://doi.org/10.1115/imece2021-71715 (accessed on 5th November 2025).

Al-Zyoud, W., Bater, R., Awad, T., Yasin, O., & Al–Zaben, A. (2018). Bioreactor for biopharmaceutical production: Simple controlled environment design. https://doi.org/10.1109/mecbme.2018.8402414 (accessed on 5th November 2025).

Baudequin, T., Nyland, R., & Ye, H. (2021). Objectives, benefits and challenges of bioreactor systems for the clinical scale expansion of T lymphocyte cells. *Biotechnology Advances, 49*, 107735. https://doi.org/10.1016/j.biotechadv.2021.107735 (accessed on 5th November 2025).

Behera, S. S., Ray, R. C., Das, U., Panda, S., & Saranraj, P. (2019). Microorganisms in fermentation. In *Learning Materials in Biosciences* (pp. 1–39). https://doi.org/10.1007/978-3-030-16230-6_1 (accessed on 5th November 2025).

Berenjian, A. (2020). Correction to: Bioreactor scale-up. In *Learning Materials in Biosciences* (p. C1). https://doi.org/10.1007/978-3-030-16230-6_11 (accessed on 5th November 2025).

Blesken, C. C., Olfers, T., Grimm, A., & Frische, N. (2016). The microfluidic bioreactor for a new era of bioprocess development. *Engineering in Life Sciences (Print), 16*(2), 190–193. https://doi.org/10.1002/elsc.201500026 (accessed on 5th November 2025).

Bosu, S., Rajamohan, N., Rajasimman, M., Raut, N., & Vasseghian, Y. (2023). Hydrogen based membrane bioreactor for environmental remediation of pollutants–Review on applications and mechanism. *International Journal of Hydrogen Energy, 48*(17), 6546–6559. https://doi.org/10.1016/j.ijhydene.2021.12.136 (accessed on 5th November 2025).

Chandra, R., Vishal, G., Sánchez, C. E. G., & Uribe, J. A. G. (2020). Bioreactor for algae cultivation and biodiesel production. In *Elsevier eBooks* (pp. 289–307). https://doi.org/10.1016/b978-0-12-821264-6.00015-2 (accessed on 5th November 2025).

Chen, L., Guttieres, D., Koenigsberg, A. L., Barone, P. W., Sinskey, A. J., & Springs, S. L. (2022). Large-scale cultured meat production: Trends, challenges and promising biomanufacturing technologies. *Biomaterials, 280*, 121274. https://doi.org/10.1016/j.biomaterials.2021.121274 (accessed on 5th November 2025).

Desobgo, S. C. Z. (2018). Modernization of fermenters for large-scale production in the food and beverage industry. In *Springer eBooks* (pp. 189–220). https://doi.org/10.1007/978-3-319-74820-7_11 (accessed on 5th November 2025).

Di Gravina, G. M., Loi, G., Auricchio, F., & Conti, M. (2023). Computer-aided engineering and additive manufacturing for bioreactors in tissue engineering: State of the art and perspectives. *Biophysics Reviews, 4*(3). https://doi.org/10.1063/5.0156704 (accessed on 5th November 2025).

Drapal, V., Gamble, J. M., Robinson, J. L., Tamerler, C., Arnold, P. M., & Friis, E. A. (2021). Integration of clinical perspective into biomimetic bioreactor design for orthopedics. *Journal of Biomedical Materials Research. Part B, Applied Biomaterials, 110*(2), 321–337. https://doi.org/10.1002/jbm.b.34929 (accessed on 5th November 2025).

Elseberg, C., Salzig, D., & Czermak, P. (2014). Bioreactor expansion of human mesenchymal stem cells according to GMP requirements. In *Methods in Molecular Biology* (pp. 199–218). https://doi.org/10.1007/7651_2014_117 (accessed on 5th November 2025).

Gerzon, G., Sheng, Y., & Kirkitadze, M. (2022). Process analytical technologies–Advances in bioprocess integration and future perspectives. *Journal of Pharmaceutical and Biomedical Analysis (Print), 207*, 114379. https://doi.org/10.1016/j.jpba.2021.114379 (accessed on 5th November 2025).

Jossen, V., Eibl, R., & Eibl, D. (2019). Single-use bioreactors–An overview (pp. 37–52). https://doi.org/10.1002/9781119477891.ch4 (accessed on 5th November 2025).

Kamali, M., Appels, L., Yu, X., Aminabhavi, T. M., & Dewil, R. (2021). Artificial intelligence as a sustainable tool in wastewater treatment using membrane bioreactors. *Chemical Engineering Journal, 417*, 128070. https://doi.org/10.1016/j.cej.2020.128070 (accessed on 5th November 2025).

Lim, D., Renteria, E. S., Sime, D. S., Ju, Y. M., Kim, J. H., Criswell, T., Shupe, T., Atala, A., Marini, F. C., Gürcan, M. N., Söker, S., Hunsberger, J., & Yoo, J. (2021). Bioreactor design and validation for manufacturing strategies in tissue engineering. *Bio-Design and Manufacturing, 5*(1), 43–63. https://doi.org/10.1007/s42242-021-00154-3 (accessed on 5th November 2025).

Mandenius, C. (2016). Challenges for bioreactor design and operation (pp. 1–34). https://doi.org/10.1002/9783527683369.ch1 (accessed on 5th November 2025).

Meena, M., Yadav, G., Sonigra, P., & Shah, M. P. (2021). A comprehensive review on application of bioreactor for industrial wastewater treatment. *Letters in Applied Microbiology, 74*(2), 131–158. https://doi.org/10.1111/lam.13557 (accessed on 5th November 2025).

Mitchell, T. C., Feng, N., Lam, Y. T., Michael, P., Santos, M., & Wise, S. G. (2023). Engineering vascular bioreactor systems to closely mimic physiological forces *in vitro*. *Tissue Engineering. Part B, Reviews, 29*(3), 232–243. https://doi.org/10.1089/ten.teb.2022.0158 (accessed on 5th November 2025).

Mitra, S., & Murthy, G. S. (2021). Bioreactor control systems in the biopharmaceutical industry: A critical perspective. *Systems Microbiology and Biomanufacturing, 2*(1), 91–112. https://doi.org/10.1007/s43393-021-00048-6 (accessed on 5th November 2025).

Morschett, H., Tenhaef, N., Hemmerich, J., Herbst, L., Spiertz, M., Doğan, D., Wiechert, W., Noack, S., & Oldiges, M. (2021). Robotic integration enables autonomous operation of laboratory scale stirred tank bioreactors with model-driven process analysis. *Biotechnology and Bioengineering, 118*(7), 2759–2769. https://doi.org/10.1002/bit.27795 (accessed on 5th November 2025).

Nikita, S., Mishra, S., Gupta, K., Runkana, V., Gomes, J., & Rathore, A. S. (2023). Advances in bioreactor control for production of biotherapeutic products. *Biotechnology and Bioengineering, 120*(5), 1189–1214. https://doi.org/10.1002/bit.28346 (accessed on 5th November 2025).

Ntwampe, S. K. O., Chowdhury, F., Sheldon, M. S., & Volschenk, H. (2010). Overview of parameters influencing biomass and bioreactor performance used for extracellular ligninase production from *Phanerochaete chrysosporium*. *Brazilian Archives of Biology and Technology, 53*(5), 1057–1066. https://doi.org/10.1590/s1516-89132010000500008 (accessed on 5th November 2025).

O'Flaherty, R., Bergin, A., Flampouri, E., Mota, L. M., Obaidi, I., Quigley, A., Xie, Y., & Butler, M. (2020). Mammalian cell culture for production of recombinant proteins: A review of the critical steps in their biomanufacturing. *Biotechnology Advances, 43*, 107552. https://doi.org/10.1016/j.biotechadv.2020.107552 (accessed on 5th November 2025).

Oh, T. H., Park, H. M., Kim, J. W., & Lee, J. M. (2022). Integration of reinforcement learning and model predictive control to optimize semi-batch bioreactor. *AIChE Journal, 68*(6). https://doi.org/10.1002/aic.17658 (accessed on 5th November 2025).

Robles, Á., Durán, F., Ruano, M., Ribes, J., Rosado, A., Seco, A., & Ferrer, J. (2015). Instrumentation, control, and automation for submerged anaerobic membrane bioreactors. *Environmental Technology, 36*(14), 1795–1806. https://doi.org/10.1080/09593330.2015.1012180 (accessed on 5th November 2025).

Rodriguez-García, E., Soto-Mendoza, A., & Guajardo, D. (2023). Serialization and data management of bioreactors through digitization: Bioprocessing 4.0–A systematic review. https://doi.org/10.23919/picmet59654.2023.10216904 (accessed on 5th November 2025).

Sarangi, P. K., & Nanda, S. (2020). Biohydrogen production through dark fermentation. *Chemical Engineering & Technology, 43*(4), 601–612. https://doi.org/10.1002/ceat.201900452 (accessed on 5th November 2025).

Schuerlein, S., Schwarz, T., Krziminski, S., Gätzner, S., Hoppensack, A., Schwedhelm, I., Schweinlin, M., Walles, H., & Hansmann, J. (2016). A versatile modular bioreactor platform for tissue engineering. *Biotechnology Journal, 12*(2). https://doi.org/10.1002/biot.201600326 (accessed on 5th November 2025).

Shanmugam, M. K., Mandari, V., Devarai, S. K., & Gummadi, S. N. (2022). Types of bioreactors and important design considerations. In *Elsevier eBooks* (pp. 3–30). https://doi.org/10.1016/b978-0-323-91167-2.00008-3 (accessed on 5th November 2025).

Szkodny, A. C., & Lee, K. H. (2022). Biopharmaceutical manufacturing: Historical perspectives and future directions. *Annual Review of Chemical and Biomolecular Engineering, 13*(1), 141–165. https://doi.org/10.1146/annurev-chembioeng-092220-125832 (accessed on 5th November 2025).

Valdiani, A., Hansen, J. K., Nielsen, U. B., Johannsen, V. K., Shariat, M., Georgiev, M. I., Omidvar, V., Ebrahimi, M., Dinanai, E. T., & Abiri, R. (2018). Bioreactor-based advances in plant tissue and cell culture: Challenges and prospects. *Critical Reviews in Biotechnology, 39*(1), 20–34. https://doi.org/10.1080/07388551.2018.1489778 (accessed on 5th November 2025).

Van Neste, C. C., Wiley, K. A., Chang, S., Borrello, J. A., Turnbull, I. C., & Costa, K. D. (2023). Designing a bioreactor to improve data acquisition and model the throughput of engineered cardiac tissues. *Journal of Visualized Experiments, 196*. https://doi.org/10.3791/64368 (accessed on 5th November 2025).

Vandermies, M., & Fickers, P. (2019). Bioreactor-scale strategies for the production of recombinant protein in the yeast *Yarrowia lipolytica*. *Microorganisms, 7*(2), 40. https://doi.org/10.3390/microorganisms7020040 (accessed on 5th November 2025).

Vasumathi, K., Premalatha, M., & Subramanian, P. (2012). Parameters influencing the design of photobioreactor for the growth of microalgae. *Renewable & Sustainable Energy Reviews, 16*(7), 5443–5450. https://doi.org/10.1016/j.rser.2012.06.013 (accessed on 5th November 2025).

Yu, H., Chong, S. K. M., Hassanbhai, A. M., Teng, Y., Balachander, G. M., Muthukumaran, P., Wen, F., & Teoh, S. H. (2020). Principles of bioreactor design for tissue engineering. In *Elsevier eBooks* (pp. 179–203). https://doi.org/10.1016/b978-0-12-818422-6.00012-5 (accessed on 5th November 2025).

Zeng, W., Guo, L., Xu, S., Chen, J., & Zhou, J. (2020). High-throughput screening technology in industrial biotechnology. *Trends in Biotechnology, 38*(8), 888–906. https://doi.org/10.1016/j.tibtech.2020.01.001 (accessed on 5th November 2025).

Zhang, J., Wehrle, E., Rubert, M., & Müller, R. (2021). 3D bioprinting of human tissues: Bio fabrication, bioinks, and bioreactors. *International Journal of Molecular Sciences, 22*(8), 3971. https://doi.org/10.3390/ijms22083971 (accessed on 5th November 2025).

Zhong, J. (2010). Recent advances in bioreactor engineering. *Korean Journal of Chemical Engineering, 27*(4), 1035–1041. https://doi.org/10.1007/s11814-010-0277-5 (accessed on 5th November 2025).

# Index

## F

## G

## N

## O

## P

## Q



## R



## S

## T

For Product Safety Concerns and Information please contact our EU representative GPSR@taylorandfrancis.com Taylor & Francis Verlag GmbH, Kaufingerstraße 24, 80331 München, Germany